The Human Placenta in Health and Disease

Editors

D. MICHAEL NELSON
LESLIE MYATT

OBSTETRICS AND GYNECOLOGY CLINICS OF NORTH AMERICA

www.obgyn.theclinics.com

Consulting Editor
WILLIAM F. RAYBURN

March 2020 • Volume 47 • Number 1

ELSEVIER

1600 John F. Kennedy Boulevard • Suite 1800 • Philadelphia, Pennsylvania, 19103-2899

http://www.theclinics.com

OBSTETRICS AND GYNECOLOGY CLINICS OF NORTH AMERICA Volume 47, Number 1
March 2020 ISSN 0889-8545, ISBN-13: 978-0-323-71097-8

Editor: Kerry Holland
Developmental Editor: Kristen Helm

Obstetrics and Gynecology Clinics (ISSN 0889-8545) is published quarterly by Elsevier Inc., 360 Park Avenue South, New York, NY 10010-1710. Months of issue are March, June, September, and December. Periodicals postage paid at New York, NY, and additional mailing offices. Subscription price per year is $325.00 (US individuals), $719.00 (US institutions), $100.00 (US students), $404.00 (Canadian individuals), $908.00 (Canadian institutions), $100.00 (Canadian students), $459.00 (international individuals), $908.00 (international institutions), and $225.00 (international students). To receive student/resident rate, orders must be accompanied by name of affiliated institution, date of term, and the signature of program/residency coordinator on institution letterhead. Orders will be billed at individual rate until proof of status is received. Foreign air speed delivery is included in all *Clinics* subscription prices. All prices are subject to change without notice. POSTMASTER: Send address changes to *Obstetrics and Gynecology Clinics*, Elsevier Health Sciences Division, Subscription Customer Service, 3251 Riverport Lane, Maryland Heights, MO 63043. **Customer Service: Telephone: 1-800-654-2452 (U.S. and Canada); 314-447-8871 (outside U.S. and Canada). Fax: 314-447-8029. E-mail: journalscustomerservice-usa@elsevier.com (for print support); journalsonlinesupport-usa@elsevier.com (for online support).**

Reprints. For copies of 100 or more of articles in this publication, please contact the Commercial Reprints Department, Elsevier Inc., 360 Park Avenue South, New York, New York 10010-1710. Tel.: 212-633-3874; Fax: 212-633-3820; E-mail: reprints@elsevier.com

Obstetrics and Gynecology Clinics of North America is also published in Spanish by McGraw-Hill Interamericana Editores S.A., P.O. Box 5-237, 06500, Mexico; in Portuguese by Reichmann and Affonso Editores, Rio de Janeiro, Brazil; and in Greek by Paschalidis Medical Publications, Athens, Greece.

Obstetrics and Gynecology Clinics of North America is covered in MEDLINE/PubMed (Index Medicus), Excerpta Medica, Current Concepts/Clinical Medicine, Science Citation Index, BIOSIS, CINAHL, and ISI/BIOMED.

Contributors

CONSULTING EDITOR

WILLIAM F. RAYBURN, MD, MBA
Associate Dean, Continuing Medical Education and Professional Development, Distinguished Professor and Emeritus Chair, Obstetrics and Gynecology, University of New Mexico School of Medicine, Albuquerque, New Mexico, USA

EDITORS

D. MICHAEL NELSON, MD, PhD
Virginia S. Lang Professor of Obstetrics and Gynecology, Department of Obstetrics and Gynecology, Washington University School of Medicine, St Louis, Missouri, USA

LESLIE MYATT, PhD, FRCOG
Bob and Charlee Moore Endowed Professor, Moore Institute of Nutrition and Wellness, Professor, Department of Obstetrics and Gynecology, Oregon Health & Science University, Portland, Oregon, USA

AUTHORS

VIKKI M. ABRAHAMS, PhD
Professor and Director, Division of Reproductive Sciences, Department of Obstetrics, Gynecology and Reproductive Sciences, Yale School of Medicine, New Haven, Connecticut, USA

ARTHUR ANTOLINI-TAVARES, MD
Department of Pathological Anatomy, School of Medicine, University of Campinas, São Paulo, Brazil

MICHAEL W. BEBBINGTON, MD, MHSc
Professor, Department of Obstetrics and Gynecology, Division of Maternal-Fetal Medicine, Washington University School of Medicine, St Louis, Missouri, USA

JANNE BOONE-HEINONEN, MPH, PhD
Associate Professor, School of Public Health, Oregon Health & Science University, Portland, Oregon, USA

GRAHAM J. BURTON, MD, DSc
Professor, Department of Physiology, Development and Neuroscience, The Centre for Trophoblast Research, University of Cambridge, Cambridge, United Kingdom

JANET M. CATOV, PhD, MS
Department of Obstetrics, Gynecology, and Reproductive Sciences, University of Pittsburgh School of Medicine, Department of Epidemiology, Graduate School of Public Health, University of Pittsburgh, Magee-Womens Research Institute, Pittsburgh, Pennsylvania, USA

MILA CERVAR-ZIVKOVIC, MD, PhD
Professor, Department of Obstetrics and Gynaecology, Medical University of Graz, Graz, Austria

KIRK P. CONRAD, MD
J. Robert and Mary Cade Professor of Physiology (Emeritus), Departments of Physiology and Functional Genomics, and Obstetrics and Gynecology, D.H. Barron Reproductive and Perinatal Biology Research Program, University of Florida College of Medicine, Gainesville, Florida, USA

MARIA LAURA COSTA, MD, PhD
Department of Obstetrics and Gynecology, School of Medicine, University of Campinas, São Paulo, Brazil

GUILHERME DE MORAES NOBREGA
Department of Obstetrics and Gynecology, School of Medicine, University of Campinas, São Paulo, Brazil

GERNOT DESOYE, PhD
Professor, Department of Obstetrics and Gynaecology, Medical University of Graz, Graz, Austria

NICOLE GRAHAM, MRCOG
Faculty of Biological, Medical and Human Sciences, Maternal and Fetal Health Research Centre, School of Medical Sciences, University of Manchester, Manchester Academic Health Science Centre, St. Mary's Hospital, Central Manchester University Hospitals NHS Foundation Trust, Manchester, United Kingdom

ALEXANDER E.P. HEAZELL, PhD, MRCOG
Faculty of Biological, Medical and Human Sciences, Professor of Obstetrics, Maternal and Fetal Health Research Centre, School of Medical Sciences, University of Manchester, Manchester Academic Health Science Centre, St. Mary's Hospital, Central Manchester University Hospitals NHS Foundation Trust, Manchester, United Kingdom

SEBASTIAN R. HOBSON, MD, PhD, MPH
Assistant Professor, Placenta Program, Maternal-Fetal Medicine Division, Department of Obstetrics and Gynaecology, Mount Sinai Hospital, University of Toronto, Toronto, Ontario, Canada

ERIC JAUNIAUX, MD, PhD, FRCOG
Professor, Academic Department of Obstetrics and Gynaecology, The EGA Institute for Women's Health, University College London (UCL), London, United Kingdom

JOHN C. KINGDOM, MD
Professor, Placenta Program, Maternal-Fetal Medicine Division, Department of Obstetrics and Gynaecology, Mount Sinai Hospital, University of Toronto, Toronto, Ontario, Canada

RAMKUMAR MENON, PhD, MS
Associate Professor, Department of Obstetrics and Gynecology, Perinatal Research Division, The University of Texas Medical Branch, Galveston, Texas, USA

ASHLEY MOFFETT, MD, MRCP, MRCPATH, FRCOG
Professor, Department of Pathology, Centre for Trophoblast Research, University of Cambridge, Cambridge, United Kingdom

JOHN J. MOORE, MD
Professor of Pediatrics and Reproductive Biology, Case Western Reserve University School of Medicine, Cleveland, Ohio, USA

W. TONY PARKS, MD
Professor, Department of Laboratory Medicine and Pathobiology, University of Toronto, Toronto, Ontario, Canada

SANJITA RAVISHANKAR, MD
Department of Pathology, Case Western Reserve University School of Medicine, University Hospitals Cleveland Medical Center, Cleveland, Ohio, USA

RAYMOND W. REDLINE, MD
Department of Pathology, Case Western Reserve University School of Medicine, University Hospitals Cleveland Medical Center, Cleveland, Ohio, USA

ANNE SØRENSEN, MD, PhD
Department of Obstetrics and Gynecology, Aalborg University Hospital, Department of Clinical Medicine, Aalborg University, Aalborg, Denmark

MATTHEW A. SHANAHAN, MD
Department of Obstetrics and Gynecology, Division of Maternal-Fetal Medicine, Washington University School of Medicine, St Louis, Missouri, USA

MARIANNE SINDING, MD, PhD
Department of Obstetrics and Gynecology, Aalborg University Hospital, Department of Clinical Medicine, Aalborg University, Aalborg, Denmark

KENT L. THORNBURG, MS, PhD
Professor, Department of Medicine, Center for Developmental Health, Knight Cardiovascular Institute, Professor, Department of Obstetrics and Gynecology, Bob and Charlee Moore Institute for Nutrition & Wellness, School of Medicine, Oregon Health & Science University, Portland, Oregon, USA

MANCY TONG, PhD
Post-doctoral Associate, Department of Obstetrics, Gynecology and Reproductive Sciences, Yale School of Medicine, New Haven, Connecticut, USA

AMY M. VALENT, DO
Assistant Professor, Department of Obstetrics and Gynecology, Oregon Health & Science University, Portland, Oregon, USA

REBECCA L. ZUR, MD
Resident, Department of Obstetrics and Gynaecology, University of Toronto, Toronto, Ontario, Canada

Contents

Birthweight is a well-known predictor of adult-onset chronic disease. The placenta plays a necessary role in regulating fetal growth and determining birth size. Maternal stressors that affect placental function and prenatal growth include maternal overnutrition and undernutrition, toxic social stress, and exposure to toxic chemicals. These stressors lead to increased vulnerability to disease within any population. This vulnerability arises from placental and fetal exposure to stressors during fetal life. The biological drivers linking various social determinants of health to compromised placental function and fetal development have been little studied.

Cardiovascular disease remains the leading killer of women, with sex-specific manifestation, mechanisms, and morbidity. Preeclampsia, fetal growth restriction, and a subset of preterm births demonstrate aberrancies in the maternal vessels supplying the placenta and damage to the placental parenchyma consistent with hypoxic/ischemic or oxidative injury. This constellation of findings, maternal vascular malperfusion (MVM) lesions, may hold the key to understanding and identifying the elevated risk for early cardiovascular disease in women who experience adverse pregnancy outcomes. This intriguing possibility has only begun to be examined, but accumulating evidence is compelling and is reviewed here.

The placenta can serve as a valuable source of information about maternal and fetal conditions during the pregnancy; however, the abilities to perform a preliminary gross examination and interpret a placental pathology report are variable among obstetricians. This article discusses the indications for placental submission to pathology; the essentials of gross examination, including elements that should be performed in the delivery suite; and the most common and clinically relevant histologic findings that may be encountered in the report.

gestations helps perinatal pathologists perform a more informed placental evaluation, allowing for better care for the mother and her children.

Primary disorders of placental implantation have immediate consequences for the outcome of a pregnancy. These disorders have been known to clinical science for more than a century, but have been relatively rare. Recent epidemiologic obstetric data have indicated that the rise in their incidence over the last 2 decades has been iatrogenic in origin. In particular, the rising numbers of pregnancies resulting from in vitro fertilization (IVF) and the increased use of caesarean section for delivery have been associated with higher frequencies of previa implantation, accreta placentation, abnormal placental shapes, and velamentous cord insertion. These disorders often occur together.

Congenital infections are an important cause of morbidity and mortality worldwide, especially in low-income settings. This review discusses the main pathways of infections and associated adverse maternal and fetal outcomes, considering the TORCH pathogens, including Zika virus; the acronym stands for Toxoplasma gondii infection, other (Listeria monocytogenes, Treponema pallidum, and parvovirus B19, among others, including Zika virus), rubella virus, cytomegalovirus, and herpes simplex viruses type 1 and type 2.

Fetal membranes (FMs) play a role in pregnancy maintenance and promoting parturition at term. The FMs are not just part of the placenta, structurally or functionally. Although attached to the placenta, the amnion has a separate embryologic origin, and the chorion deviates from the placenta by the first month of pregnancy. Other than immune protection, these FM functions are not those of the placenta. FM dysfunction is associated with and may cause adverse pregnancy outcomes. Ongoing research may identify biomarkers for pending preterm premature rupture of the FMs as well as therapeutic agents, to prevent it and resulting preterm birth.

Preeclampsia may arise from impaired decidualization in some women. Transcriptomics of mid-secretory biopsy endometrial stromal cells decidualized in vitro and of early gestation choriodecidua from women who experienced preeclampsia with severe features overlapped significantly with the classical endometrial disorders giving rise to the concept of "endometrium spectrum disorders". That is, recurrent implantation failure and miscarriage, endometriosis, normotensive intrauterine growth restriction, preeclampsia and preterm birth may all lie on a continuum of decidual dysregulation, in which phenotypic expression is determined by the specific molecular pathway(s) disrupted and severity of disruption. Women conceiving by programmed IVF protocols showed widespread dysregulation of cardiovascular function and increased rates of adverse pregnancy outcomes including preeclampsia. Programmed cycles preclude development of a corpus luteum (CL), a major regulator of endometrial function. Lack of circulating CL product(s) that are not replaced in programmed cycles (eg, relaxin) could adversely impact the maternal cardiovascular system directly and/or compromise decidualization, thereby increasing preeclampsia risk.

Because of the critical role that placental structure and function plays during pregnancy, abnormal placental structure and function is closely related to stillbirth: when an infant dies before birth. However, understanding the role of the placental and specific lesions is incomplete, in part because of the variation in definitions of lesions and in classifying causes of stillbirths. Nevertheless, placental abnormalities are seen more frequently in stillbirths than live births, with placental abruption, chorioamnionitis, and maternal vascular malperfusion most commonly reported. Critically, some placental lesions affect the management of subsequent pregnancies. Histopathological examination of the placenta is recommended following stillbirth.

This article describes the use of placental magnetic resonance imaging (MRI) relaxation times in the in vivo assessment of placental function. It focuses on T2*-weighted placental MRI, the main area of the authors' research over the past decade. The rationale behind T2*-weighted placental MRI, the main findings reported in the literature, and directions for future research and clinical applications of this method are discussed. The article concludes that placental T2* relaxation time is an easily obtained and robust measurement, which can discriminate between normal and dysfunctional placenta. Placenta T2* is a promising tool for in vivo assessment of placental function.

OBSTETRICS AND GYNECOLOGY CLINICS

SERIES OF RELATED INTEREST

Clinics in Perinatology
www.perinatology.theclinics.com

Foreword

The Placenta: Its Importance from Womb to Tomb

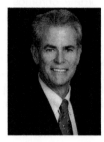

William F. Rayburn, MD, MBA
Consulting Editor

The placenta is a fantastic organ that provides the indispensable interface between mother and fetus. Discoveries from the study of placental implantation, anatomy, and function apply from the earliest stages of pregnancy until delivery of the baby and, in some circumstances, may predict eventual human morbidity and mortality (*from Womb to Tomb*). This issue, edited with expertise from D. Michael Nelson, MD, PhD and Leslie Myatt, PhD, brings to our attention how much we have to learn about both normal placental function and the abnormal function that accompanies many complications of pregnancy. The issue consists of contributions from individuals who are leaders in placentology. Mentioned throughout the issue is The Human Placenta Project, sponsored by the National Institute of Child Health and Human Development. Reference to this rich resource is appropriate in understanding the role of the placenta in health and disease.

Implantation disorders of the placenta are recognized in this issue as events in early gestation that could jeopardize both maternal and fetal health. The fetoplacental unit is nature's transplant. Immune dysfunction or a mismatch may underlie a whole spectrum of pregnancy outcomes, including failure of implantation, early and late pregnancy loss, preeclampsia, and preterm birth. Pregnancies resulting from artificial reproductive technologies are predisposed to placental developmental abnormalities leading to adverse outcomes.

High-resolution ultrasound visualization of placental anatomy and blood flow is now routine. Most pregnancies are well dated, permitting a more complete and timely assessment of fetal growth and anatomy. Visualization of a placenta previa, placental abruption, and adherent placenta presumably results from disturbed trophoblast-decidual interactions. Knowing the specialized anatomy in the dichorionic or monochorionic placentas of multifetal gestations helps obstetricians to optimize outcomes.

Obstet Gynecol Clin N Am 47 (2020) xiii–xiv
https://doi.org/10.1016/j.ogc.2020.01.002
0889-8545/20/© 2020 Published by Elsevier Inc.

obgyn.theclinics.com

Other technologies, such as MRI, are employed much less often but offer new insights into blood flow and transport of some nutrients.

Suboptimal placental function directly impacts fetal growth. As an example, gestational diabetes is the direct result of diabetogenic placental hormones, stressing insulin reserves in a pregnant woman. As more reproductive age women are obese, we are finding that obesity contributes to the increasing incidence of gestational diabetes and is itself associated with placental dysfunction and its impact on fetal growth. Intrauterine growth restriction derives from several placental disorders: chromosomal mosaicism, impaired placental development, uteroplacental hypoperfusion, or inadequate placental transport of nutrients.

Although a placental examination by the obstetrician is recommended, by consensus, routine pathologic examination is not mandatory. As a minimum, the placenta and umbilical cord should be inspected in the delivery room. Requested examinations of the placenta by a pathologist are often an afterthought following a complicated delivery. Histopathologic diagnoses offer explanations about some suboptimal outcomes for counseling couples and their families about the recent or any future pregnancy. The chorioamnionic fetal membranes play essential roles in regulating amniotic fluid volume and in signaling events associated with term and preterm birth with or without premature rupture of the membranes. Placental infections are a major source of unfavorable pregnancy outcomes. Understanding the routes by which infections gain access to the fetoplacental unit can aid obstetricians in recommending what tests to order and what infections may be most likely involved.

This issue introduces the concept that fetuses are susceptible to "in utero developmental programming," which predisposes to subsequent clinically apparent maladies in children and adults. The role of the placenta in the in utero mechanisms that predispose to metabolic syndrome, hypertension, cardiovascular disease, cerebrovascular accidents, and other disorders in later life regardless of fetal genetic constitution cannot be ignored .

Placental anatomy, physiology, and molecular structure remain some of the most intriguing and understudied topics in obstetrics. A broad range of basic science and clinicial contributors to this issue has aided in uncovering secrets about this unique organ. I appreciate the efforts of coeditors, Dr Nelson and Dr Myatt, and desire to direct our readers to issues of placental function. It is hoped that the practical information provided herein will aid in the design, development, and implementation of placental investigations for optimizing care of all pregnant women.

William F. Rayburn, MD, MBA
Department of Obsterics and Gynecology
University of New Mexico School of Medicine
MSC 10 5580, 1 University of New Mexico
Albuquerque, NM 87131-0001, USA

E-mail address:
wrayburn@salud.unm.edu

Preface

The Human Placenta in Health and Disease

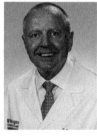 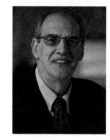

D. Michael Nelson, MD, PhD   Leslie Myatt, PhD, FRCOG
Editors

The placenta is arguably the most important organ for continued survival of *Homo sapiens*. The human placenta is the director of pregnancy, performing many diverse functions that control maternal metabolism and fetal growth and development that mediate survival of the offspring. Despite the biological importance of this organ, we have only begun to scratch the surface of understanding both normal placental function and, to an even lesser extent, the placental dysfunction that accompanies many disorders of pregnancy. This knowledge deficit was the rationale underpinning The Human Placenta Project, which is sponsored by the National Institute of Child Health and Human Development as a collaborative research effort to understand the role of the placenta in health and disease. This endeavor aims to develop new tools to study the organ in real time, to dissect placental development from the earliest stages of implantation onward, and to elucidate mechanisms that maintain optimal function throughout pregnancy. Contributions from a broad range of scientists and clinicians synergize to pursue the secrets of this unique organ.

The following articles target key disorders associated with placental pathology and dysregulated pathophysiology. We give an overview of the topics below, bolding the subjects covered. We introduce the series with a hot topic in the literature, the *Developmental Origins of Health and Disease*, commonly dubbed *DOHaD*.

Our knowledge of *DOHaD* has flourished over the 2 decades since the Barker Hypothesis described a *thrifty phenotype* in babies who were born growth restricted. The small size of such fetuses reflected placental dysfunction that was associated first with subsequent hypertension in adult men, and later, with a constellation of adult diseases irrespective of sex, including hypertension, cardiovascular disease, and strokes. Extensive research into the in utero mechanisms that predispose to these maladies in later life led to the concept of in utero programming of some fetuses, independent of their genetic constitution. Mechanisms underlying the epigenetic programming of

Obstet Gynecol Clin N Am 47 (2020) xv–xviii
https://doi.org/10.1016/j.ogc.2020.01.001
0889-8545/20/© 2020 Published by Elsevier Inc.

offspring exposed to in utero stress via placental dysfunction have been identified in a variety of organs, notably the kidneys, heart, and pancreas, among others.[1] Such dysfunction commonly results from implantation disorders that yield a placenta that exhibits inadequate nutrient transport, hypoxia, or enhanced oxidative stress, but also the effect of other conditions that may be encountered during a pregnancy, including obesity, diabetes, and environmental pollutants. Collectively, the DOHaD studies indicate that fetuses are susceptible to developmental programming during gestation, which predisposes to clinically apparent maladies in childhood or adult ages.

If babies are affected by their placentas, how about mothers? In the last 2 decades, follow-up studies of women with pregnancy complications associated with placental maldevelopment, dysfunction, or both have shown a number of common disorders that occur with advancing age in the parturient and which link in part to a history of a pregnancy disorder. These observations have evolved into an area of research targeting *Cardiovascular Health After Maternal Placental Syndromes*, commonly dubbed *CHAMPS*. Preeclampsia, intrauterine growth restriction (IUGR), and preterm birth, among other placenta-related issues, associate with a 2- to 10-fold increased future risk for a woman to develop diabetes mellitus, chronic hypertension, cardiovascular disease, cerebrovascular disease, or metabolic syndrome, compared with women with uncomplicated pregnancy outcomes.[2] This burgeoning association suggests that pregnancy complications secondary to placental dysfunction provide a window into the future health of the affected individual.

DOHaD and CHAMPS underscore the importance of recognition that placental function contributes to the future health of some individuals from *womb to tomb*. It is now apparent that the sex of the fetus and its associated placenta affect adverse outcomes from fetal programming and also later life events in the mother and therefore need to be considered in all basic science and clinical scenarios. Together, this knowledge sets the stage to consider 2 important topics related to placental development and evolution over gestation. Placental *pathology* is all too often an afterthought following a high-risk delivery, yet histopathologic diagnoses offer retrospective explanations for some suboptimal outcomes while also offering data for counseling couples about their risk for future pregnancies. *Immunology* is pivotal in determining the success or failure of every pregnancy, as the fetoplacental unit is nature's transplant. Immune dysfunction or mismatch may underlie a whole spectrum of pregnancy outcomes, including failure of implantation, early and late pregnancy loss, preeclampsia, and preterm birth. Clinicians with basic knowledge in these 2 areas will serve patients better in both preconception counseling and pregnancy management.

Multiple disease phenotypes emanate from the normal function or suboptimal performance of the human placenta. Gestational *diabetes* is the direct result of diabetogenic placental hormones stressing insulin reserves in a pregnant woman. The growing obesity epidemic contributes to the increasing incidence of gestational diabetes and is itself associated with placental dysfunction and adverse pregnancy outcomes, including large- and small-for-gestational-age babies. *IUGR* derives from several sources, which includes placental chromosomal mosaicism, inadequacy of placental development of uteroplacental perfusion, and inadequate placental transport of nutrients.

Patients and families are commonly ecstatic when told that there is not 1, but 2, fetuses present in the uterus when scanned by ultrasound. Two for the price of one! This said, *twins* can certainly be "double trouble," whether there are 2 separate placentas or 1 placenta supplying both babies. Indeed, the advent of high-resolution ultrasound and fetal surgery has revolutionized the management of both dichorionic and monochorionic placentas. Knowing the specialized anatomy present in the placenta(s) of multifetal gestations, from early gestation through the third trimester, helps clinicians to optimize outcomes of this especially high-risk group.

Implantation disorders of the placenta are gaining expanded recognition among practitioners, especially those without tertiary care facilities readily available, as antenatal transfer for potentially life-threatening events has become increasingly important to optimize both maternal and fetal care. The diagnosis of placenta *previa* in the third trimester and the marked rise in incidence of placenta *accreta* secondary to previous cesarean-section scars are implantation disorders with high morbidity, especially due to hemorrhage. Preterm birth requiring acute response teams, massive transfusion protocols, and complicated abdominopelvic surgery with cesarean-hysterectomy are commonly the result of abnormal placental location or invasion into the uterus.

The *chorioamnionic* fetal membranes play vital, if underappreciated, roles in regulation of amniotic fluid volume and in signaling cascades that are associated with both term and preterm birth. Preterm premature rupture of membranes is an ominous condition. *Infections* of the chorionic villi or within the chorioamnion may lay dormant for days or weeks before clinical signs or diagnostic tests can determine the nature of a patient's problem among a panoply of findings, such as suboptimal fetal growth, diffuse nonspecific clinical signs, or fetal abnormalities. Placental infections are a major source for poor pregnancy outcomes, and understanding the routes by which infectious agents gain access to the fetoplacental unit helps clinicians to predict what tests to run and what agents are involved.

Imaging of the human placenta has been revolutionized by high-resolution ultrasound, including 3-dimensional imaging and Doppler flow studies. Management of all pregnancies have benefited from this revolution, as dating is rarely a question and high-risk pregnancies are monitored for growth and to provide reassurance of fetal well-being. Newer technologies are now being implemented to assess functional and structural parameters not available from ultrasound assessments. Importantly, MRI is increasingly applied to study of the placenta, as this offers new insights into blood flow and transport of some nutrients. The article on imaging offers insights into the future tools that will be available to clinicians to enhance assessment of pregnancy progression.

Artificial reproductive technologies (ART) are now standard of care throughout the westernized world. ART has been a boon for women with a number of fertility disorders, yet pregnancies that result from some of the manipulations employed are predisposed to an increased risk for placental developmental abnormalities and poor outcomes, including preeclampsia. ART pregnancies show significantly increased placental thickness and a higher incidence of hematomas, with both linked to an increased perinatal risk.[3] A recent metaanalysis identified that pregnancies of ART patients, compared with those conceived without ART, exhibited a higher incidence of placenta previa, placental abruption, and morbidly adherent placenta. The mechanisms by which ART adds risk to placental development are generally unknown, but disturbed trophoblast-decidual interactions in early pregnancy after ART conception may predispose to later complications in the pregnancies.

Few events are more devastating than experiencing a *stillbirth*. Many questions arise. Why has this happened? What did I do to cause this? Did my provider miss something? Is this punishment for my previous actions? Guilt and remorse characterize the patient and family of a pregnancy ending with a stillbirth. The article on stillbirth addresses the issues related to stillbirth and outlines key components for clinicians to consider in managing all pregnancies, high risk or not. Placental dysfunction, particularly associated with obesity and gestational diabetes, is high on the list.

Importantly, the future pregnancies of such individuals carry substantial risks for placental dysfunction, whether this be stillbirth or placental dysfunction associated with preterm birth, IUGR, or preeclampsia.

We hope you enjoy reading the articles in this issue. The placenta is clearly important *from womb to tomb*. Stay tuned for new developments as The Human Placenta Project in particular, and placental research in general, elucidates new discoveries about this important organ.

D. Michael Nelson, MD, PhD
Department of Obstetrics and Gynecology
Washington University
School of Medicine
660 South Euclid Avenue
Mail Stop: 8064-37-1005
St. Louis, MO 63110, USA

Leslie Myatt, PhD, FRCOG
Department of Obstetrics and Gynecology
Oregon Health & Science University
3181 SW Sam Jackson Park Road
Portland, Oregon 97239-3098, USA

E-mail addresses:
NelsonDM@wustl.edu (D.M. Nelson)
MyattL@ohsu.edu (L. Myatt)

REFERENCES

1. McMillen IC, Robinson JS. Developmental origins of the metabolic syndrome: prediction, plasticity, and programming. Physiol Rev 2005;85(2):571–633.
2. Staff AC, Redman CW, Williams D, et al. Pregnancy and long-term maternal cardiovascular health: progress through harmonization of research cohorts and biobanks. Hypertension 2016;67(2):251–60.
3. Joy J, Gannon C, McClure N, et al. Is assisted reproduction associated with abnormal placentation? Pediatr Dev Pathol 2012;15(4):306–14.

Social Determinants of Placental Health and Future Disease Risks for Babies

Kent L. Thornburg, MS, PhD[a,b,c,d,*],
Janne Boone-Heinonen, MPH, PhD[e], Amy M. Valent, DO[c]

KEYWORDS

- Placental health • Maternal stress • Social determinants of health • Maternal obesity
- Pregnancy outcomes

KEY POINTS

- Maternal stressors that are associated with fetal growth include maternal diet, toxic social stress, and exposure to harmful chemicals, each of which affects fetal organ structure and epigenetic status.
- The social determinants of health represent the social environment in which people live. Adverse social conditions are associated with poor pregnancy outcomes.
- The role of social factors in determining the health of the placenta has not been thoroughly investigated.
- Maternal social factors likely stimulate release of stress molecules such as cortisol to modify placental function and modify growth of fetal organs.

If people remember the placenta at all, it is as the unseemly and insignificant afterbirth that follows the delivery of a baby. Even among medical scientists, the placenta remains the forgotten organ, explaining why it has been understudied relative to other organs over the era of modern medicine. It is now becoming possible to build a story around each newly born baby that has predictive value regarding health risks that follow that individual through infancy, childhood, adolescence, and adulthood. The

[a] Moore Institute, Oregon Health & Science University, 3030 SW Moody Avenue, MDYMI, Portland, OR 97239, USA; [b] Center for Developmental Health, Knight Cardiovascular Institute, Oregon Health & Science University, 3030 SW Moody Avenue, MDYMI, Portland, OR 97239, USA; [c] Department of Obstetrics and Gynecology, Oregon Health & Science University, 3181 SW Sam Jackson Road, Portland, OR 97239, USA; [d] Bob and Charlee Moore Institute for Nutrition & Wellness, School of Medicine, Oregon Health & Science University, 3030 SW Moody Avenue, MDYMI, Portland, OR 97239, USA; [e] School of Public Health, Oregon Health & Science University, 3181 SW Sam Jackson Park Road, Portland, OR 97239, USA
* Corresponding author. Knight Cardiovascular Institute, School of Medicine, Oregon Health & Science University, 3030 SW Moody Avenue, MDYMI, Portland, OR 97239.
E-mail address: thornbur@ohsu.edu

Obstet Gynecol Clin N Am 47 (2020) 1–15
https://doi.org/10.1016/j.ogc.2019.11.002
0889-8545/20/© 2019 Elsevier Inc. All rights reserved.

obgyn.theclinics.com

story includes biological indicators of how the baby grew before birth, the physical attributes of the mother, and the social world that influenced the mother's and father's health. In addition, it is becoming clear that the health of the placenta is also an important determinant of the health risks of offspring. The authors propose that the placenta, in contrast with its unappreciated status heretofore, plays a key role in the health of all human populations.

Both the father and the mother have important influences on placental growth and function and consequent fetal outcomes. In an Indian study, maternal, but not paternal, body mass index, and paternal, but not maternal, height were positively associated with placental volume.[1] These transgenerational effects are suspected to be, in part, epigenetic. This article focuses primarily on mothers because of their required relationship with the placenta; fathers are slighted herein because of the paucity of information on specific paternal stressors that lead to a placental outcome. This article is designed to build a theoretic framework for the relationship between the human maternal social environment and placental growth and function. In it, human data are emphasized. That limitation should not detract from the outstanding animal research that explores biological factors through which maternal influences drive the role of the placenta in the developmental origins of disease. These data have been reviewed recently.[2,3] The premise underlying this article is that social conditions of the mother before and during pregnancy strongly affect the fetus through the placenta and, as such, have transgenerational importance.

Since Barker and colleagues first showed that birthweight was a predictor of cardiovascular disease, the discovery has been dramatically expanded.[4] In some cases, such as the effects of starvation during the Dutch Hunger Winter, birthweight was not affected in babies exposed to famine when restricted to early gestation.[5] For some chronic conditions, placental size and shape along with maternal phenotype are even better predictors of future disease than birthweight.[3,6] For example, among people in the Helsinki Birth Cohort, a small maternal surface area of the placenta was associated with coronary heart disease, but only in mothers taller than the median height (160 cm) of the cohort.[7] In contrast, among people whose mothers were less than the median height, the prevalence of hypertension was reduced from 38% if the placental area was less than 200 cm^2, to 21% if the area was greater than 320 cm^2 ($P = .0007$).[8] Thus, the risks for both coronary heart disease and hypertension are related to placental size. In men, hypertension was associated with placental width.[9] In women, offspring hypertension was linked to the mother's height, an indicator of the mother's diet and protein metabolism.[9] These examples suggest that the growth patterns of the placenta, under specific conditions of maternal phenotype, are powerful determinants of disease risk in offspring. However, the biological links between maternal physiologic condition and placentation have been little studied.

THE WORSENING HEALTH OF UNITED STATES POPULATIONS

Over the last 3 generations, obesity and type 2 diabetes have been increasing in prevalence in the United States.[10] In apparent contrast, the mortality from heart disease has decreased by more than half, beginning in the late 1960s. More people with diagnosed heart disease are now surviving for a length of time sufficient to die of other causes. The decrease in cardiac death rates should bring optimism to those so diagnosed. However, mortality data obscure the fact that the numbers of people with heart disease have been increasing in recent years.[11] Young people, including women 35 to 54 years old, are among those now affected by cardiac disease.[12]

The prevalence of diagnosed diabetes mellitus has been increasing at an accelerated rate beginning in the mid-1990s. In 2015, some 30 million people in the United States were estimated to have acquired diabetes.[13] Of these, more than 70% will acquire cardiovascular disease,[14] the most prevalent and expensive disease worldwide. At present, the cost of health care in the United States is about $3.3 trillion.[15] The American Heart Association predicted in 2017 that total heart disease costs would increase from the current ~$500 billion per year to some $1.1 trillion by the year 2035.[16] This massive increase would be required to cover costs for cardiovascular disease alone. It would add to the current $3.3 trillion[17] annual cost of health care as the population ages and more highly expensive drugs become available. Epidemiologic studies and secular trends in disease rates support the view that the US population has become increasingly vulnerable to expensive diseases over the last 3 generations.[17] Social factors are likely to be important drivers of this trend.

SOCIAL DETERMINANTS OF HEALTH AND DISEASE

The social determinants of health concept is defined by the social and environmental contexts in which people "are born, grow, live, work, and age"[18] and make lifestyle decisions. The topic has gained popularity over the past 2 decades and has become its own field of study. The social determinants of health is a complex concept because sociology includes multiple interacting factors (**Fig. 1**), ranging from economic stability and safe housing to access to medical care, each influenced by economic and social policies and cultural conditions.[19,20] The importance of social determinants as influencers of health is highlighted by the World Health Organization,[20] Centers for Disease Control and Prevention, and the Institute of Medicine.[21–23] Healthy People 2020

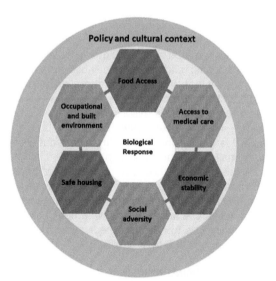

Fig. 1. The elements that comprise the social determinants of health include all social factors in a person's environment, with examples noted in the hexagonal boxes. Social adversity can lead to psychological and behavioral changes that elicit biological responses that affect a pregnant mother, her placenta, and ultimately the developmental integrity of fetal organs. These social determinants must be placed in cultural context, molded by public health policy, to understand how each one leads to a biological outcome among different ethnic groups.

developed 5 key determinants that influence health outcomes: economic stability, education, social and community context, health and health care, and neighborhood and built environment.[24] Each has the potential to influence pregnancy outcomes.

Geographic differences in life expectancy, as seen in the counties across the United States, are evidence of the social determinants of disease.[25] When reported in 2014, there was a 20-year difference in life expectancy at birth between Oglala Lakota County in South Dakota and Eagle County in Colorado, a mere 805 km (500 miles) away.[26] These two counties represented the shortest (66 years) and longest (86 years) life expectancy in the United States. The former county is within an Indian reservation where native people live under adverse conditions and have the lowest per-capita income in the country. In contrast, Eagle County has high levels of educational attainment, income, and access to medical care. Most people who reside in the county are physically active, trim, and well off. Differences in life expectancy up to some 16 years may also characterize different neighborhoods within a given city. Chicago is an example.[27] The differences in health status between those who live well and those who live with adversity 1.6 km (1 mile) away are profound and drive home the powerful impact of social circumstances as substrate for disease and compromised longevity.

OUTCOMES OF PREGNANCIES AFFLICTED BY MATERNAL SOCIAL ADVERSITIES

Poor diet, chemical exposures, and psychosocial stress are each consistently linked with adverse reproductive and child outcomes.[28] Women with low incomes are less likely to have access to medical care, to afford safe housing, or have access to healthy foods.[29–32] They are more likely to work in jobs with chemical exposure risk,[33,34] live in neighborhoods with high levels of pollution and crime,[35–37] and experience abuse or violence.[38,39] Women with minority race or ethnicity additionally face persistent discrimination and adverse social interactions.[40–42] Social circumstances such as incarceration, homelessness, and toxic stress at work have been little studied in pregnancy even though they are common.[43–45] Inadequate access to basic needs such as food, medical care, safe housing, and money to pay bills also has direct biological effects on pregnant women by inducing a chronic stress response, increasing cortisol levels, and eliciting other stress responses.[46–48]

Low socioeconomic status (SES) is associated with teen pregnancy, small-for-gestational-age (SGA) infants, gestational diabetes, preterm birth,[49–51] and preeclampsia. Low SES is further correlated with lower education levels, increased substance use,[52] food insecurity, and poor mental health,[53] all of which have been associated with increased rates of childhood obesity, poor psychosocial development, and perinatal mortality. Women facing these challenges are more likely to have inadequate prenatal care,[54] to be younger, and to belong to minority populations. Difficulty accessing the resources necessary to live a healthy life (eg, transportation, quality food, safe neighborhoods to exercise, medication costs) further perpetuates health disadvantages for women and their families.

SOCIAL FACTORS AFFECT OFFSPRING HEALTH

As indicated earlier, the Helsinki Birth Cohort was valuable in making associations between biological traits and disease outcomes. Several examples show the relationship between social conditions and chronic disease risk. Eriksson and colleagues[7,9] and Barker and colleagues[55] found that sudden cardiac death was associated with low SES of the victim's father. In addition, low educational status among offspring was highly associated with sudden cardiac death, with a hazard ratio (HR) of 3.4 (95%

confidence interval [CI], 2.0–5.8) in men and HR 4.7 (1.1–20.0) in women, compared with those with high levels of attainment (P for trend, 0.0001 and 0.01, respectively). Other medical conditions were also related to social conditions. In addition, lifespan was reduced by some 8 years in boys who were born small but who grew rapidly in childhood in a compensatory manner.[56] Reduced lifespan was associated with low maternal SES and slow intrauterine growth. The influence of such environmental conditions on fetal growth has been noted by others.[57]

MATERNAL OBESITY AS A CONSEQUENCE OF SOCIAL ADVERSITY

The prevalence of obesity among pregnant women is increasing throughout the United States. Maternal obesity is associated with several adverse pregnancy outcomes, including SGA, macrosomia, gestational diabetes, preeclampsia, cesarean delivery, and childhood obesity.[58] The obese condition affects placental growth and function.[58] There is evidence that high-SES women are less likely to become obese than low-SES women. In Finland's Helsinki Health Study Cohort, women 40 to 60 years old were studied. After adjustment for educational level, baseline obesity was associated with poverty (odds ratio [OR], 1.23; 95% CI, 1.05–1.44), frequent economic difficulties (OR, 1.74; 95% CI, 1.52–1.99), low household net income (OR, 1.23; 95% CI, 1.07–1.41), low household wealth (OR, 1.90; 95% CI, 1.59–2.26), and low personal income (OR, 1.22; 95% CI, 1.03–1.44).[59] This finding shows the well-known link between social status and health over the life course. These social issues also affect women who become pregnant.

RACISM AND PREGNANCY OUTCOMES

Racism is a known cause of health disparities[60] and has a profound effect on pregnancy outcomes,[61,62] including increased rates of preterm birth and infant mortality. The health of American women of African descent has been worsening over the past generation. African American women experience worse pregnancy outcomes than do non-Hispanic white women. Non-Hispanic black women have higher rates of preterm birth that are more than 50% higher than those of non-Hispanic white women.[63] Although the role of racism on placental growth and function has not been studied directly, increases in diastolic pressure in combination with racism lead to lower birthweight, which has a placental component and an increased risk of preterm birth.[64]

DEVELOPMENTAL ORIGINS OF HEALTH AND DISEASE

An understanding of the developmental origins of disease offers an added and often neglected perspective on social status and disease prevalence. Maternal exposure to poor diet, chemical exposures, and psychosocial stress influence fetal development such that babies affected are more biologically susceptible to further social adversities (so-called second hits) that lead to disease throughout the life course.[28]

Through what mechanisms could social factors affect the placenta? The most compelling among many possibilities are the powerful stressors known to be associated with early-life adversities and adult-onset chronic disease. These stressors include toxic social stress, maternofetal malnutrition, and exposure to chemical toxins (**Fig. 2**). In addition to social stress, several medical conditions, including diabetes mellitus[65] and preeclampsia,[66,67] affect placental function and lead to maternal physiologic abnormalities such as hyperglycemia and hyperlipidemia. These factors along

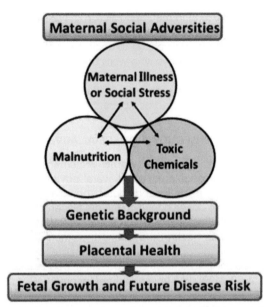

Fig. 2. Maternal social adversities act through stressors, including social stress, illness, poor nutrition, and toxic chemicals, that detrimentally affect placental health in accordance with epigenetic drivers and genetic predispositions. Robust fetal growth and unfettered organ development depend on a well-constructed and healthy placenta that is able to perform optimal transport, endocrine, and gas exchange functions.

with disturbances in the maternal intestinal microbiome are likely causes that affect placental function and pregnancy outcome.

There is increasing evidence that epigenetic modifications of expression of genes that are associated with a poor environment and that lead to disease risk are influenced by an individual's genetic background.[3] Weinberger's laboratory showed that, among people with genetic propensities for schizophrenia, those who were affected by the disease more often had mothers with adverse conditions in pregnancy, such as preeclampsia or intrauterine growth restriction. These conditions resulted in higher expression of risk genes in their placentas compared with people in whom the disease did not manifest.[68] These data suggest that maternal stressors affect gene activity in the placenta and influence susceptibility for disease states in the offspring.

THE MATERNAL INTESTINAL MICROBIOME AND THE PLACENTA

Based on previous studies, the maternal intestinal microbiome could have an important role in pregnancy at least 2 ways:

1. The microbial community in the gut may provide important nutritive substances, such as unique short-chain fatty acids, that cross the placenta and nourish the fetus.[69]
2. Bacterial species derived from the maternal gut could find their way to the fetus via the placenta and affect fetal health.[70,71]

Evidence is mounting that living microbes can be found in the normal placenta. However, research is needed to determine the degree to which such findings are laboratory specific. Because it is known from animal[72] and human[73] studies that social stressors affect the gut microbiome, there is reason to suspect that maternal stress may affect 1 or both of the processes mentioned earlier and these could affect placental function.

NUTRITIONAL STRESS IN PREGNANCY AND PLACENTAL FUNCTION

Pregnant women are different from hibernating pregnant bears. Pregnant bears are able to store fat before winter and "sleep" for months while pregnant without eating. While hibernating, their offspring grow normally even though their body temperature decreases by 7°C to 8°C and their respiration and heart rate decrease substantially.[74] Surprisingly, they stay fit during their rest period. They do not lose much muscle because they recycle urea from fat to make protein.[75,76]

In contrast, human fetuses require a constant supply of nutrients in order to grow normally, especially in the last 2 trimesters. Fetuses acquire their nutrients from maternal muscle and fat turnover, which supplies amino acids and lipids, respectively. In addition, they acquire a host of nutrients gleaned from their mothers' diets. Babies whose mothers were starved in midgestation or late gestation during the Dutch Hunger Winter were lighter than babies unexposed, but not by much.[5] Thus, it is clear that human babies can benefit from maternal tissue turnover, although less so than bears. There is evidence that pregnancy outcomes are better if women consume a nutritious diet before they become pregnant. In studies among 1962 at-risk Indian women who started supplementation 3 months or longer before pregnancy, mean birthweight increased by 48 g and the incidence of low birth weight was reduced by 24%.[77] Women who consumed the supplement only during pregnancy did not show the same benefit. It seems that prepregnancy nutrition is equally, if not more, important than nutrient consumption during pregnancy.

On average, people in the United States have been increasing their consumption[78] of calories from fast foods and highly processed industrial foods over recent decades. These foods have high inflammatory potential.[79] This eating pattern has become part of the food culture in the United States. Women do not eat worse diets than men and are thus not to blame for changes in disease patterns within the US population. Men and women alike consume poor diets according to the culture in which they live.

MATERNAL SOCIAL STRESS AND PLACENTAL FUNCTION

The varied forms of social stress were described earlier (see **Fig. 1**). Although toxic chemicals and poor diets are forms of physiologic stress, social stress can be synergistic to those stressors through an insidious process that alters normal physiologic processes over weeks to months. Most reproductive scientists and clinicians are aware that social stress is related to poor pregnancy outcomes. However, the role of the placenta in mediating those outcomes has not received enough attention. Although it is well known that maternal adversities are associated with preterm birth, intrauterine growth retardation, and later-life disease risk, neurologic outcomes are only now coming to light.[80] They include developmental delays, anxiety, hyperactivity, attention deficits, and compromised cognitive function in offspring children.[81]

One way to evaluate the impact of stress on pregnancy outcomes is to study women who were pregnant during a significant disaster. Studies include natural disasters such as an ice storm[82,83] or flooding,[84] and human-made disasters such as the 9/11 terrorist attacks in New York City[85] and the Dutch Hunger Winter.[5] Among the findings of these studies was a reduction in birthweight, increased weight of offspring during childhood, and cognitive deficits. Women who experienced violence during pregnancy also have smaller babies and increased rates of preterm delivery.[86] These studies fit well with outcomes following stress in pregnant animals. The maternal-placental-fetal neuroendocrine axis is well known to be important in normal fetal development and it is likely to be the driver of placental contributions to maternal stress responses that affect the fetus.[87] The full axis is complicated because it involves maternal pituitary, adrenal, placental, fetal pituitary, and fetal adrenal tissues. Other hormone-related actions are involved, including the renin-angiotensin system, atrial natriuretic system, as well as catecholamine neurotransmitters. Corticotropin-releasing hormone (CRH) derived from the placenta is particularly interesting: like cortisol, it seems to be a stress response hormone associated with premature delivery.[87,88]

There is strong evidence that maternal stress leads to increased plasma levels of maternal CRH and glucocorticoids. Cortisol stimulates the placenta to increase its production of CRH in a feed-forward fashion. Thus, when maternal cortisol levels are high, CRH levels increase as well. Cortisol inhibits fetal growth (except for the heart and kidney) so that even babies born at term in highly stressed mothers are smaller and have an increased risk for disease. The placenta generates the enzyme 11β-hydroxysteroid dehydrogenase-2, which chemically modifies cortisol to its inactive form, cortisone. However, this protective mechanism is compromised under highly stressful conditions so that excess cortisol can traverse the placenta and affect the fetus.

MATERNAL SOCIAL STATUS, TOXICANT EXPOSURE, AND THE PLACENTA

People who live at a social disadvantage are more commonly exposed to toxic chemicals and are subjected to higher plasma concentrations.[89] Toxicants range from pesticides, polycyclic aromatic hydrocarbons, particulate matter, and toxic metals to plasticizers and multiple toxins in cigarette smoke. Pregnant women who live in poorer areas are also exposed to more toxicants than people in better social circumstances. Preterm birth is more common in mothers of low SES, in part because of exposure to environmental pollutants during pregnancy.[90] Maternal toxicants are taken up by the placenta. Some are expelled back into the maternal circulation, whereas others are passed to the fetus in varying degrees.[91] In the placenta, redox-inactive metals, including cadmium, lead, and mercury, deplete cellular antioxidants, particularly thiol-containing antioxidants and enzymes.[92] This process leads to high levels of oxidative stress within the placenta and fetus. Plasticizers are known to be endocrine disruptors that are found commonly in the blood of pregnant women. When the concentration is high enough, toxicants cause enduring physiologic and epigenetic effects in offspring.[93]

P-glycoproteins (P-gps) are members of a group of transporters in the ATP binding cassette superfamily. Some P-gps members impart multidrug resistance by the active extrusion of toxic substances from many different types of cells. They function as plasma membrane proteins of 170 kDa encoded by the ABCB1 gene.[94] These proteins that protect against toxic substances are functional within the trophoblast layers of the placenta but gradually reduce their expression over the course of gestation.[95] There is reason to believe that they are compromised in stressed placentas by general inflammatory processes[96] or by specific cytokines.[97] They may also be downregulated by augmentation of histone deacytelases.[98] There is evidence that multidrug resistance proteins protect the placenta to some degree from high circulating cortisol levels experienced under conditions of chronic maternal stress.[99,100] It can reasonably be hypothesized that fetuses carried by mothers with metabolic disease and who are exposed to chronic social stresses are more likely to experience toxin exposures because they are exposed to higher levels of toxicants consequent to reduced P-gps–derived protection.

CAN HEALTH CARE PRACTITIONERS PREDICT THE LIFELONG HEALTH OF BABIES?

This article makes the case that social determinants should be included in an assessment of a baby's risk for future disease. The scientific community has known for decades that low birthweight predicts disease and that food deprivation during pregnancy is a cause of developmental programming even if birthweight is not affected.[5] It is only recently that scientists have discovered that the placental and maternal phenotypes are also predictors of chronic health conditions in adults. Obstetricians can observe the growth of the babies and placentas in real time, both are important indicators of later disease. However, the predictive power of biological observations would be more robust if the parents' exposures to toxic chemicals, nutritional histories, and social adversities were known.

Is there a link between the maternal social environment, placental function, and the epidemic of chronic disease? The placenta is present for less than 300 days out of some 30,000 days in an average lifetime, or about 1% of the lifespan. How could it carry such biological significance? This question is especially important at this time because of the aforementioned rapid deterioration of the health of US populations and the prospect of facing a financial crisis in health care. The answer to the question lies in the intended function of the placenta; in a mere 9 months, the placenta provides all of the nutrient building blocks of the fetal body, which are the foundation for a life of health or disease. If, because of poor social circumstances, placental function is compromised, babies born in such conditions will carry increased disease risks for a lifetime.

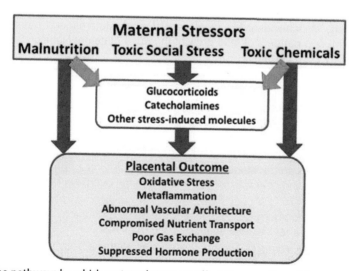

Fig. 3. The pathways by which maternal stressors affect the growth and function of the human placenta are little understood. Inadequate nutrition and toxic chemicals affect the placenta directly. However, both join with toxic social stress in causing the maternal release of stress-induced factors that include glucocorticoids and catecholamines. The sum of these maternal stressors leads to inflammation, oxidative stress, and consequent compromised placenta function.

BY WHAT BIOLOGICAL MECHANISMS DOES THE SOCIAL ENVIRONMENT MOLD THE GROWTH AND FUNCTION OF THE PLACENTA AND DETERMINE THE HEALTH OF THE BABY?

Although some aspects of maternal stress and fetal outcomes have been investigated, most have not. **Fig. 3** shows the interactions between the types of stress and the pathways that affect placental growth and function. Uncovering the intricacies of placental biology is of the same importance as investigations in any other field of medicine because of the placenta's potential impact on the health of human populations. Scientists, clinicians, and funding agencies should devise strategies to expedite research on the link between the social drivers that lead to compromised placentas and babies, not only to relieve human suffering but also to avert dramatic reductions in health care financial support that will otherwise accompany the predicted increase in the prevalence of chronic disease in the United States. Now is an appropriate time for reproductive scientists and funding agencies to invest in the social determinants of health and disease and discover the role of the placenta in linking the two.

ACKNOWLEDGMENTS

The authors thank Kim Rogers, Lisa Rhuman, and Bernadette Battilega for help in preparing the article.

DISCLOSURE

The authors thank the National Institutes of Health: PO1 HD34430 (KLT), R21 HD090529 (KLT), R01 AG032339 NIH/NIA, K01 DK102857 (JBH), K12 WRHR OHSU (AMV).

REFERENCES

1. Wills AK, Chinchwadkar MC, Joglekar CV, et al. Maternal and paternal height and BMI and patterns of fetal growth: the Pune Maternal Nutrition Study. Early Hum Dev 2010;86(9):535–40.
2. Sferruzzi-Perri AN, Camm EJ. The programming power of the placenta. Front Physiol 2016;7:33.
3. Burton GJ, Fowden AL, Thornburg KL. Placental origins of chronic disease. Physiol Rev 2016;96(4):1509–65.
4. Barker DJ, Winter PD, Osmond C, et al. Weight in infancy and death from ischaemic heart disease. Lancet 1989;2(8663):577–80.
5. Roseboom T, van der Meulen J, Ravelli A, et al. Effects of prenatal exposure to the Dutch famine on adult disease in later life: an overview. Mol Cell Endocrinol 2001;185:93–8.
6. Barker DJ, Thornburg KL. Placental programming of chronic diseases, cancer and lifespan: a review. Placenta 2013;34(10):841–5.
7. Eriksson JG, Kajantie E, Thornburg KL, et al. Mother's body size and placental size predict coronary heart disease in men. Eur Heart J 2011;32(18):2297–303.
8. Barker DJ, Thornburg KL, Osmond C, et al. The surface area of the placenta and hypertension in the offspring in later life. Int J Dev Biol 2010;54(2–3): 525–30.
9. Eriksson JG, Kajantie E, Osmond C, et al. Boys live dangerously in the womb. Am J Hum Biol 2010;22(3):330–5.

10. Boyle JP, Honeycutt AA, Narayan KM, et al. Projection of diabetes burden through 2050: impact of changing demography and disease prevalence in the U.S. Diabetes care 2001;24(11):1936–40.
11. Benjamin EJ, Virani SS, Callaway CW, et al. Heart disease and stroke statistics-2018 update: a report from the American Heart Association. Circulation 2018; 137(12):e67–492.
12. Arora S, Stouffer GA, Kucharska-Newton AM, et al. Twenty year trends and sex differences in young adults hospitalized with acute myocardial infarction. Circulation 2019;139(8):1047–56.
13. More than 100 million Americans have diabetes or prediabetes. Centers for Disease Control and Prevention Press Release; 2017. Available at: https://www.cdc.gov/media/releases/2017/p0718-diabetes-report.html.
14. Cardiovascular Disease and Diabetes American Heart Association Center for Health Metrics and Evaluation, 2015. This is a website report by the American Heart Association. https://www.heart.org/en/health-topics/diabetes/why-diabetes-matters/cardiovascular-disease–diabetes.
15. Health and Economic Costs of Chronic Disease. National Center for Chronic Disease Prevention and Health Promotion. 2019. Available at: https://www.cdc.gov/chronicdisease/about/costs/index.htm.
16. Cardiovascular disease: a costly burden for America, projections through 2035. American Heart Association Center for Health Metrics and Evaluation; 2017. Available at: https://healthmetrics.heart.org/cardiovascular-disease-a-costly-burden/.
17. National health expenditure fact sheet. Centers for Medicare & Medicaid Services; 2019. Available at: https://www.cms.gov/research-statistics-data-and-systems/statistics-trends-and-reports/nationalhealthexpenddata/nhe-fact-sheet.html.
18. Doyle SK, Chang AM, Levy P, et al. Achieving health equity in hypertension management through addressing the social determinants of health. Curr Hypertens Rep 2019;21(8):58.
19. Braveman P, Gottlieb L. The social determinants of health: it's time to consider the causes of the causes. Public Health Rep 2014;129(Suppl 2):19–31.
20. Braveman P, Egerter S, Williams DR. The social determinants of health: coming of age. Annu Rev Public Health 2011;32:381–98.
21. Adler NE, Stead WW. Patients in context–EHR capture of social and behavioral determinants of health. N Engl J Med 2015;372(8):698–701.
22. Institute of Medicine. Capturing social and behavioral domains in electronic health records: phase 1. Washington, DC: The National Academic Press; 2014.
23. National Academies of Sciences, Engineering, and Medicine. A framework for educating health professionals to address the social determinants of health. Washington (DC): National Academies Press (US); 2016.
24. Social Determinants of Health. Office of disease prevention and health promotion, Healthy Peoplegov. 2019;2020 Topics & Objectives. Available at: https://www.healthypeople.gov/2020/topics-objectives/topic/social-determinants-of-health.
25. Dwyer-Lindgren L, Bertozzi-Villa A, Stubbs RW, et al. Inequalities in life expectancy among US counties, 1980 to 2014: temporal trends and key drivers. JAMA Intern Med 2017;177(7):1003–11.
26. Achenbach J. U.S. life expectancy varies by more than 20 years from county to county. Washington Post May 9, 2017.
27. Mapping life expectancy: 16 years in Chicago, Illinois. Center on Society and Health, Virginia Commonwealth University; 2019. Available at: https://societyhealth.vcu.edu/work/the-projects/mapschicago.html.

28. Messer LC, Boone-Heinonen J, Mponwane L, et al. Developmental programming: priming disease susceptibility for subsequent generations. Curr Epidemiol Rep 2015;2(1):37–51.
29. Wheeler SM, Bryant AS. Racial and ethnic disparities in health and health care. Obstet Gynecol Clin North Am 2017;44(1):1–11.
30. Dodson RE, Udesky JO, Colton MD, et al. Chemical exposures in recently renovated low-income housing: influence of building materials and occupant activities. Environ Int 2017;109:114–27.
31. Gross RS, Mendelsohn AL, Arana MM, et al. Food insecurity during pregnancy and breastfeeding by low-income hispanic mothers. Pediatrics 2019;143(6) [pii: e20184113].
32. Leung CW, Epel ES, Ritchie LD, et al. Food insecurity is inversely associated with diet quality of lower-income adults. J Acad Nutr Diet 2014;114(12): 1943–53.e2.
33. Holmes LM, Ling PM. Workplace secondhand smoke exposure: a lingering hazard for young adults in California. Tob Control 2017;26(e1):e79–84.
34. Moyce SC, Schenker M. Occupational exposures and health outcomes among immigrants in the USA. Curr Environ Health Rep 2017;4(3):349–54.
35. Harris KM. Mapping inequality: childhood asthma and environmental injustice, a case study of St. Louis, Missouri. Soc Sci Med 2019;230:91–110.
36. Payne-Sturges D, Gee GC. National environmental health measures for minority and low-income populations: tracking social disparities in environmental health. Environ Res 2006;102(2):154–71.
37. Yu H, Stuart AL. Exposure and inequality for select urban air pollutants in the Tampa Bay area. Sci Total Environ 2016;551-552:474–83.
38. Holliday CN, McCauley HL, Silverman JG, et al. Racial/ethnic differences in women's experiences of reproductive coercion, intimate partner violence, and unintended pregnancy. J Womens Health (Larchmt) 2017;26(8):828–35.
39. Sumner SA, Mercy JA, Dahlberg LL, et al. Violence in the United States: status, challenges, and opportunities. JAMA 2015;314(5):478–88.
40. Panza GA, Puhl RM, Taylor BA, et al. Links between discrimination and cardiovascular health among socially stigmatized groups: a systematic review. PLoS One 2019;14(6):e0217623.
41. Cuevas AG, Ho T, Rodgers J, et al. Developmental timing of initial racial discrimination exposure is associated with cardiovascular health conditions in adulthood. Ethn Health 2019. [Epub ahead of print].
42. Dominguez TP. Race, racism, and racial disparities in adverse birth outcomes. Clin Obstet Gynecol 2008;51(2):360–70.
43. Clarke JG, Adashi EY. Perinatal care for incarcerated patients: a 25-year-old woman pregnant in jail. JAMA 2011;305(9):923–9.
44. Sufrin C, Kolbi-Molinas A, Roth R. Reproductive justice, health disparities and incarcerated women in the United States. Perspect Sex Reprod Health 2015; 47(4):213–9.
45. Chisholm CA, Bullock L, Ferguson JEJ 2nd. Intimate partner violence and pregnancy: epidemiology and impact. Am J Obstet Gynecol 2017;217(2):141–4.
46. Hertzman C, Boyce T. How experience gets under the skin to create gradients in developmental health. Annu Rev Public Health 2010;31:329–47, 323p following 347.
47. McEwen BS. Brain on stress: how the social environment gets under the skin. Proc Natl Acad Sci U S A 2012;109(Suppl 2):17180–5.

48. Laraia BA, Leak TM, Tester JM, et al. Biobehavioral factors that shape nutrition in low-income populations: a narrative review. Am J Prev Med 2017;52(2s2): S118–26.
49. Kim MK, Lee SM, Bae SH, et al. Socioeconomic status can affect pregnancy outcomes and complications, even with a universal healthcare system. Int J Equity Health 2018;17(1):2.
50. Leppalahti S, Gissler M, Mentula M, et al. Is teenage pregnancy an obstetric risk in a welfare society? A population-based study in Finland, from 2006 to 2011. BMJ open 2013;3(8):e003225.
51. Bo S, Menato G, Bardelli C, et al. Low socioeconomic status as a risk factor for gestational diabetes. Diabetes Metab 2002;28(2):139–40.
52. Mulia N, Schmidt L, Bond J, et al. Stress, social support and problem drinking among women in poverty. Addiction 2008;103(8):1283–93.
53. Atif N, Lovell K, Rahman A. Maternal mental health: the missing "m" in the global maternal and child health agenda. Semin Perinatol 2015;39(5):345–52.
54. Osterman MJK, Martin JA. Timing and adequacy of prenatal care in the United States, 2016. Natl Vital Stat Rep 2018;67(3):1–14.
55. Barker DJ, Larsen G, Osmond C, et al. The placental origins of sudden cardiac death. Int J Epidemiol 2012;41(5):1394–9.
56. Barker DJ, Osmond C, Thornburg KL, et al. The lifespan of men and the shape of their placental surface at birth. Placenta 2011;32(10):783–7.
57. Dimasuay KG, Boeuf P, Powell TL, et al. Placental responses to changes in the maternal environment determine fetal growth. Front Physiol 2016;7:12.
58. Howell KR, Powell TL. Effects of maternal obesity on placental function and fetal development. Reproduction 2017;153(3):R97–108.
59. Hiilamo A, Lallukka T, Manty M, et al. Obesity and socioeconomic disadvantage in midlife female public sector employees: a cohort study. BMC Public Health 2017;17(1):842.
60. Williams DR, Collins C. Racial residential segregation: a fundamental cause of racial disparities in health. Public Health Rep 2001;116(5):404–16.
61. Chae DH, Clouston S, Martz CD, et al. Area racism and birth outcomes among Blacks in the United States. Soc Sci Med 2018;199:49–55.
62. Bower KM, Geller RJ, Perrin NA, et al. Experiences of racism and preterm birth: findings from a pregnancy risk assessment monitoring system, 2004 through 2012. Womens Health Issues 2018;28(6):495–501.
63. McKinnon B, Yang S, Kramer MS, et al. Comparison of black-white disparities in preterm birth between Canada and the United States. CMAJ 2016;188(1): E19–26.
64. Hilmert CJ, Dominguez TP, Schetter CD, et al. Lifetime racism and blood pressure changes during pregnancy: implications for fetal growth. Health Psychol 2014;33(1):43–51.
65. Pantham P, Aye IL, Powell TL. Inflammation in maternal obesity and gestational diabetes mellitus. Placenta 2015;36(7):709–15.
66. Myatt L. Role of placenta in preeclampsia. Endocrine 2002;19(1):103–11.
67. Roberts JM, Escudero C. The placenta in preeclampsia. Pregnancy Hypertens 2012;2(2):72–83.
68. Ursini G, Punzi G, Chen Q, et al. Convergence of placenta biology and genetic risk for schizophrenia. Nat Med 2018;24(6):792–801.
69. Tan J, McKenzie C, Potamitis M, et al. The role of short-chain fatty acids in health and disease. Adv Immunol 2014;121:91–119.

70. Walker RW, Clemente JC, Peter I, et al. The prenatal gut microbiome: are we colonized with bacteria in utero? Pediatr Obes 2017;12(Suppl 1):3–17.

71. Yu K, Rodriguez MD, Paul Z, et al. Proof of principle: physiological transfer of small numbers of bacteria from mother to fetus in late-gestation pregnant sheep. PLoS One 2019;14(6):e0217211.

72. Cui B, Gai Z, She X, et al. Effects of chronic noise on glucose metabolism and gut microbiota-host inflammatory homeostasis in rats. Sci Rep 2016;6:36693.

73. Hemmings SMJ, Malan-Muller S, van den Heuvel LL, et al. The microbiome in posttraumatic stress disorder and trauma-exposed controls: an exploratory study. Psychosom Med 2017;79(8):936–46.

74. Stenvinkel P, Jani AH, Johnson RJ. Hibernating bears (Ursidae): metabolic magicians of definite interest for the nephrologist. Kidney Int 2013;83(2):207–12.

75. Nelson RA, Jones JD, Wahner HW, et al. Nitrogen metabolism in bears: urea metabolism in summer starvation and in winter sleep and role of urinary bladder in water and nitrogen conservation. Mayo Clin Proc 1975;50(3):141–6.

76. Nelson RA. Protein and fat metabolism in hibernating bears. Fed Proc 1980; 39(12):2955–8.

77. Potdar RD, Sahariah SA, Gandhi M, et al. Improving women's diet quality preconceptionally and during gestation: effects on birth weight and prevalence of low birth weight–a randomized controlled efficacy trial in India (Mumbai Maternal Nutrition Project). Am J Clin Nutr 2014;100(5):1257–68.

78. Briefel RR, Johnson CL. Secular trends in dietary intake in the United States. Annu Rev Nutr 2004;24:401–31.

79. Ryu S, Shivappa N, Veronese N, et al. Secular trends in Dietary Inflammatory Index among adults in the United States, 1999-2014. Eur J Clin Nutr 2019;73(10): 1343–51.

80. Rondo PH, Ferreira RF, Nogueira F, et al. Maternal psychological stress and distress as predictors of low birth weight, prematurity and intrauterine growth retardation. Eur J Clin Nutr 2003;57(2):266–72.

81. Wadhwa PD, Sandman CA, Garite TJ. The neurobiology of stress in human pregnancy: implications for prematurity and development of the fetal central nervous system. Prog Brain Res 2001;133:131–42.

82. King S, Dancause K, Turcotte-Tremblay AM, et al. Using natural disasters to study the effects of prenatal maternal stress on child health and development. Birth Defects Res C Embryo Today 2012;96(4):273–88.

83. King S, Laplante DP. The effects of prenatal maternal stress on children's cognitive development: project Ice Storm. Stress 2005;8(1):35–45.

84. Dancause KN, Laplante DP, Hart KJ, et al. Prenatal stress due to a natural disaster predicts adiposity in childhood: the Iowa Flood Study. J Obes 2015; 2015:570541.

85. Eskenazi B, Marks AR, Catalano R, et al. Low birthweight in New York City and upstate New York following the events of September 11th. Hum Reprod 2007; 22(11):3013–20.

86. Nesari M, Olson JK, Vandermeer B, et al. Does a maternal history of abuse before pregnancy affect pregnancy outcomes? A systematic review with meta-analysis. BMC Pregnancy Childbirth 2018;18(1):404.

87. Petraglia F, Imperatore A, Challis JR. Neuroendocrine mechanisms in pregnancy and parturition. Endocr Rev 2010;31(6):783–816.

88. Weinstock M. The potential influence of maternal stress hormones on development and mental health of the offspring. Brain Behav Immun 2005;19(4): 296–308.

89. Tyrrell J, Melzer D, Henley W, et al. Associations between socioeconomic status and environmental toxicant concentrations in adults in the USA: NHANES 2001-2010. Environ Int 2013;59:328–35.
90. Anand M, Agarwal P, Singh L, et al. Persistent organochlorine pesticides and oxidant/antioxidant status in the placental tissue of the women with full-term and pre-term deliveries. Toxicol Res 2015;4(2):326–32.
91. Chen Z, Myers R, Wei T, et al. Placental transfer and concentrations of cadmium, mercury, lead, and selenium in mothers, newborns, and young children. J Expo Sci Environ Epidemiol 2014;24(5):537–44.
92. Ahamed M, Mehrotra PK, Kumar P, et al. Placental lead-induced oxidative stress and preterm delivery. Environ Toxicol Pharmacol 2009;27(1):70–4.
93. Manikkam M, Tracey R, Guerrero-Bosagna C, et al. Plastics derived endocrine disruptors (BPA, DEHP and DBP) induce epigenetic transgenerational inheritance of obesity, reproductive disease and sperm epimutations. PLoS One 2013;8(1):e55387.
94. Devault A, Gros P. Two members of the mouse mdr gene family confer multidrug resistance with overlapping but distinct drug specificities. Mol Cell Biol 1990; 10(4):1652–63.
95. Sun M, Kingdom J, Baczyk D, et al. Expression of the multidrug resistance P-glycoprotein, (ABCB1 glycoprotein) in the human placenta decreases with advancing gestation. Placenta 2006;27(6–7):602–9.
96. Goralski KB, Hartmann G, Piquette-Miller M, et al. Downregulation of mdr1a expression in the brain and liver during CNS inflammation alters the in vivo disposition of digoxin. Br J Pharmacol 2003;139(1):35–48.
97. Sukhai M, Yong A, Pak A, et al. Decreased expression of P-glycoprotein in interleukin-1beta and interleukin-6 treated rat hepatocytes. Inflamm Res 2001; 50(7):362–70.
98. Duan H, Zhou K, Zhang Y, et al. HDAC2 was involved in placental P-glycoprotein regulation both in vitro and vivo. Placenta 2017;58:105–14.
99. Yates CR, Chang C, Kearbey JD, et al. Structural determinants of P-glycoprotein-mediated transport of glucocorticoids. Pharm Res 2003;20(11):1794–803.
100. Benediktsson R, Calder AA, Edwards CR, et al. Placental 11 beta-hydroxysteroid dehydrogenase: a key regulator of fetal glucocorticoid exposure. Clin Endocrinol 1997;46(2):161–6.

The Placenta as a Window to Maternal Vascular Health

W. Tony Parks, MD[a], Janet M. Catov, PhD, MS[b,c,d],*

KEYWORDS

- Placenta • Maternal vascular malperfusion • Women • Cardiovascular

KEY POINTS

- The placenta is evaluated to understand fetal health, and emerging evidence indicates that maternal vascular malperfusion (MVM) features may provide clues to women's later life cardiovascular risk.
- Pathologic changes that directly involve the maternal vascular supply to the placenta, collectively termed decidual vasculopathy, develop early in gestation, and their effects on maternal blood flow to the placenta may be etiologic for the other MVM findings.
- A second group of MVM lesions includes those entities that likely arise subsequently in the pregnancy as a result of hypoxic/ischemic injury and oxidative damage to the placenta (small placental size, villous infarction, retroplacental hemorrhage, accelerated villous maturation, and distal villous hypoplasia).
- MVM lesions are detected in each of the great obstetric syndromes, and emerging evidence suggests that decidual vasculopathy may be linked to future pregnancy complications, maternal dyslipidemia, higher blood pressure, and increased vascular resistance years after delivery.
- Identification of the mechanisms leading to decidual vasculopathy may improve pregnancy health and contribute new sex-specific insights regarding the etiology of cardiovascular disease in women.

Sources of Funding: This work was funded by the American Heart Association Go Red for Women Strategically Focused Research Network, contracts AHA 16SFRN27810001 and 16SFRN28930000, The Placenta as a Window to Maternal Microvascular Disease Risk (Catov).
^a Department of Laboratory Medicine and Pathobiology, University of Toronto, 600 University Avenue, Toronto, Ontario M5G 1X5, Canada; ^b Department of Obstetrics, Gynecology, and RS, University of Pittsburgh School of Medicine, 204 Craft Avenue, Pittsburgh, PA 15213, USA; ^c Department of Epidemiology, Graduate School of Public Health, University of Pittsburgh, Pittsburgh, PA, USA; ^d Magee-Womens Research Institute, 204 Craft Avenue, Suite A208, Pittsburgh, PA 15213, USA
* Corresponding author. Magee-Womens Research Institute, 204 Craft Avenue, Suite A208, Pittsburgh, PA 15213.
E-mail address: catovjm@upmc.edu

INTRODUCTION

Cardiovascular disease (CVD) in women remains a major health concern. Although it is now known that CVD manifests differently in women than in men, exploration of these differences is ongoing and incomplete. Optimal treatment regimens for women also remain to be determined. Despite an overall decline in the CVD death rate in the United States, the rate of decline has been slower for women compared with men. In addition, racial disparities in CVD in women stubbornly persist. CVD mortality is 70% higher in African American women compared with white women.[1]

A generation ago, many pregnancy complications were considered to be isolated occurrences with limited recurrence risks and essentially no impact on the later life health of the mother. This comforting fiction began to unravel with the discovery that women with a history of preeclampsia have an increased risk for the early development of cardiovascular disease. It is now known that women with pregnancy complications including preeclampsia, preterm birth, and fetal growth restriction are at twofold to eightfold higher risk of CVD compared to women with uncomplicated pregnancies,.[2] Although the mechanisms that may explain this excess risk are unknown, the connection to preeclampsia may provide a clue. It has long been known that a subset of the placentas from women with preeclampsia will show aberrancies in the maternal vessels supplying the placenta and damage to the placental parenchyma consistent with hypoxic/ischemic or oxidative injury. This constellation of findings is termed maternal vascular malperfusion (MVM), and these lesions may hold the key to understanding and identifying the elevated risk for early CVD in women who experience adverse pregnancy outcomes. This intriguing possibility has only begun to be examined, but accumulating evidence is compelling. The authors review this new body of work and propose that understanding the etiology of MVM in the placenta may provide new mechanistic insight into the development of CVD in women.

MATERNAL VASCULAR MALPERFUSION

Proper development and function of the hemochorial human placenta is critically dependent on pregnancy-induced adaptations of the maternal vascular system to the growing conceptus. Foremost among these is the remodeling of the decidual and inner myometrial segments of the maternal spiral arteries. From early in gestation through the first several weeks of the second trimester, specialized subsets of extravillous trophoblast (EVT) migrate from the fetomaternal interface into the maternal tissues.[3] These cells are involved in a variety of functions, including modulation of the maternal immune response, promoting the attachment of the placenta to the uterus, and fostering the transfer of endometrial glandular secretions from the mother to the placenta.[4–7]

Arguably their most important task, however, is altering the structure and flow properties of the maternal spiral arteries. Embryonic and fetal oxygen requirements and tolerances vary throughout the gestation, and EVT-induced vascular alterations serve to modulate the oxygen and nutrient flow to the conceptus. Spiral arteries are the most distal uterine vasculature that enters the placenta, extending through the inner myometrium and the entirety of the decidua. Two or 3 spiral arteries generally run together, often coiling tightly around each other. In their native, un-remodeled state, these vessels have modest lumens maintained by a surrounding smooth muscle wall. This vascular smooth muscle wall retains the ability to constrict in response to neurogenic or hormonal signals, potentially endangering the blood flow to the placenta and fetus. To mitigate this risk, the invading EVTs initiate and promote the remodeling of the spiral arteries, a task likely dependent on interactions with uterine NK cells.[4] Remodeling

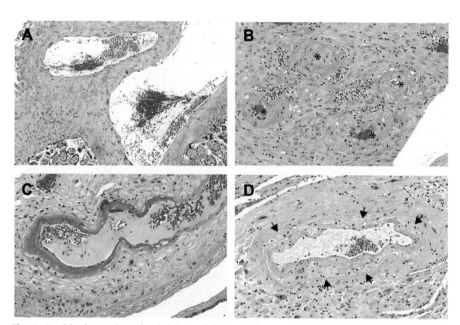

Fig. 1. Decidual vasculopathy. (*A*) Remodeled spiral artery. This image shows adjacent spiral artery cross-sections from the basal plate, with loss of vascular smooth muscle, fibrinoid deposition in the walls, and EVT in the fibrinoid. (*B*) Mural hypertrophy. This image shows 4 vascular cross-sections, each identified by an asterisk. The smooth muscle walls show prominent muscular hypertrophy with a minimal luminal diameter. (*C*) Fibrinoid necrosis. This spiral artery shows replacement of the vascular wall by dense, deep red fibrinoid necrosis. (*D*) Atherosis with foamy macrophages. The lumen of this spiral artery also shows fibrinoid replacement of the vessel wall. Large numbers of foamy macrophages are also present in the vessel wall outside of the fibrinoid necrosis. Arrows point to some of the foamy macrophages.

leads to the complete dissolution of the smooth muscle wall, with replacement by fibrinoid[8] (**Fig. 1**A). With the smooth muscle gone, spiral artery blood flow can no longer be directly controlled by the mother or the growing fetus. Remodeling also alters the arterial shapes. The narrow, tightly coiled spiral arteries widen along the remodeled segments, with the distal end developing a funnel shape. The opening of the remodeled spiral artery into the placenta is 5 to 10 times the diameter of an unaltered spiral artery.[9] These changes significantly increase the amount of blood that can flow into the placenta, while the funnel shape of the terminal arterial segment slows and smooths the flow of blood into the placenta.[9]

Early in gestation, the developing embryo is susceptible to oxidative damage.[10,11] To help protect the embryo and early fetus, an additional subset of EVT invades the lumens of the spiral arteries, and these cells aggregate to form endovascular trophoblastic plugs that occlude or at least significantly obstruct the spiral arteries.[12,13] Plasma, containing dissolved oxygen and nutrients, continues to reach the placental intervillous spaces, but maternal erythrocytes are excluded. This early feature of vascular remodeling maintains the oxygen concentration in the placenta at less than 20 mm Hg (3%–5%) through the first trimester,[10,14] while the surrounding maternal decidual oxygen concentration is 50 to 70 mm Hg (8%–10%).[15] After the endovascular trophoblastic plugs dissolve at around 12 weeks of gestation, the oxygen concentration in the placenta rises to 40 to 50 mm Hg.[10,14,15]

Remodeling of the spiral arteries can be considered as occurring in 2 waves. The first, described previously, takes place in the first trimester. This initial wave remodels the more superficial aspects of the spiral arteries. Vascular remodeling continues through the first half of the second trimester,[3,16] however, with deeper invasion of the EVT. This second trimester remodeling can eliminate the vascular smooth muscle through the full thickness of the decidua and the inner one-third of the myometrium. Remodeling does not occur uniformly, however, with the vessels beneath the placental periphery less efficiently remodeled than those beneath the central placenta. Spiral arteries in the decidua adherent to the extraplacental membranes are only invaded minimally if at all by EVT. The smooth muscle walls of these vessels become thin and may disappear, but the extensive remodeling noted beneath the placental parenchyma does not occur. Failure of the maternal spiral arteries to remodel leaves the placenta susceptible to hypoxic damage or hypoxia/reperfusion injury with oxidative damage.[17–19] The failure of spiral arteries to remodel and the resulting damage patterns collectively comprise MVM.

Individual MVM lesions fall into 2 broad categories. The first group includes those pathologic changes that directly involve the maternal vascular supply to the placenta. Collectively termed decidual vasculopathy, these lesions likely develop early in gestation, and their effects on maternal blood flow to the placenta may be etiologic for the other MVM findings. Although decidual vasculopathy has long been described as a feature of placental pathology, the significance of these lesions came into focus through the histologic examination placental bed biopsies.[20] These studies evaluated the spiral arteries in myometrial and lower decidual segments of the uterus, areas not normally accessible on delivered placentas. In placental bed biopsies, most spiral artery segments from preeclamptic women show absent or incomplete remodeling, while nearly 90% of the spiral artery segments from normal pregnancies are completely remodeled.[21] Moreover, as reported by Brosens, these disorders of deep placentation are more common in each of the great obstetric syndromes.[20] Delivered placentas, containing no myometrium and only the most superficial portion of the decidua, show these changes far less frequently.

DEDICUAL VASCULOPATHY

Four distinct manifestations of decidual vasculopathy have been identified.[22,23] These include absent or incomplete remodeling of a basal plate spiral artery, mural hypertrophy, fibrinoid necrosis, and atherosis. Absent or incomplete remodeling of a basal plate spiral artery (alternatively termed persistence of a muscularized basal plate artery) is the most basic of these lesions.[23] The name is entirely descriptive of the pathologic findings. EVT invasion is focally inadequate to remodel a spiral artery beneath the placenta, resulting in the retention of at least part of the vascular smooth muscle wall. Although complete absence of remodeling is the most striking and definitive appearance for this entity, incomplete remodeling is more common; only a portion of the vessel remains un-remodeled, with retention of a segment of the smooth muscle wall. Because the spiral arteries of the extraplacental membranes may retain a small amount of smooth muscle in their walls, absent or incomplete remodeling cannot be identified in these vessels and can only be diagnosed in the basal plate arteries.

Mural hypertrophy manifests as a thickening of the smooth muscle wall of a spiral artery (**Fig. 1**B). Although this entity can occur either in the placental basal plate or in the extraplacental membranes, it is found more commonly in the spiral arteries of the extraplacental membranes. The extensive remodeling that occurs in the placental basal plate generally removes all smooth muscle from the spiral arteries, precluding the development of mural hypertrophy. Uncommonly, a basal plate vessel with absence of vascular remodeling will additionally undergo mural hypertrophy. Although thickening of the smooth muscle wall of a small artery or arteriole may be found in response to chronic hypertension elsewhere in the body, mural hypertrophy can occur in relation to the placenta even in the absence of chronic hypertension.

Like mural hypertrophy, fibrinoid necrosis may occur either in the arteries of the placental basal plate or the extraplacental membranes. Fibrinoid necrosis has a striking appearance, with replacement of the normal vessel wall by a prominent layer of waxy, deep red material (**Fig. 1**C). Normal fibrinoid replacement of a spiral artery wall may at times appear similar to fibrinoid necrosis, but normal fibrinoid has a lighter pink-red color, and EVT will often be found within the fibrinoid. Confusingly, fibrinoid in this context may refer to either of 2 entirely different entities. The fibrinoid that is deposited in spiral artery walls as a consequence of normal vascular remodeling is comprised of extracellular matrix type material. Fibrinoid necrosis represents the remnant degenerated debris of the vascular smooth muscle wall.

Atherosis, the final subtype of decidual vasculopathy, has features strikingly similar to large vessel atherosclerosis (**Fig. 1**D). Atherosis is characterized by the presence of foamy macrophages within the walls of the spiral arteries. These foamy macrophages are frequently embedded within or adjacent to the fibrinoid material of fibrinoid necrosis, and atherosis and fibrinoid necrosis commonly co-occur. Fibrinoid necrosis may actually develop first, with atherosis appearing later in the course of the disease.[24]

Atherosis is found in only 0.4% of placentas from uncomplicated pregnancies.[25] The incidence is increased in pregnancies with adverse outcomes, occurring in 10.2% of placentas from preeclamptic pregnancies, 9% of placentas following a fetal death, 1.7% of pregnancies with a small for gestational age fetus, and 1.2% of pregnancies with spontaneous preterm labor.[25] The presence of atherosis in a placenta results in a sixfold higher likelihood of that placenta showing other evidence of MVM.[26] Perhaps first hypothesized by Staff and colleagues,[17] this maternal vessel pathology in a transient organ, the placenta, requires only a few months of gestation to form and may provide an accelerated life course model of vessel susceptibility to metabolic and vascular impairments later in life in the face of challenges such as aging and weight gain.

OTHER MATERNAL VASCULAR MALPERFUSION LESIONS

The second group of individual MVM lesions includes those entities that likely arise subsequently in the pregnancy as a result of hypoxic/ischemic injury and oxidative damage to the placenta. Those entities included in the Amsterdam criteria for MVM include small placental size, villous infarction, retroplacental hemorrhage, accelerated villous maturation, and distal villous hypoplasia.[23]

Villous infarction (**Fig. 2**D) is one of the most easily recognized MVM lesions.[22,23] Thirty to 60 spiral arteries typically supply a placenta with maternal blood.[9] Occlusion of one or more of these arteries results in the death of the villi overlying the spiral artery opening. The zone of infarction extends laterally and vertically from the occluded vessel, ending where the mixing of blood from adjacent spiral arteries is sufficient to maintain the viability of the villi. Infarcts thus usually occur along the basal plate and are broad-based with wedge or pyramidal shapes. A gradient of hypoxic damage will often extend from the infarcted tissue into the nearby surviving villi.

One of the most frequent MVM lesions is accelerated villous maturation (**Fig. 2**A, B). The placenta is a short-lived organ that undergoes near-continuous change throughout its limited lifespan. The placental villi correspondingly vary in a predictable

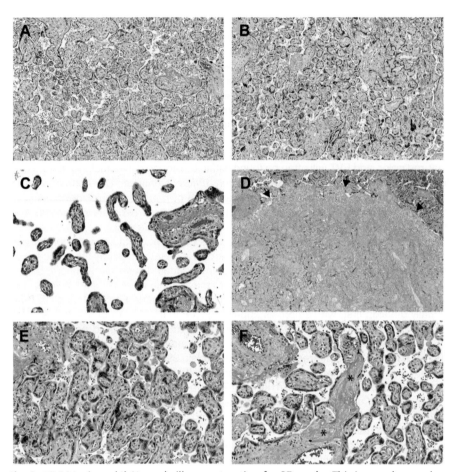

Fig. 2. MVM Lesions. (*A*) Normal villous maturation for 37 weeks. This image shows a low power view of normal villi in a 37-week placenta. (*B*) Accelerated villous maturation for 37 weeks. This image shows a low power view of accelerated villous maturation in a 37-week placenta. The villi are notably smaller than the normal villi, and a high percentage of the villi contain at least 1 syncytial knot. (*C*) Distal villous hypoplasia. The villi in this image are narrow and elongated with minimal branching. This architecture leaves the villi widely spaced and easily recognized. (*D*) Old (remote) villous infarction. This image shows a remote infarct filling nearly the entirety of the panel. The affected villous structures show degeneration with loss color intensity. Arrows highlight the border with the viable villi present along the upper border of the image. (*E*) Increased syncytial knots. This image contains numerous small terminal villi, most harboring at least one densely basophilic syncytial knot. (*F*) Increased intervillous fibrin. This image shows an elongated aggregate of intervillous fibrin that adheres to several viable villi. Asterisks indicate the intervillous fibrin.

pattern throughout a normal gestation, a process termed villous maturation. Several different types of villi have been described, and their proportions change as the gestation progresses. Estimating the appropriateness of the villous proportions to the gestational age provides 1 means of assessing villous maturation. More generally, placental villi undergo several unidirectional changes during a pregnancy. First trimester villi are large, with abundant loose stroma, centrally placed vessels and 2 complete circumferential layers of surrounding trophoblast (an inner cytotrophoblast layer and an outer syncytiotrophoblast layer). As the pregnancy progresses, each of these characteristics is altered. With increasing gestational age, the villi become smaller. Their stroma becomes denser, particularly for the larger villi. The villous vessels come to predominate at the villous periphery, where they dilate into sinusoidal vessels. And the trophoblast layers thin, with aggregation of the syncytiotrophoblast nuclei. These changes serve to optimize gas and nutrient exchange as the pregnancy progresses. Under hypoxic stress, this orderly maturational process can be accelerated, so that the villi take on the appearance (and functional properties) of villi older than their gestational age. The assessment of villous maturation is considerably easier in a preterm placenta, where the accelerated villi match the villous appearance of a later gestational age, than in a term placenta, where the features of hypermaturation are more subtle.

Distal villous hypoplasia (**Fig. 2**C) is an entity that typically arises only after prolonged fetal hypoxia, often in a placenta showing other evidence of accelerated villous maturation. Distal villous hypoplasia is characterized by nonbranching angiogenesis of the villi. The villi appear long and thin with little branching. The intervillous space is open, with widely scattered villi. Syncytial knots are generally increased. Distal villous hypoplasia has been associated with absent or reversed end-diastolic flow in the umbilical artery, an increased pulsatility index in the uterine artery, and fetal growth restriction.[27–29]

Several additional MVM lesions often co-occur with accelerated villous maturation, and some of these features in the past have been tabulated as independent markers for MVM. Increased syncytial knots (**Fig. 2**E) have long been recognized as a feature of accelerated villous maturation and MVM. The syncytiotrophoblast comprises the outer layer covering the placental villi. This layer, which is a true syncytium, functions as the endothelium for the placenta, and is the primary zone of contact between maternal blood and the placenta. Syncytiotrophoblast nuclei often group together, and this clustering becomes more pronounced with increasing gestational age. When 5 or more syncytiotrophoblast nuclei cluster and form a rounded bulge above the villous surface, this entity is termed a syncytial knot.[30] Norms have been developed for the percentage of terminal villi containing a syncytial knot at each week of gestation, and these values can be employed to detect increased syncytial knotting.[30]

Increased amounts of fibrinoid (**Fig. 2**F) may also be deposited in placentas with accelerated villous maturation. Fibrinoid in this context consists of a mixture of extracellular matrix type material and products of the coagulation cascade. These small foci are usually found within and extending from a villus, often contacting and cementing adjacent villi. Fibrinoid is also often deposited along the surfaces of larger stem villi.

MATERNAL VASCULAR MALPERFUSION LESIONS AND MATERNAL VASCULAR HEALTH

In the context of maternal later life CVD, the various forms of decidual vasculopathy likely provide the most direct and compelling evidence that a mother's vasculature may be abnormal and therefore more susceptible to early CVD. Their rarity in delivered placentas, however, limits their utility in individual cases. The secondary MVM lesions, although providing only indirect evidence for maternal vascular proclivity for early CVD, are more readily and frequently detected, and they may therefore function better as a screening test for an increased risk of early maternal CVD.

The maternal prepregnancy cardiometabolic profile is likely related to both placental health and long-term CVD. The few studies that evaluate the trajectory of prepregnancy factors, pregnancy complications, and progression to long-term cardiometabolic disease reveal that the risk identified by pregnancy complications is not well explained by prepregnancy features. The authors have reported that preterm birth is linked to maternal metabolic syndrome after delivery even after accounting for metabolic features measured before conception (blood pressure, waist circumference, triglycerides, fasting glucose, and high-density lipoprotein cholesterol).[31] Remarkably similar results have been reported in a Scandinavian cohort, where blood pressure was higher after delivery in women with hypertension in pregnancy, accounting for prepregnancy blood pressure.[32] There are several limitations with these studies that the placenta may help resolve. Pregnancy complications are heterogeneous, and the placenta may distinguish subtypes. Second, although traditional CVD risk factors may be antecedents to MVM and these complications, they are themselves imprecise. Like occult CVD risk that is not apparent until patients are challenged on a treadmill, pregnancy is a biologic stressor that may more successfully separate high- and low-risk women than risk factors measured before conception. Further, the placenta, with its own 9-month life course, may catalog maternal vascular impairments and mark cardiometabolic risk after pregnancy. If true, MVM lesions in the placenta may represent perhaps the earliest evidence of CVD risk in women. In addition, while prepregnancy blood pressure, lipids, and insulin resistance are often unavailable to clinicians, the placenta is accessible at every delivery. Thus, even if risk identified by the placenta was pre-existing, the placenta offers an efficient, cost-effective, and potentially robust tissue-specific indicator of this risk revealed at delivery.

Although MVM lesions have a well-established association with preeclampsia and growth restriction,[33] and perhaps up to one-third of spontaneous preterm births,[34] there are few epidemiologic studies regarding prevalence of these lesions in the setting of normal and complicated pregnancies. Decidual bed biopsies, which suggested that almost all cases of severe pre-eclampsia involved profound maternal spiral artery impairments[35] are not feasible on a population level. Instead, newer cohort studies have shed new light upon the prevalence and consequences of MVM lesions. In a cohort of 944 healthy women with uncomplicated pregnancies, Romero and colleagues reported that 35.7% had evidence of MVM lesions, with 7.6% having multiple vascular pathologies.

Hauspurg has recently reported that MVM lesions in otherwise uncomplicated pregnancies were related to a 1.6-fold excess risk of adverse pregnancy complications in a subsequent pregnancy.[36] Indeed, decidual vasculopathy accounted for much of this association, and was related to a 2.5-fold excess risk for subsequent pregnancy complications. Another report using this same clinical cohort of more than 20,000 births with placental histology data indicated that black women were 14% more likely to have MVM lesions and 58% more likely to have decidual vasculopathy compared with white women.[37] These race differences were detected in term and preterm births, and in complicated as well as uncomplicated pregnancies. Evidence of race/ethnicity associations with MVM is, however, equivocal, perhaps due to study differences. For example, the Romero cohort was 81% black and thus likely lacking the population diversity needed to detect race differences. A re-examination of Collaborative Perinatal Project data from more than 50,000 placentas delivered in the early 1960s also did not detect race differences in MVM. Pathology approaches from more than 50 years ago, however, included only fibrinoid necrosis of the vessel walls the definition of decidual vasculopathy, while contemporary criteria include absence of vascular remodeling and mural hypertrophy of decidual arterioles as additional key diagnostic features.[23] The Pregnancy Outcomes and Community Health (POUCH) Study, a pregnancy cohort recruited from 5 Michigan communities (1998–2004, n = 1039), reported that black compared with white/other women (20% vs 7%).and obese compared with normal weight women (17% vs 6%) were more likely to have evidence of poor spiral artery remodeling.[38] Taken together, these race- and obesity-related findings are consistent with the notion that MVM, and decidual vasculopathy in particular, may be related to a prepregnancy maternal susceptibility that persists or exacerbates after pregnancy. If true, MVM may identify a high-risk group of women in the years after delivery.

There are only a handful of studies to pursue the cardiovascular determinants and sequelae of MVM. Stevens and colleagues[39] studied women with preeclampsia with and without decidual vasculopathy 7 months, on average, after delivery. Preeclampsia with DV was associated with higher diastolic blood pressure, lower left ventricular stroke volume (71 vs 76 mL, P=.032), higher total peripheral vascular resistance (1546 vs 1385, P=.009), and a higher percentage of low plasma volume (34% vs 19%, P=.030) compared with preeclampsia without DV. Two other studies have attempted to improve the decidual characterization of spiral artery impairments by including research biopsy specimen collection approaches. One demonstrated that at delivery, women older than 35 with acute atherosis had higher low-density lipoprotein cholesterol (LDL-C) and higher concentrations of apolipoprotein-B, the most atherogenic lipid component, compared to women without atherosis.[40] Another study of women the day after delivery indicated women with atherosis (n = 3) had higher triglycerides and LDL-C compared to those without atherosis.[41]

Because a minority of preeclampsia cases have evidence of DV, it is possible that the placental vascular lesion rather than the clinical presentation of preeclampsia may be an important CVD risk marker. If true, then non-PE births with MVM may also mark women at higher CVD risk. The authors' group tested this possibility in a study of women with prior non-preeclamptic preterm births with and without MVM and inflammatory lesions. Not only was the presence of both lesions associated with the worst neonatal outcomes,[42] co-occurrence of MVM and inflammatory lesions was also associated with a higher maternal cardiovascular risk burden in the decade after delivery compared to both women with term births and women with preterm births without these placental pathology findings.[43]

SUMMARY

More studies are needed to identify the mechanisms leading to impaired spiral artery remodeling. For example, studies that characterize decidual features more susceptible to MVM are needed. This tissue is remote and not easily accessed at delivery. Liquid biopsy approaches may help, as might novel imaging developments. This knowledge can then be leveraged to understand mechanisms that may link this pathology in the placenta to future pregnancy health and long-term maternal health. A recent review suggested that a sequence of endothelial injury, fragmentation, and repair in the vessel wall was implicated in DV, with the possibility that a parallel process in the systemic vasculature may also occur.[44] This may be due to activation of a local or systemic renin-angiotensin system,[45] immune-mediated injury,[46] or other unknown mechanisms. For example, higher concentrations of circulating angiogenic factors are detected in women with placental evidence of malperfusion, raising the possibility that impaired angiogenesis may be either a precursor or consequence of these pathologies.[47,48]

Although the placenta has been studied for decades as critical for fetal and newborn health, what it may reveal regarding maternal health is an emerging question. The standardization of placental histology evaluations, increased effort to characterize the developing placenta using noninvasive molecular methods, and development of novel imaging techniques to understand impairments in placental perfusion de novo now also make feasible the possibility that clues to maternal vascular health may also be detected in the placenta.

DISCLOSURE

The authors have nothing to disclose.

REFERENCES

1. Mosca L, Manson JE, Sutherland SE, et al. Cardiovascular disease in women: a statement for healthcare professionals from the American Heart Association. Writing Group. Circulation 1997;96(7):2468–82.
2. Rich-Edwards JW, Fraser A, Lawlor DA, et al. Pregnancy characteristics and women's future cardiovascular health: an underused opportunity to improve women's health? Epidemiol Rev 2014;36:57–70.
3. Pijnenborg R, Dixon G, Robertson WB, et al. Trophoblastic invasion of human decidua from 8 to 18 weeks of pregnancy. Placenta 1980;1(1):3–19.
4. Velicky P, Knöfler M, Pollheimer J. Function and control of human invasive trophoblast subtypes: Intrinsic vs. maternal control. Cell Adh Migr 2016;10(1–2):154–62.
5. Moser G, Gauster M, Orendi K, et al. Endoglandular trophoblast, an alternative route of trophoblast invasion? Analysis with novel confrontation co-culture models. Hum Reprod 2010;25(5):1127–36.
6. Moser G, Weiss G, Gauster M, et al. Evidence from the very beginning: endoglandular trophoblasts penetrate and replace uterine glands in situ and in vitro. Hum Reprod 2015;30(12):2747–57.
7. Burton GJ, Watson AL, Hempstock J, et al. Uterine glands provide histiotrophic nutrition for the human fetus during the first trimester of pregnancy. J Clin Endocrinol Metab 2002;87(6):2954–9.
8. Pijnenborg R, Vercruysse L, Hanssens M. The uterine spiral arteries in human pregnancy: facts and controversies. Placenta 2006;27(9–10):939–58.
9. Burton GJ, Woods AW, Jauniaux E, et al. Rheological and physiological consequences of conversion of the maternal spiral arteries for uteroplacental blood flow during human pregnancy. Placenta 2009;30(6):473–82.
10. Jauniaux E, Watson AL, Hempstock J, et al. Onset of maternal arterial blood flow and placental oxidative stress. A possible factor in human early pregnancy failure. Am J Pathol 2000;157(6):2111–22.
11. Jauniaux E, Hempstock J, Greenwold N, et al. Trophoblastic oxidative stress in relation to temporal and regional differences in maternal placental blood flow in normal and abnormal early pregnancies. Am J Pathol 2003;162(1):115–25.
12. Roberts VHJ, Morgan TK, Bednarek P, et al. Early first trimester uteroplacental flow and the progressive disintegration of spiral artery plugs: new insights from contrast-enhanced ultrasound and tissue histopathology. Hum Reprod 2017; 32(12):2382–93.
13. Hustin J, Schaaps JP. Echographic [corrected] and anatomic studies of the maternotrophoblastic border during the first trimester of pregnancy. Am J Obstet Gynecol 1987;157(1):162–8.
14. Rodesch F, Simon P, Donner C, et al. Oxygen measurements in endometrial and trophoblastic tissues during early pregnancy. Obstet Gynecol 1992;80(2):283–5.
15. Huppertz B, Weiss G, Moser G. Trophoblast invasion and oxygenation of the placenta: measurements versus presumptions. J Reprod Immunol 2014; 101-102:74–9.

16. Pijnenborg R, Bland JM, Robertson WB, et al. Uteroplacental arterial changes related to interstitial trophoblast migration in early human pregnancy. Placenta 1983;4(4):397–413.
17. Staff AC, Dechend R, Redman CW. Review: preeclampsia, acute atherosis of the spiral arteries and future cardiovascular disease: two new hypotheses. Placenta 2013;34(Suppl):S73–8.
18. Burton GJ. Oxygen, the Janus gas; its effects on human placental development and function. J Anat 2009;215(1):27–35.
19. Redman CW, Sargent IL. Placental stress and pre-eclampsia: a revised view. Placenta 2009;30(Suppl A):S38–42.
20. Brosens I, Pijnenborg R, Vercruysse L, et al. The "great obstetrical syndromes" are associated with disorders of deep placentation. Am J Obstet Gynecol 2011;204(3):193–201.
21. Brosens K. Placenta bed disorders. Cambridge (United Kingdom): Cambridge University Press; 2010.
22. Redline RW, Boyd T, Campbell V, et al. Maternal vascular underperfusion: nosology and reproducibility of placental reaction patterns. Pediatr Dev Pathol 2004;7(3):237–49.
23. Khong TY, Mooney EE, Ariel I, et al. Sampling and definitions of placental lesions: amsterdam placental workshop group consensus statement. Arch Pathol Lab Med 2016;140(7):698–713.
24. Khong TY. Acute atherosis in pregnancies complicated by hypertension, small-for-gestational-age infants, and diabetes mellitus. Arch Pathol Lab Med 1991; 115(7):722–5.
25. Kim YM, Chaemsaithong P, Romero R, et al. The frequency of acute atherosis in normal pregnancy and preterm labor, preeclampsia, small-for-gestational age, fetal death and midtrimester spontaneous abortion. J Matern Fetal Neonatal Med 2015;28(17):2001–9.
26. Kim YM, Chaemsaithong P, Romero R, et al. Placental lesions associated with acute atherosis. J Matern Fetal Neonatal Med 2015;28(13):1554–62.
27. Krebs C, Macara LM, Leiser R, et al. Intrauterine growth restriction with absent end-diastolic flow velocity in the umbilical artery is associated with maldevelopment of the placental terminal villous tree. Am J Obstet Gynecol 1996;175(6): 1534–42.
28. Veerbeek JH, Nikkels PG, Torrance HL, et al. Placental pathology in early intrauterine growth restriction associated with maternal hypertension. Placenta 2014;35(9):696–701.
29. Orabona R, Donzelli CM, Falchetti M, et al. Placental histological patterns and uterine artery Doppler velocimetry in pregnancies complicated by early or late pre-eclampsia. Ultrasound Obstet Gynecol 2016;47(5):580–5.
30. Loukeris K, Sela R, Baergen RN. Syncytial knots as a reflection of placental maturity: reference values for 20 to 40 weeks' gestational age. Pediatr Dev Pathol 2010;13(4):305–9.
31. Catov J, Althouse A, Lewis C, et al. Preterm delivery and metabolic syndrome in women followed from prepregnancy through 25 years later. Obstet Gynecol 2016; 127:1127–34.
32. Romundstad PR, Magnussen EB, Smith GD, et al. Hypertension in pregnancy and later cardiovascular risk: common antecedents? Circulation 2010;122(6): 579–84.
33. Parks WT. Placental hypoxia: the lesions of maternal malperfusion. Semin Perinatol 2015;39(1):9–19.

34. Romero R, Dey SK, Fisher SJ. Preterm labor: one syndrome, many causes. Science 2014;345(6198):760–5.
35. Brosens IA, Robertson WB, Dixon HG. The role of the spiral arteries in the pathogenesis of preeclampsia. Obstet Gynecol Annu 1972;1:177–91.
36. Hauspurg A, Redman EK, Assibey-Mensah V, et al. Placental findings in non-hypertensive term pregnancies and association with future adverse pregnancy outcomes: a cohort study. Placenta 2018;74:14–9.
37. Assibey-Mensah V, Parks WT, Gernand AD, et al. Race and risk of maternal vascular malperfusion lesions in the placenta. Placenta 2018;69:102–8.
38. Kelly R, Holzman C, Senagore P, et al. Placental vascular pathology findings and pathways to preterm delivery. Am J Epidemiol 2009;170(2):148–58.
39. Stevens DU, Al-Nasiry S, Fajta MM, et al. Cardiovascular and thrombogenic risk of decidual vasculopathy in preeclampsia. Am J Obstet Gynecol 2014;210(6):545.e1-6.
40. Moe K, Alnaes-Katjavivi P, Storvold GL, et al. Classical cardiovascular risk markers in pregnancy and associations to uteroplacental acute atherosis. Hypertension 2018;72(3):695–702.
41. Veerbeek JH, Brouwers L, Koster MP, et al. Spiral artery remodeling and maternal cardiovascular risk: the spiral artery remodeling (SPAR) study. J Hypertens 2016;34(8):1570–7.
42. Catov JM, Scifres CM, Caritis SN, et al. Neonatal outcomes following preterm birth classified according to placental features. Am J Obstet Gynecol 2017;216(4):411.e1-14.
43. Catov JM, Muldoon MF, Reis SE, et al. Preterm birth with placental evidence of malperfusion is associated with cardiovascular risk factors after pregnancy: a prospective cohort study. BJOG 2018;125(8):1009–17.
44. Hecht JL, Zsengeller ZK, Spiel M, et al. Revisiting decidual vasculopathy. Placenta 2016;42:37–43.
45. Morgan T, Craven C, Ward K. Human spiral artery renin-angiotensin system. Hypertension 1998;32(4):683–7.
46. Sones JL, Lob HE, Isroff CE, et al. Role of decidual natural killer cells, interleukin-15, and interferon-γ in placental development and preeclampsia. Am J Physiol Regul Integr Comp Physiol 2014;307(5):R490–2.
47. Baltajian K, Hecht JL, Wenger JB, et al. Placental lesions of vascular insufficiency are associated with anti-angiogenic state in women with preeclampsia. Hypertens Pregnancy 2014;33(4):427–39.
48. Schmella MJ, Assibey-Mensah V, Parks WT, et al. Plasma concentrations of soluble endoglin in the maternal circulation are associated with maternal vascular malperfusion lesions in the placenta of women with preeclampsia. Placenta 2019;78:29–35.

What Obstetricians Need to Know About Placental Pathology

Sanjita Ravishankar, MD, Raymond W. Redline, MD*

KEYWORDS

- Placenta • Pathology • Chorioamnionitis • Fetal vascular • Maternal vascular
- Villitis

KEY POINTS

- The Amsterdam consensus classification provides a common framework for obstetricians and pathologists alike to understand placental pathology.
- The criteria for submission of placentas for pathologic examination include maternal, neonatal, and placental indications.
- A careful, systematic gross examination of the placenta, including the membranes, umbilical cord, fetal surface, and maternal surface, is key. Much of this can also be performed by the obstetrician at delivery.
- The major categories of placental lesions include vascular or perfusion abnormalities, both maternal and fetal; inflammatory or infectious abnormalities, both acute and chronic; and assorted other lesions, 2 of which (massive perivillous fibrin deposition and chronic histiocytic intervillositis) are rare but have a high risk of recurrence.

INTRODUCTION

The placenta is a unique organ that sits at the interface of, and facilitates nearly all interactions between, maternal and fetal physiology. It is the sole source of oxygen and nutrition for the fetus, and provides a protective barrier against external insults. The placenta is also a highly adaptable organ that is capable of showing a wide range of pathologic changes in response to various maternal and fetal factors and stressors. Many of these changes can be observed with gross and microscopic examination of the placenta after delivery, thus providing a unique opportunity to inform both maternal and fetal clinical management.

This article examines the indications for submission, the essentials of gross examination, and the major histologic findings for 3 broad diagnostic categories of placental lesions:

Department of Pathology, Case Western Reserve University School of Medicine, University Hospitals Cleveland Medical Center, 11100 Euclid Avenue, Cleveland, OH 44106, USA
* Corresponding author.
E-mail address: Raymondw.redline@uhhospitals.org

Obstet Gynecol Clin N Am 47 (2020) 29–48
https://doi.org/10.1016/j.ogc.2019.10.007
0889-8545/20/© 2019 Elsevier Inc. All rights reserved.

- Vascular/perfusion abnormalities
  - Maternal vascular malperfusion
  - Fetal vascular malperfusion
- Inflammatory/infectious processes
  - Histologic acute chorioamnionitis
  - Villitis of unknown cause
  - Villitis caused by infectious organisms
- Rare lesions with high risk of recurrence
  - Massive perivillous fibrin deposition/maternal floor infarction
  - Chronic histiocytic intervillositis

Other important lesions, including morbidly adherent placenta (creta), delayed villous maturation, villous capillary proliferative lesions, meconium myonecrosis, and specific findings indicating specific genetic/chromosomal abnormalities, are discussed in 2 recently published placental textbooks.[1,2]

INDICATIONS FOR PLACENTAL EXAMINATION

In most cases, tissue that is removed or spontaneously expressed from the body is routinely sent for pathologic evaluation, but the placenta is a notable exception. Because many placentas are normal, it is impractical to submit all placentas to pathology, particularly at large hospitals with busy labor and delivery centers. As such, the College of American Pathologists and Royal College of Pathologists have each developed guidelines for the placentas that should be submitted to pathology.[3,4] An adapted version is shown in **Table 1**.

In addition, there are also a few conditions in which placental submission to pathology is not considered to be likely to be high yield, and may not be a practical use of limited resources. These include placentas from cesarean deliveries without any other indications,[3] cholestasis/pruritus of pregnancy,[4] and normal pregnancies. However, these are simply guidelines, and submission of the placenta to pathology is ultimately at the discretion of the clinician.

In some institutions, placentas are selected for pathologic examination, and the remainder are stored in a refrigerator at 4°C for approximately 1 week. During the storage period, if any previously unrecognized complications arise, including those involving the neonate, the placenta may be retrieved and submitted for pathologic examination. Placentas are well preserved when refrigerated, and meaningful examination can be performed in these conditions.[5]

In addition, it is essential to develop a mechanism to indicate to the pathologist what specific indications and questions prompted submission of a given placenta to pathology. Knowledge of this information helps guide the gross and histologic examination of the placenta and generally results in a more comprehensive and clinically useful interpretation of any disorder that may be present. Findings that may be nonspecific in one clinical context may have enormous clinical significance in another. This communication may be facilitated in any number of ways, depending on the institution, using either the electronic medical record or paper forms.

GENERAL PLACENTAL EXAMINATION
Gross Examination

The first step of placental pathologic examination is gross examination: essentially, what does the placenta look like? Although this examination will be performed and documented more formally in the pathology laboratory, obstetricians can perform at

Table 1		
Indications for placental submission to pathology		
Maternal Indications	Essential	Prematurity ($\leq$34 wk of gestation) or postmaturity (>42 wk)
		Systemic disorders with concern for mother or infant (eg, diabetes, hypertension)
		Peripartum fever or infection
		Unexplained or excessive third-trimester bleeding
		Severe oligohydramnios/polyhydramnios
		Thick and/or viscid meconium
		Invasive procedures with suspected placental injury
		Unexplained or recurrent pregnancy complications
	Optional	Premature delivery, 34–37 wk of gestation
		Maternal substance abuse
Fetal/Neonatal Indications	Essential	Stillbirth or neonatal death
		NICU admission
		Birth depression (cord blood pH<7.0, Apgar score $\leq$6 at 5 min, assisted ventilation >10 min, hematocrit <35%)
		Neonatal seizures
		Suspected infection or sepsis
		Small or large for gestational age (<10th or >90th percentile)
		Hydrops fetalis
		Major congenital anomalies or abnormal karyotype
		Multiple gestation with same-sex infants and fused placentas, or discordant growth
	Optional	Multiple gestation without other indication
		Fetal distress or nonreassuring fetal status
Placental Indications	Essential	Structural abnormalities of the placental disk or membranes (eg, mass, thrombosis, hematoma, abnormal coloration or odor)
		Small or large placental size or weight for gestational age
		Umbilical cord lesions (eg, long/short/hypercoiled/ abnormal insertion/single artery)

Abbreviation: NICU, neonatal intensive care unit.

Adapted from Langston C, Kaplan C, Macpherson T, et al. Practice guideline for examination of the placenta: Developed by the placental pathology practice guideline development task force of the College of American Pathologists. Arch Pathol Lab Med 1997;121(5):449-76 and Cox P, Evans C. Tissue pathway for histopathological examination of the placenta. The Royal College of Pathologists 2017.

least a cursory examination of the placenta at delivery. If there is any question of an abnormality, the placenta should be submitted to pathology, with a corresponding note on the requisition indicating the observation that was made.

Gross examination of the placenta can be divided into 4 anatomic categories:

1. Membranes
2. Umbilical cord
3. Fetal surface
4. Maternal surface

The membranes are composed of 3 layers: the amnion, the chorion, and a variable amount of adherent decidua. The membranes are normally tan to slightly yellow and translucent. If meconium staining is present, they may be green stained. If there is hemosiderin deposition in the membranes secondary to chronic bleeding/abruption, the membranes may be brown stained. If severe chorioamnionitis is present, they may be opaque. These changes may extend to involve the membranes on the fetal surface of the placenta, and may be easier to observe in that location.

The umbilical cord is normally white to pale yellow, contains 2 arteries and 1 vein, and shows a certain degree of twisting or coiling, most commonly in a left or counter-clockwise direction.[6] Normal ranges for umbilical cord length have been published,[7-9] with the caveat that these are generally based on measurement at the time of delivery, and measurements taken by the pathology laboratory are often shorter, because portions of the cord are used for cord gases and so forth, and may not be received with the specimen. Several important abnormalities of the cord can be recognized grossly:

- Number of vessels
  - Single umbilical artery
  - Cysts or other abnormal enlargements of embryologic remnants
- Length
  - Long cord (generally >70 cm, as measured during examination in pathology)
  - Short cord (generally <35 cm, with the caveat mentioned earlier regarding lack of availability of the entire cord in pathology)[10]
- Coiling
  - Hypercoiling (>3 coils/10 cm)[11]
  - Hypocoiling (<1 coil/10 cm)
- Diameter
  - Thin/strictured cord
- Knots
  - False knots (redundancy of the umbilical vein: no clinical significance)
  - True knots
- Cord insertion
  - Marginal (cord inserts at the margin of the placenta)
  - Velamentous (cord inserts in the membranes, with unprotected membranous fetal vessels)
  - Furcate (cord divides into vessels with loss of Wharton's jelly, before insertion into the placenta: results in unprotected fetal vessels)

The fetal surface is covered by a continuation of the peripheral membranes, and often reflects the same changes seen in that location. There are often scattered deposits of subchorionic fibrin that can be seen on the fetal surface grossly, which tend to increase with gestational age. The membranes normally insert marginally, meaning at the peripheral margin of the placenta. Extrachorial placentation refers to the presence of villous tissue beyond the apparent site of membrane insertion, and classically has been separated into 2 forms: circumvallation and circummargination. Various definitions distinguishing these two forms have been suggested, but the only clinically significant distinction is the presence of entrapped old hemorrhage and hemosiderin adjacent to the circumvallate form. Therefore, sections should be taken in all placentas with foci of so-called extrachorial placentation to document those cases with evidence of hemorrhage.

Other findings that can be observed grossly on the fetal surface include amnion nodosum and squamous metaplasia. Squamous metaplasia of the amnionic epithelium is an extremely common, benign finding that can be grossly visualized as irregularly shaped, small, tan-white lesions near the umbilical cord insertion site and that cannot be manually removed. Amnion nodosum presents as diffusely distributed, rounded, yellow-white lesions that contain fetal hair and superficial squamous cells.

Unlike the nodules of squamous metaplasia, amnion nodosum can be removed by scraping the nodules gently. Amnion nodosum is a pathologic finding and is associated with severe oligohydramnios.

The maternal surface, although not nearly as photogenic as the fetal surface, is also an important element of placental gross examination. One of the most important parts of its evaluation, which obstetricians should perform with each placenta that is delivered, is to check it for completeness. If the placenta is torn or fragmented and cannot be reconstructed, or if any cotyledons are missing, the placenta is deemed incomplete, and the possibility of retained placental tissue, and the consequences of this possibility, must be raised. The maternal surface should also be evaluated for the presence and size of any adherent blood clots, which may represent evidence of placental abruption. These clots are described as marginal or central, and the presence or absence of indentation of the underlying placental parenchyma is also noted. It should be noted that it may be impossible to differentiate between the blood clots that can be frequently seen loosely attached to the maternal surface and those found in a recent acute abruption, and the lack of definitive pathologic evidence of acute abruption does not preclude the diagnosis in the context of a supportive clinical impression.

Specimen Processing

In most institutions in the United States, at least 4 to 5 microscopic slides are examined for routine placentas. These slides include sections of the umbilical cord, membrane roll, and 3 sections of the placental parenchyma, to include both the maternal and fetal surfaces. Additional sections may be examined if gross lesions are identified.

Placental Pathology Reporting

Historically, there has been a great deal of heterogeneity in the style and quality of placental pathology reporting. Recently, attempts have been made to encourage standardization of terminology, through the efforts of the Amsterdam Placental Workshop Group Consensus Statement.[11] A synoptic reporting format has also recently been proposed, and has been suggested by the authors as a method to enhance the comprehensiveness and quality of placental pathology reporting.[12]

In general, the placental pathology report is composed of the same basic sections that are used in reporting the pathology of other organ systems in a particular institution, which includes a section for the clinical history, provided by the obstetrician on the specimen requisition; a gross description, including a summary of the sections that were taken for histologic examination; and a final diagnosis. Other sections that may be used as appropriate include a microscopic description and a diagnostic comment. The final diagnosis section should include the placental weight, and a note about whether it is small or large for the stated gestational age, which should be communicated by the obstetrician to the pathologist with the clinical history. Clinically significant gross findings may also be integrated in the final diagnosis, particularly if there are histologic correlates, and if the gross lesions are supportive of a particular diagnostic category.[13] Note that most placental disease processes are not confined to, or defined by, a single pathologic lesion, an idea that has been termed the constellation-of-findings concept. If possible, attempts should be made in the report to classify relevant lesions under a diagnostic heading. In general, the number and magnitude of the relevant findings parallel the level of confidence in the diagnosis, and the potential clinical relevance. An example report from our institution is shown in **Box 1**.

Box 1
Example placental pathology report showing the constellation-of-findings concept of reporting

Final diagnosis

A placenta:
- Small, histologically mature placenta (208 g; less than fifth percentile for 33 weeks)
- Findings consistent with maternal vascular malperfusion:
    Accelerated villous maturation
    Decidual vasculopathy (mural hypertrophy, fibrinoid necrosis. and acute atherosis of decidual arterioles)
    Increased syncytial knots and perivillous fibrin deposition

MATERNAL VASCULAR MALPERFUSION

This category is defined as a group of placental lesions that reflect abnormal maternal perfusion of the placenta, primarily caused by defects in trophoblast invasion and remodeling of maternal spiral arterioles. The lesions associate with increased vascular tone in uterine arteries, failure to increase circulating blood volume, and implantation in a region with poor arterial supply.[14] Maternal vascular malperfusion (MVM) can conceptually be separated into 2 categories of histologic findings: global/partial (partial interruption of perfusion to the entire placenta) and segmental/complete (complete interruption of blood flow to a portion/segment of the placenta), further described here.

Gross Findings

Placentas with MVM are usually small for gestational age and have an increased fetal/placental weight ratio. The umbilical cord may be thin. Villous infarction is often seen, represented by firm, tan-white to tan-yellow lesions within the placental parenchyma. Although infarcts are often better visualized grossly after formalin fixation, they can usually be palpated as firm areas, even if they are not obviously visible in fresh placentas.

Microscopic Findings

The underlying disorder affecting the maternal spiral arterioles can be visualized on placental examination in the form of decidual vasculopathy/arteriopathy. These changes are usually able to be visualized in the marginal decidua of the membrane roll, which is prepared as part of routine placental examination. The earliest form of decidual arteriopathy is mural hypertrophy, which refers to a concentric thickening of the vessel wall, such that the lumen of the vessel occupies 30% or less of the total diameter of the arteriole, caused by a combination of medial and/or myointimal hyperplasia and hypertrophy. This lesion may progress to early degenerative changes of the wall, associated with a chronic perivascular inflammatory infiltrate, termed chronic perivasculitis. This condition can further progress to fibrinoid necrosis of the arteriolar wall, with or without acute atherosis, the accumulation of lipid laden macrophages within the vessel wall[15] (**Fig. 1**).

Global/partial MVM is manifested microscopically as accelerated villous maturation, which refers to regions of the placenta with villous underdevelopment and paucity, alternating with regions with villous crowding, with increased syncytial knots, perivillous fibrin deposition, and villous agglutination.[14] Alternatively stated, it is the presence of small or short hypermature villi for the gestational age, usually

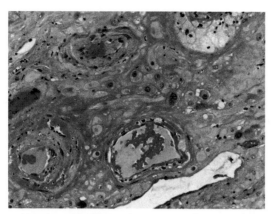

Fig. 1. Decidual arteriopathy, with fibrinoid necrosis and acute atherosis of the wall of a decidual arteriole, from the membrane roll (H&E stain, original magnification ×20).

accompanied by increased syncytial knots.[11] This change is a reflection of variable narrowing of uterine arteries caused by defective remodeling and decidual arteriopathy, which leads to uneven and high-velocity maternal perfusion of the placenta.

Segmental/complete MVM manifests as villous infarction. Villous infarcts have well-defined margins and are often localized to the basal plate. They represent a region of the placenta that has undergone death caused by complete loss of maternal perfusion. Depending on the age of the infarct, they show similar histologic features to infarcts in other organ systems; the trophoblast loses nuclear basophilia, followed by luminal obliteration of the fetal vessels, stromal fibrosis, and complete involution of both the trophoblast and fetal vessels. There is collapse of the intervillous space, and the villi become surrounded by fibrin. In advanced/remote infarcts, only the "ghosts" of the villous structure can be seen (**Fig. 2**).

Clinical Associations

Decidual arteriopathy is most common in cases of preeclampsia that are accompanied by fetal growth restriction and abnormal pulsed flow Doppler testing. It is also

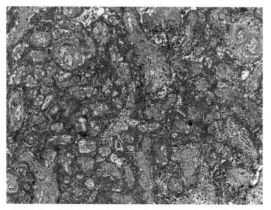

Fig. 2. Villous infarction showing loss of nuclear basophilia of the trophoblast, collapse of the intervillous space, and replacement with fibrin (H&E stain, original magnification ×10).

seen in cases of preeclampsia without fetal growth restriction, including chronic hypertension, gestational hypertension, and gestational diabetes.

Accelerated villous maturation and villous infarction are associated with preeclampsia, fetal growth restriction, pregestational diabetes, and maternal autoimmune disease, including antiphospholipid syndrome. Less severe changes can be seen with chronic or gestational hypertension, obesity, sleep-disordered breathing, and pregnancy at high altitudes. Villous infarction limited to the marginal region of the placenta can be seen in otherwise normal placentas, and, by themselves, may not indicate maternal vascular disorder. However, any infarction seen in a preterm placenta, and involvement of more than 5% of nonmarginal placental parenchyma at term, is generally considered to be abnormal.[11]

FETAL VASCULAR MALPERFUSION

This category is defined by a group of placental lesions that serve as evidence of reduced or absent perfusion between the villous parenchyma and the fetus. This condition is most commonly caused by obstruction of blood flow through the umbilical cord; however, other contributing factors include fetal cardiac insufficiency, hyperviscosity, and thrombophilias. Like MVM, fetal vascular malperfusion (FVM) can be conceptually subdivided into 2 histologic patterns: global/partial and segmental/complete, which are further described here.

Gross Findings

By far the most commonly associated gross findings seen in FVM are abnormalities of the umbilical cord. Several anatomic lesions and some clinical conditions can lead to partial or complete umbilical cord obstruction, and subsequently FVM (**Table 2**).[16] This concept has been termed the umbilical cord at risk. Note that the potentially obstructing clinical conditions, such as nuchal cord, body cord, or cord prolapse, may leave only subtle or no pathologic evidence of their occurrence, and therefore it is vital that this information is transmitted to the pathologist in the clinical history provided with the placenta when it is submitted for examination.

Abnormalities of the chorionic plate vessels are less commonly seen on gross examination. These abnormalities may show ectasia or organized thrombi, indicating partial or complete occlusion. Rarely, the final downstream product of FVM is a focus

Table 2 Macroscopic umbilical cord abnormalities associated with fetal vascular malperfusion	
Obstructive Anatomic Lesions	Long UC
	True knot of UC
	Hypercoiled UC (>4 coils/10 cm)
	UC stricture (diameter<5 mm)
Potentially Obstructing Anatomic Lesions	Marginal/membranous insertion of UC
	Furcate insertion of UC
	Thin UC (<8 mm)
	Tethered UC
Potentially Obstructing Clinical Conditions	UC entanglement (nuchal cord, body cord)
	UC prolapse

Abbreviation: UC, umbilical cord.
Adapted from Redline RW, Ravishankar S. Fetal vascular malperfusion, an update. APMIS 2018;126(7):562; with permission.

of avascular villi, large enough to be visible by gross examination. Selected examples of these findings are shown in **Fig. 3**.

Microscopic Findings

FVM can be subdivided into 2 histologic patterns: global/partial and segmental/complete. Global/partial FVM is so named because it is the result of a chronic, partial, or intermittent obstruction of the entire fetal vascular tree. The microscopic findings seen in association with this pattern include vascular ectasia, defined as a vessel that is at least 4 times the luminal diameter of its neighbors; fibrin deposition in the walls of large fetal vessels, designated intramural fibrin deposition; and small foci of either partially or entirely ischemic terminal chorionic villi, each consisting of only 2 to 4 villi (**Fig. 4A**). These villi are described as either being entirely avascular or they may show the earlier stage of ischemia, termed villous stromal-vascular karyorrhexis, in which they show fragmentation of the fetal vessels with extravasated fetal red cells and karyorrhectic debris. Segmental/complete FVM is the pattern of FVM seen in association with complete obstruction of a segment of the fetal vascular tree. The microscopic findings seen in association with this pattern include thrombi within the large chorionic plate or stem villous fetal vessels, which may be recent (composed only of fibrin) or remote

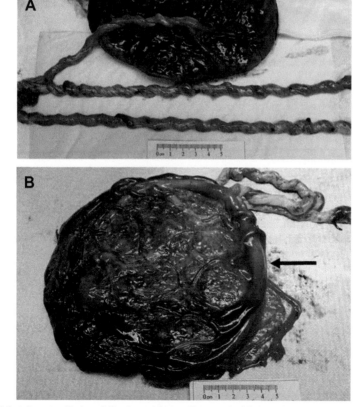

Fig. 3. (*A*) A hypercoiled umbilical cord (>4 coils/10 cm). (*B*) Grossly visible chorionic vessel thrombus (*arrow*).

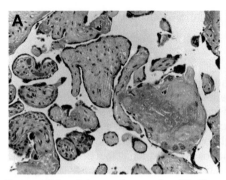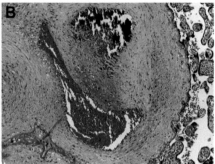

Fig. 4. (*A*) Small focus of avascular villi. Note the contrast between the small cluster in the center with hyalinized stroma and complete lack of fetal vessels and the surrounding, normally vascularized villi (original magnification ×20). (*B*) Remote (calcified) nonocclusive thrombus within a stem villous vessel (H&E stain, original magnification ×10).

(with calcification, **Fig. 4**B); chorionic or stem vessel obliteration; and intermediate or large foci of avascular villi or villous stromal-vascular karyorrhexis. Of note, the global/partial and segmental/complete patterns of FVM are not mutually exclusive, and significant overlap or progression from one pattern to the other may occur, particularly because the predisposing anatomic abnormalities (the umbilical cord at risk) are common to both patterns.

High-grade FVM is defined as 45 or more avascular villi seen over 3 examined sections of placental parenchyma, or an average of more than 15 avascular villi per section, or 2 or more occlusive or nonocclusive thrombi within chorionic plate or major stem vessels.[11,16]

As might be expected, FVM often leads to significant fetal stress, and the major placental findings that are nonspecifically associated with fetal stress (increased circulating fetal nucleated red blood cells, and evidence of prolonged meconium exposure) may also be seen in association with FVM.

Clinical Associations

Global/partial FVM is associated with neonatal encephalopathy.[17] Elements of both global and segmental FVM have been associated with nonreassuring fetal heart rate, intrauterine fetal demise, intrauterine growth restriction, chronic fetal monitoring abnormalities, neonatal coagulopathies, and fetal cardiac abnormalities.[18–21] High-grade FVM has the highest rate of associated adverse outcomes, particularly cerebral palsy and neonatal encephalopathy.[22,23]

In general, the recurrence risk for FVM is considered to be small. The major exception to this is inherited coagulopathy, and the risk of recurrence is increased in cases with a history of maternal or neonatal thromboembolic disease.[24]

HISTOLOGIC ACUTE CHORIOAMNIONITIS

This histopathology is an inflammatory response in the chorionic plate of the placenta and amniochorial membranes, usually in response to the presence of microorganisms in the amniotic fluid. These microorganisms reach the placenta via the ascending route of infection from the cervicovaginal flora and then breach the amniochorial membrane and infect the amniotic fluid. The resulting inflammatory response may have both a maternal component and fetal component.[25,26]

Gross Findings

Inflammation of the membranes and chorionic plate results in an opaque appearance, rather than the normal translucent appearance. The chorionic plate may also become yellow or cream colored, similar to the color of pus (**Fig. 5A**). The fetal inflammatory response, if severe, may cause yellow discoloration of the umbilical cord, with concentric rings around the vessels on cross section. Candida infection in particular results in a characteristic appearance of the umbilical cord, with pale yellow microabscesses visible on the surface (**Fig. 5B**).

Microscopic Findings

Histologic acute chorioamnionitis (HCA) comprises a maternal component and a fetal component, which frequently coexist. Note that both the maternal and fetal inflammatory responses may be patchy in their distribution in the placenta. The maternal inflammatory response begins as an aggregation of neutrophils in the subchorionic fibrin, and, with increasing severity, these cells can be found in the chorion and the overlying amnion (**Fig. 6**). The fetal inflammatory response generally begins in the chorionic

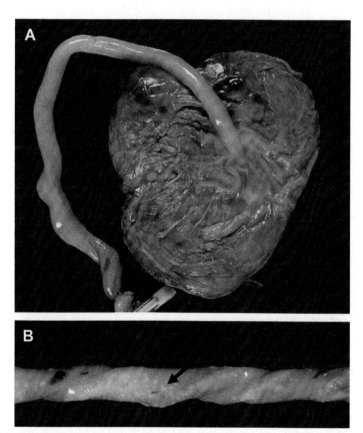

Fig. 5. (*A*) Gross appearance of acute chorioamnionitis. Note the opacity and slightly yellow to creamy discoloration of the fetal surface. (*B*) Gross appearance of Candida in umbilical cord. Note the small yellow-white plaques scattered on the surface of the umbilical cord (*arrow*); these correspond with microabscesses containing the Candida organisms. (*Courtesy of* H. Pinar, MD, Providence, RI.)

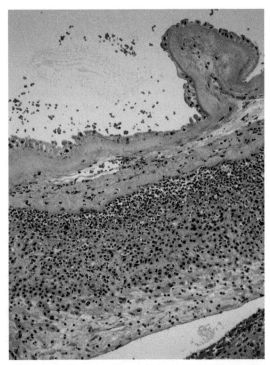

Fig. 6. Acute chorioamnionitis. Maternal inflammatory response; neutrophils extend from the subchorion, through the chorion, and into the amnion at the top (H&E stain, original magnification ×20).

plate vessels, as neutrophils sometimes admixed with eosinophils, which marginate and then migrate through the vessel wall and into the overlying stroma. This inflammatory response is usually oriented toward the overlying amniotic epithelium and the amniotic cavity. In severe cases, this process also affects the umbilical cord, generally involving the umbilical vein (umbilical phlebitis) first, followed by the umbilical arteries (umbilical arteritis). If all 3 umbilical vessels are involved, it is termed umbilical panvasculitis. If the acute inflammation significantly extends into the Wharton jelly, it is termed necrotizing funisitis or perivasculitis. A grading and staging system for HCA has been developed (**Table 3**).[27] Whether or not this particular system is used, placental pathology reports should always comment on the extent and severity of the maternal and fetal responses.

Clinical Associations

Acute chorioamnionitis can be considered a clinical diagnosis or a histologic diagnosis, and the correlation between the two is not perfect. The incidence of HCA tends to be the highest among preterm deliveries, and prolonged rupture of membranes is an important risk factor. The clinical sequelae of HCA can be caused by the infectious organism or by the immune response. HCA is associated with a myriad of perinatal morbidities, including neonatal sepsis,[28] increased risk for respiratory complications, necrotizing enterocolitis, and neurodisability (including cerebral palsy).[23,25,29] Severe (grade 2) fetal inflammatory response in particular is associated with cerebral palsy.

Table 3
Staging and grading of histologic acute chorioamnionitis

Maternal Inflammatory Response		
Stage 1 (early)	Acute subchorionitis or chorionitis	Neutrophils in the subchorionic fibrin and/or membrane trophoblast
Stage 2 (intermediate)	Acute chorioamnionitis	Neutrophils in fibrous chorion and/or amnion
Stage 3 (advanced)	Necrotizing chorioamnionitis	Amniocyte necrosis, neutrophil karyorrhexis
Grade 1 (mild to moderate)	Not severe	
Grade 2 (severe)	Severe acute chorioamnionitis	Confluent microabscesses between the chorion and decidua
Fetal Inflammatory Response		
Stage 1 (early)	Chorionic vasculitis or umbilical phlebitis	Intramural neutrophils in the chorionic vessels and/or umbilical vein
Stage 2 (intermediate)	Umbilical arteritis ± phlebitis or panvasculitis	Intramural neutrophils in the umbilical artery or arteries, ± umbilical vein
Stage 3 (advanced)	Necrotizing funisitis/ perivasculitis	Neutrophils in concentric rings around 1 or more umbilical vessels
Grade 1 (mild to moderate)	Not severe	
Grade 2 (severe)	Severe fetal inflammatory response	Confluent intramural neutrophils in fetal vessels with degeneration of vascular smooth muscle

Adapted from Redline RW, Faye-Petersen O, Heller D, et al. Amniotic infection syndrome: nosology and reproducibility of placental reaction patterns. Pediatr Dev Pathol 2003;6(5):435-48; with permission.

HCA can also lead to placental abruption.[30] Chorioamnionitis associates with maternal sequelae, including endometritis and sepsis.[31]

VILLITIS OF UNKNOWN ETIOLOGY/CHRONIC VILLITIS

Villitis of unknown etiology (VUE) is an infiltration of the chorionic villi by maternal T-cells and histiocytes, in the absence of an identifiable infectious cause. Although the lack of an infectious cause is a prerequisite for the diagnosis, there is no standard protocol for work-up for infectious causes. Importantly, the histologic pattern of VUE is fairly distinct, and different from that seen in common infectious causes[32] (discussed later).

Gross Findings

There are no specific gross findings associated with VUE. However, VUE can be associated with avascular villi or increased perivillous fibrin deposition, both of which can be seen grossly if they involve large regions of the placenta.

Microscopic Findings

VUE is characterized by a focal or patchy infiltrate of lymphocytes and histiocytes involving the chorionic villi, with intervening normal placental parenchyma (**Fig. 7**). The infiltrate is usually mixed, and occasionally rare neutrophils and giant cells may be seen. Extensive involvement with neutrophils, plasma cells, or true necrotizing granulomatous inflammation should raise suspicion for an infectious cause. The pattern of involvement of VUE can be subdivided into 3 types:

1. Exclusive involvement of the distal/terminal villi.
2. Involvement of the more proximal/stem villi, or occasionally the chorionic plate. This type can be associated with obliterative fetal vasculopathy, in which the inflammation extends into the stem villous or chorionic plate vessels and results in luminal obliteration, with downstream avascular villi.
3. Exclusive or predominant involvement of the basal plate anchoring villi and the adjacent terminal villi. This type is frequently associated with chronic deciduitis with plasma cells, yielding lymphoplasmacytic deciduitis.

VUE is graded by the number of contiguous villi that are involved in each focus. Low-grade chronic villitis contains fewer than 10 involved villi per focus, and can be either focal, defined as only 1 slide showing the lesion, or multifocal with more than 1 slide showing the lesion. High-grade chronic villitis contains more than 10 involved villi per focus, and this lesion can be patchy or diffuse, with the latter showing greater than 30% of the terminal villi involved.[11] High-grade, diffuse chronic villitis is also commonly associated with perivillous fibrin deposition.

Clinical Associations

VUE in general is a fairly common placental lesion, affecting 5% to 15% of third-trimester placentas, and those with low-grade histology may have no recognizable clinical sequela.[33] However, high-grade chronic villitis, particularly with obliterative fetal vasculopathy, is associated with increased risk of adverse neurologic outcomes.[22,23] High-grade VUE also has a 10% to 25% recurrence risk and is associated with intrauterine growth restriction.

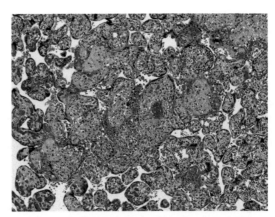

Fig. 7. Chronic villitis. Focus of distal/terminal villi with a lymphohistiocytic infiltrate, and mild, patchy surrounding fibrin deposition (H&E stain, original magnification ×10).

VILLITIS CAUSED BY SPECIFIC INFECTIOUS ORGANISMS

There are several clinically significant specific infectious organisms that are associated with characteristic histologic patterns of villitis in the placenta and that bear mentioning. This list is not meant to be comprehensive, it simply highlights some of the classic or common associations of which obstetricians should be aware.

Listeria

Acute villitis is an overall uncommon finding in the placenta, but, when it occurs, it is most commonly in the setting of either maternal sepsis with acute chorioamnionitis (discussed earlier) or caused by infection by *Listeria monocytogenes*. Unlike acute chorioamnionitis, which results from ascending intrauterine infection, acute villitis results from direct infection of the villi via maternal blood. Neutrophilic intervillous abscesses, which may be large enough to be seen grossly, are characteristic of listeria placentitis. There is also usually a necrotizing acute chorioamnionitis, with the organisms identifiable with a silver or tissue Gram stain, usually in the centers of the abscesses.[25,34]

Cytomegalovirus

Cytomegalovirus placentitis is most commonly seen in the setting of primary infection. A characteristic "TORCH (toxoplasmosis, other [syphilis, varicella-zoster, parvovirus B19], rubella, cytomegalovirus, and herpes)–like pattern of chronic villitis is seen. The villi are diffusely involved but to an uneven degree compared with the pattern in VUE. The villitis characteristically includes plasma cells in addition to abundant histiocytes, occasional lymphocytes, and prominent tissue damage, which includes fibrosis, edema, hemosiderin deposition, or some combination of these. Characteristic owl's-eye nuclear and cytoplasmic inclusions may be seen (**Fig. 8**A), particularly

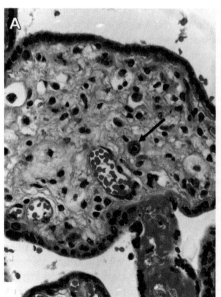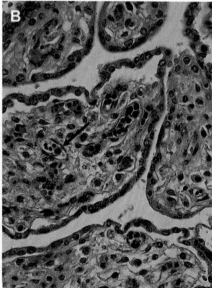

Fig. 8. (A) Characteristic owl's-eye inclusion of cytomegalovirus infection in villous stromal cell (*arrow*) (original magnification ×40). (B) Placenta with parvovirus inclusion in a fetal normoblast (*arrow*); note the marked increase in circulating fetal nucleated red blood cells and villous edema, consistent with hydrops (H&E stain, original magnification ×60).

in the fetal vascular endothelial cells and villous stromal cells. However, this finding is not seen in all cases, and the placental findings may vary depending on the duration and gestational age at the time of infection.[35] Increased perivillous fibrin deposition, and even massive perivillous fibrin deposition (discussed later), have also been observed (S. Ravishankar, unpublished data, 2018). Immunohistochemistry can be a useful tool to show the infection, particularly in cases in which the viral inclusions are rare or difficult to find.

Parvovirus

Parvovirus B19 is an important cause of second-trimester miscarriage and hydrops caused by fetal anemia. On gross and low-power microscopic examination of the placenta, the findings are similar to those seen in any case of fetal hydrops: the placenta is often enlarged and pale, with diffuse villous edema. On closer examination, a significant increase in circulating fetal normoblasts and erythroid precursors is seen in the fetal circulation. The diagnosis can be confirmed with identification of the typical ground-glass nuclear inclusions within these cells (**Fig. 8**B). Immunohistochemistry and appropriate serologic testing of maternal blood also aid in the diagnosis.[25]

Syphilis

Placentas with congenital syphilis grossly tend to be large and heavy. Necrotizing funisitis limited to the area around the umbilical vein is a rare, but fairly specific finding. Microscopically, there is villous enlargement and chronic villitis with plasma cells, along with endothelial and fibroblastic proliferation. Chronic deciduitis with plasma cells has also been described, but is nonspecific.[36]

Zika

Zika virus is an arthropod-borne infection that has recently been the cause of an epidemic in South and Central America. When the infection occurs in pregnancy, there is an increased risk for significant fetal anomalies, most notably microcephaly, and poor clinical outcomes. The pathogenic mechanisms of congenital transmission and placental disorder are continuing to be defined. Early reports with limited numbers of cases have fairly consistently shown hyperplasia of Hofbauer cells as a prominent finding, without significant acute or chronic villitis.[37,38] A recent review of placentas from 87 mothers infected with Zika virus generally showed mild, nonspecific changes, with the exception of placentas from fetuses and infants with congenital anomalies, which were more likely to show a high-grade TORCH-like pattern of villitis, along with other abnormalities, including villous stromal alterations (Redline and Ravishankar, unpublished data, 2019).

RARE LESIONS WITH A HIGH RISK OF RECURRENCE
Massive Perivillous Fibrin Deposition/Maternal Floor Infarction

Massive perivillous fibrin deposition (MPVFD) and maternal floor infarction (MFI) are related, uncommon, idiopathic placental lesions with characteristic gross and histopathologic features. They are important to recognize because of their association with poor pregnancy outcomes and increased risk of recurrence in subsequent pregnancies. Although perivillous fibrin deposition is a normal physiologic process that increases with gestational age, in MPVFD and MFI there is a pathologic increase in deposition. MPVFD is defined as gross involvement of greater than or equal to 25% to 50% of the placental parenchyma and/or microscopic involvement of greater than or equal to 25% to 50% on a single slide, spanning the fetal to the maternal surfaces (**Fig. 9**A). MFI grossly resembles a rind of fibrin that encases the basal villi, and

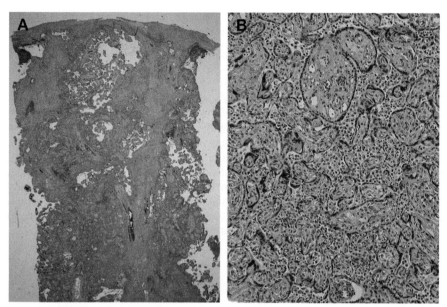

Fig. 9. (*A*) Massive perivillous fibrin deposition. Full-thickness involvement of more than 50% of the placental parenchyma on the slide with perivillous fibrin deposition, with only small islands of viable placental parenchyma remaining (H&E stain, original magnification ×2). (*B*) Chronic histiocytic intervillositis. Macrophages fill the intervillous space, surrounding distal villi (H&E stain, original magnification ×20).

microscopically must involve at least 3.0 mm of the parenchyma, adjacent to the maternal floor.[39] MPVFD and MFI have been reported in association with infections such as coxsackievirus; maternal autoimmune disease; and coagulopathy, such as antiphospholipid syndrome.[40] It has also been associated with mutations resulting in long-chain 3-hydroxyacyl coenzyme A dehydrogenase deficiency.[41] Significant fetal associations include intrauterine growth restriction and intrauterine fetal demise. The recurrence rate in subsequent pregnancies is approximately 40%.[39] A recent case report has suggested that treatment with intravenous immunoglobulin, heparin, and aspirin can result in a healthy pregnancy after recurrent MPVFD.[42]

Chronic Histiocytic Intervillositis

Chronic histiocytic intervillositis (CHI) is an uncommon, idiopathic inflammatory process that is associated with poor reproductive outcomes, including fetal growth restriction and pregnancy loss. Like MPVFD/MFI, CHI has an increased risk of recurrence in subsequent pregnancies. CHI is characterized by a diffuse infiltrate of maternal histiocytes involving the intervillous space, with a variable amount of associated perivillous fibrin deposition (**Fig. 9**B). There is no involvement of the villi, and the diagnosis should not be made in the presence of a significant admixed component of chronic villitis (discussed earlier).[43] CHI is associated with maternal immunologic conditions, including systemic lupus erythematosus and antiphospholipid syndrome. An association with neonatal alloimmune thrombocytopenia has also been reported,[44] along with increased levels of maternal serum alkaline phosphatase.[45] As previously mentioned, CHI is associated with poor pregnancy outcomes, with an overall recurrence rate of 67% to 100% without treatment, and a high incidence of intrauterine fetal demise and intrauterine growth restriction in affected pregnancies. Treatments have included aspirin, corticosteroids, heparin, and hydroxychloroquine, alone or in combination, with some success.[46]

SUMMARY

The placenta is the common link that brings obstetricians, neonatologists, and pathologists together in an attempt to understand the maternal, fetal, and neonatal physiologic and pathologic processes that determine the outcomes of pregnancies. A common understanding among all parties as to the indications, basic gross examination, and histologic patterns of injury is important to maximize the diagnostic, prognostic, and therapeutic benefit of placental examination. Critical for advancement in this field is a common language between pathologists to bring uniformity to and improve the clinician's understanding of placental pathology reports. The Amsterdam consensus terminology[11] has served as an important step in this direction, and will aid in future communication and collaborations between clinicians and pathologists.

DISCLOSURE

The authors have nothing to disclose.

REFERENCES

1. Khong TY, Mooney EE, Nikkels PGJ, et al, editors. Pathology of placenta: a practical guide. Cham (Switzerland): Springer; 2019.
2. Redline RW, Boyd TK, Roberts DJ, editors. Placental and gestational pathology. Cambridge (United Kingdom): Cambridge University Press; 2018.
3. Langston C, Kaplan C, Macpherson T, et al. Practice guidelines for examination of the placenta. Developed by the placental pathology practice guideline development task force of the College of American Pathologists. Arch Pathol Lab Med 1997;121:449–76.
4. Cox P, Evans C. Tissue pathway for histopathological examination of the placenta. London: The Royal College of Pathologists; 2017. Available at: https://www.rcpath.org/resourceLibrary/tissue-pathway-histopathological-placenta.html.
5. Baergen RN. Indications for submission and macroscopic examination of the placenta. APMIS 2018;126:544–50.
6. Kaplan C. Umbilical cord. In: Color atlas of gross placental pathology. 2nd edition. New York: Springer; 2007. p. 25–44.
7. Mills JL, Harley EE, Moessinger AC. Standards for measuring umbilical cord length. Placenta 1983;4:423–6.
8. Georgiadis L, Keski-Nisula L, Harju M, et al. Umbilical cord length in singleton gestations: a Finnish population-based retrospective register study. Placenta 2014;35:275–80.
9. Linde LE, Rasmussen S, Kessler J, et al. Extreme umbilical cord lengths, cord knot and entanglement: risk factors and risk of adverse outcomes, a population-based study. PLoS One 2018;13(3):e0194814.
10. Ukazu A, Ravikumar S, Roche N, et al. Are short umbilical cords seen in pathology really short? Fetal Pediatr Pathol 2018;37(5):359–62.
11. Khong YT, Mooney EE, Ariel I, et al. Sampling and definitions of placental lesions: Amsterdam placental working group consensus statement. Arch Pathol Lab Med 2016;140:698–713.

12. Benton SJ, Lafreniere AJ, Grynspan D, et al. A synoptic framework and future directions for placental pathology reporting. Placenta 2019;77:46–57.

13. Turowski G, Parks WT, Arbuckle S, et al. The structure and utility of the placental pathology report. APMIS 2018;126:638–46.

14. Redline RW. Maternal vascular malperfusion. In: Redline RW, Boyd TK, Roberts DJ, editors. Placental and gestational pathology. Cambridge (United Kingdom): Cambridge University Press; 2018. p. 62–9.

15. Redline RW. Maternal vascular/trophoblastic developmental abnormalities. In: Redline RW, Boyd TK, Roberts DJ, editors. Placental and gestational pathology. Cambridge (United Kingdom): Cambridge University Press; 2018. p. 49–57.

16. Redline RW, Ravishankar S. Fetal vascular malperfusion, an update. APMIS 2018; 126:561–9.

17. Vik T, Redline R, Nelson KB, et al. The placenta in neonatal encephalopathy: a case-control study. J Pediatr 2018;202:77–85.

18. Redline RW, Pappin A. Fetal thrombotic vasculopathy: the clinical significance of extensive avascular villi. Hum Pathol 1995;26:80–5.

19. Redline RW. Clinical and pathological umbilical cord abnormalities in fetal thrombotic vasculopathy. Hum Pathol 2004;35:1494–8.

20. Parast MM, Crum CP, Boyd TK. Placental histologic criteria for umbilical blood flow restriction in unexplained stillbirth. Hum Pathol 2008;39:948–53.

21. Saleemuddin A, Tantbirojin P, Sirois K, et al. Obstetric and perinatal complications in placentas with fetal thrombotic vasculopathy. Pediatr Dev Pathol 2010;13: 459–64.

22. Redline RW. Severe fetal placental vascular lesions in term infants with neurologic impairment. Am J Obstet Gynecol 2005;192:452–7.

23. Redline RW, O'Riordan MA. Placental lesions associated with cerebral palsy and neurologic impairment following term birth. Arch Pathol Lab Med 2000;124: 1785–91.

24. Vern TZ, Alles AJ, Kowal Vern A, et al. Frequency of factor V-Leiden and prothrombin G20210A in placentas and their relationship with placental lesions. Hum Pathol 2000;31:1036–43.

25. Roberts D. Placental infections. In: Redline RW, Boyd TK, Roberts DJ, editors. Placental and gestational pathology. Cambridge (United Kingdom): Cambridge University Press; 2018. p. 115–36.

26. Cox P, Cohen MC, Scheimberg IB. Acute chorioamnionitis. In: Khong TY, Mooney EE, Nikkels PGJ, et al, editors. Pathology of placenta: a practical guide. Cham (Switzerland): Springer; 2019. p. 103–7.

27. Redline RW, Faye-Petersen O, Heller D, et al. Amniotic infection syndrome: nosology and reproducibility of placental reaction patterns. Pediatr Dev Pathol 2003;6:435–48.

28. Ji H, Bridges M, Pesek E, et al. Acute funisitis correlates with the risk of early-onset sepsis in term newborns assessed using the Kaiser Sepsis Calculator. Pediatr Dev Pathol 2019. https://doi.org/10.1177/1093526619855467.

29. Chisholm K, Heerema-McKenney A, Tian L, et al. Correlation of preterm infant illness severity with placental histology. Placenta 2016;39:61–9.

30. Nath CA, Ananth CV, Smulian JC, et al. Histologic evidence of inflammation and risk of placental abruption. Am J Obstet Gynecol 2007;197:319.e1-6.

31. DeNoble AE, Heine RP, Dotters-Katz SK. Chorioamnionitis and infectious complications after vaginal delivery. AM J Perinatol 2019. https://doi.org/10.1055/s-0039-1692718.

32. Redline RW. Villitis of unknown etiology: noninfectious chronic villitis in the placenta. Hum Pathol 2007;38:1439–46.
33. Parast M. Chronic villitis/villitis of unknown etiology. In: Redline RW, Boyd TK, Roberts DJ, editors. Placental and gestational pathology. Cambridge (United Kingdom): Cambridge University Press; 2018. p. 137–44.
34. Heerema-McKenney A. Defense and infection of the human placenta. APMIS 2018;126:570–88.
35. Garcia AG, Fonseca EF, Marques RL, et al. Placental morphology in cytomegalovirus infection. Placenta 1989;10:1–18.
36. Sheffield JS, Sanchez PJ, Wendel GD Jr, et al. Placental histopathology of congenital syphilis. Obstet Gynecol 2002;100:126–33.
37. Rosenberg AZ, Yu W, Hill DA, et al. Placental pathology of Zika virus: viral infection of the placenta induces villous stromal macrophage (Hofbauer cell) proliferation and hyperplasia. Arch Pathol Lab Med 2017;141:43–8.
38. Schwartz DA. Viral infection, proliferation, and hyperplasia of Hofbauer cells and absence of inflammation characterize the placental pathology of fetuses with congenital Zika virus infection. Arch Gynecol Obstet 2017;295(6):1361–8.
39. Katzman PJ, Genest DR. Maternal floor infarction and massive perivillous fibrin deposition: histological definitions, association with intrauterine fetal growth restriction, and risk of recurrence. Pediatr Dev Pathol 2002;5:159–64.
40. Katzman PJ, Ernst LM, Scheimberg IB. Massive perivillous fibrinoid deposition and maternal floor infarct. In: Khong TY, Mooney EE, Nikkels PGJ, et al, editors. Pathology of the placenta: a practical guide. Cham (Switzerland): Springer; 2019. p. 77–82.
41. Griffin AC, Strauss AW, Bennett MJ, et al. Mutations in long-chain 3-hydroxyacyl coenzyme A dehydrogenase are associated with placental maternal floor infarction/massive perivillous fibrin deposition. Pediatr Dev Pathol 2012;15:368–74.
42. Abdulghani S, Moretti F, Gruslin A, et al. Recurrent massive perivillous fibrin deposition and chronic intervillositis treated with heparin and intravenous immunoglobulin: a case report. J Obstet Gynaecol Can 2017;39(8):676–81.
43. Redline RW. Chronic histiocytic intervillositis. In: Redline RW, Boyd TK, Roberts DJ, editors. Placental and gestational pathology. Cambridge (United Kingdom): Cambridge University Press; 2018. p. 152–5.
44. Dubruc E, Lebreton F, Giannoli C, et al. Placental histological lesions in fetal and neonatal alloimmune thrombocytopenia: a retrospective cohort study of 21 cases. Placenta 2016;48:104–9.
45. Marchaudon V, Devisme L, Petit S, et al. Chronic histiocytic intervillositis of unknown etiology: clinical features in a consecutive series of 69 cases. Placenta 2010;32:140–5.
46. Mekinian A, Costedoat-Chalumeau N, Masseau A, et al. Chronic histiocytic intervillositis: outcome, associated diseases and treatment in a multicenter prospective study. Autoimmunity 2015;48:40–5.

Immunology of the Placenta

Mancy Tong, PhD[a], Vikki M. Abrahams, PhD[b],*

KEYWORDS

- Immune adaptation • Innate immune • Pattern recognition • Pregnancy loss
- Preeclampsia • Preterm birth • Tolerance • Trophoblast

KEY POINTS

- Maternal immune cells with a supportive phenotype crosstalk with the placenta, and this is necessary for successful placentation and pregnancy outcome.
- The placenta uses several mechanisms to regulate maternal immune tolerance and adaptation.
- The placenta has the ability to sense infectious and non-infectious triggers and generate innate, immune-like responses.
- Disruption in these regulatory and protective mechanisms is associated with pregnancy complications, such as pregnancy loss, preeclampsia, and preterm birth.

INTRODUCTION

Pregnancy is an immune paradox in which the mother must tolerate the fetus, a semi-allograft, while at the same time maintain immune defense against pathogens. From the time of implantation at the very start of pregnancy, placental trophoblast cells directly interact with cells of the maternal immune system that are either circulating, resident in the endometrium of pregnancy, the decidua, or recruited to the maternal-fetal interface. Despite significant research advancements, it still remains incompletely understood how placental cells expressing paternal (non-self) antigens evade immune attack by the mother and how they transform the uterus into an immune-rich, yet propregnancy, site in which the placenta and fetus are able to thrive for the duration of pregnancy.

This review provides a broad overview of the immunology of the placenta, summarizing the key mechanisms used by the placenta to modulate immune function at the maternal-fetal interface such that local immune tolerance and adaptation is induced without global systemic immune suppression. Instead, both systemic and local innate immunity remains intact throughout gestation to protect the mother against infection,

[a] Department of Obstetrics, Gynecology and Reproductive Sciences, Yale School of Medicine, 310 Cedar Street, LSOG 309A, New Haven, CT 06510, USA; [b] Division of Reproductive Sciences, Department of Obstetrics, Gynecology and Reproductive Sciences, Yale School of Medicine, 310 Cedar Street, LSOG 305C, New Haven, CT 06510, USA
* Corresponding author.
E-mail address: vikki.abrahams@yale.edu

Obstet Gynecol Clin N Am 47 (2020) 49–63
https://doi.org/10.1016/j.ogc.2019.10.006
0889-8545/20/© 2019 Elsevier Inc. All rights reserved.

obgyn.theclinics.com

and locally innate immune cells may also play a role in promoting successful placentation and parturition.

IMMUNE CELLS AT THE MATERNAL-FETAL INTERFACE

The maternal-fetal interface primarily consists of maternal decidual stromal, invading placental trophoblast, and maternal immune cells. The presence and appropriate phenotype/function of these maternal immune cells is absolutely necessary for a successful pregnancy[1] (**Fig. 1**). During the first trimester of pregnancy, most of the maternal leukocytes present in the decidua are natural killer (NK) cells, with the remaining being macrophages, T cells, and dendritic cells.[2,3] Other immune cells such as mast cells, B cells, and innate lymphoid cells are also present at low numbers.[1,4] Although the numbers of NK cells remain relatively stable throughout gestation, there is an expansion of regulatory T cells (Tregs) with gestation that accumulate around invading trophoblasts.[5] The potential roles of the dominant immune cells at the maternal-fetal interface are briefly described.

Natural Killer Cells

Innate immune NK cells are present in both the non-pregnant (endometrial NK cells) and the pregnant uterus (uterine or decidual NK cells). During pregnancy, decidual NK (dNK) cells account for ~70% of all immune cells in the decidua, are found surrounding invading extravillous trophoblasts,[6] and have a phenotype (CD56^{bright}CD16$^-$) distinct from peripheral NK cells.[7,8] The origin of dNK cells remains controversial, as it is unclear whether these cells are recruited from the periphery, or if the local environment drives their unique phenotype, or both. One study reported that

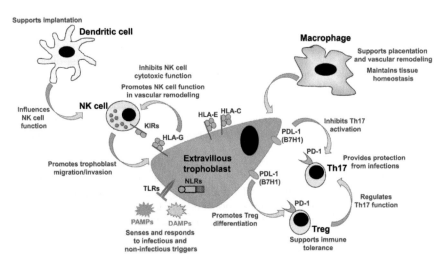

Fig. 1. The presence and appropriate phenotype/function of decidual maternal immune cells, such as natural killer (NK) cells, regulatory T cells (Tregs), macrophages, and dendritic cells is necessary for a successful pregnancy, and this is regulated in part by the extravillous trophoblast. In addition, the placenta through its expression of innate immune Toll-like receptors (TLRs) and Nod-like receptors (NLRs) provides a protective response against pathogens and danger signals that helps to maintain and promote a healthy pregnancy. DAMPs, damage-associated molecular patterns; HLA, human leukocyte antigen; KIR, killer immunoglobulin-like receptor; PAMPs, pathogen-associated molecular patterns; PD-1, programmed cell death protein 1; PDL-1, programmed death ligand 1.

decidual stromal expression of transforming growth factor (TGF)-β and interleukin 15 (IL-15) promotes the conversion of circulating CD56[dim] CD16+ NK cells into a dNK-like cell phenotype.[7] More recently, a population of dNK cells that are found in repeated pregnancies has been identified; and these "memory-like" NK cells may be involved in promoting placentation.[9] Indeed, the function of dNK cells is also unique. Although these dNK cells express cytotoxic factors such as perforin and granzyme A and B, they fail to exert cytolytic effects against the trophoblast, although these factors may be important during infection.[10] Instead, dNK cells support implantation, trophoblast migration and invasion, and remodeling of uterine spiral arteries, a key process to allow adequate perfusion of the growing placenta and fetus[6,11,12] (see **Fig. 1**). In mice, these processes are mediated by dNK cell secretion of interferon-γ and angiogenic factors, whereas in humans, these processes are mediated by NK cell–derived IL-8, inducible protein 10 (IP-10), and angiogenic factors.[6,11] dNK cells have also been reported to induce apoptosis of vascular smooth muscle cells and endothelial cells to aid in spiral artery remodeling.[13] NK cell depletion compromises pregnancy in mice, underscoring their importance during pregnancy.[14]

Macrophages

Macrophages are antigen-presenting cells that can respond and adapt to the local microenvironment, participating in a wide range of physiologic processes from implantation to parturition.[1] Both placental (fetal) macrophages (Hofbauer cells) and decidual (maternal) macrophages are present during normal pregnancy. Macrophages classically exist as an M1 (proinflammatory) or M2 (antiinflammatory) phenotype, although other subsets have been reported.[15] M1 macrophages typically respond to proinflammatory cytokines to propagate inflammation, whereas M2 macrophages are involved in tissue repair and resolution of inflammation. Hofbauer cells exhibit an M2 phenotype and may play a role in placental physiology.[16] However, these cells are also able to generate inflammatory responses toward infectious triggers, suggesting that they may also play a role in microbial-driven placental inflammation.[17] In contrast, decidual macrophages exhibit a high level of phenotypic plasticity. During the periimplantation period, these macrophages are typically M1, whereas during placentation, there is a mixture of M1 and M2 macrophages that accumulate around the spiral arteries,[18] where they are thought to be involved in placental development, vascular remodeling, and tissue homeostasis[19] (see **Fig. 1**). Once the placenta is established, most uterine macrophages are M2 for the remainder of gestation. Conversely, near parturition, M1 macrophages accumulate.[15]

T Cells

T cells are a diverse population of adaptive immune cells, some of which may be involved in promoting successful implantation, maternal tolerance, and remodeling of the spiral arteries.[20] Many subsets of T cells exist, each with different antigen specificity and functions at the maternal-fetal interface, including CD4+ T cells (30%–45%) and CD8+ cells (45%–75%).[21,22] Of the CD4+ cells, 5% to 30% are Th1 cells, ~5% are Th2 cells, and ~5% are Tregs; Tregs are the most important for inducing tolerance and placentation.[21] In addition to Tregs, CD4+ Th17 cells that produce IL-17 have also been described in pregnancy (see **Fig. 1**). The activity of these inflammatory Th17 cells is regulated by Tregs and dNK cells, and it is proposed that these cells may play a role in defense against pathologic infection.[23] Thus, a fine balance between Th17 cells and Tregs seems to be important in normal pregnancy, and an imbalance may lead to pregnancy complications.[24] Although activated Th1 and cytotoxic T cells are actively excluded from the mouse decidua via epigenetic changes in decidual stromal cells causing reduced expression of chemotactic signals,[20] low numbers of cytotoxic T cells can also be found in the human decidua; however, they express less degradative perforin and granzyme B than circulating cytotoxic T cells.[5]

T cells are activated by interacting with antigen-presenting cells that induce their proliferation and differentiation.[20] Although T cells with fetal/paternal antigen specificity have been reported during pregnancy, they are infrequent because several mechanisms exist at the maternal-fetal interface to reduce the formation of these reactive T cells as will be discussed later.[22] Thus, it has been proposed that T-cell activation during pregnancy occurs predominately through antigen-independent mechanisms via cytokine exposure rather than antigen-dependent T-cell receptor engagement.[22]

T Regulatory Cells

Tregs are responsible for the maintenance of immunologic self-tolerance by secreting immunosuppressive cytokines such as IL-10 and TGF-β that can suppress alloreactive/self-reactive lymphocytes.[25,26] During pregnancy, CD4+CD25^{high}FoxP3+ Tregs readily increase in number and are thought to play a key role in inducing maternal tolerance to the fetus.[25,26] The specific factors that induce Treg expansion during pregnancy are not well understood and may involve hormonal changes as well as exposure to paternal antigens in the seminal fluid. Indeed, Tregs specific for paternal-derived antigens have been observed.[26] Other studies have reported that interactions with trophoblasts may also induce Treg differentiation[27] (see **Fig. 1**). In the mouse, Tregs play a key role in limiting uterine inflammation during implantation, and reduced Treg numbers reduce fertility in murine allogeneic matings.[26] Furthermore, fetal-specific Treg cells can persist after parturition and rapidly reaccumulate in subsequent pregnancies that suggest a memory response.[28]

Dendritic Cells

Dendritic cells are antigen-presenting cells that after exposure to pathogens or inflammatory stimuli migrate via the lymphatic system to lymph nodes where they can present antigens to naïve T cells to direct their expansion, polarization, and activation.[29] Low numbers of dendritic cells can be found in the human decidua from the first trimester; however, it is thought that those present cannot migrate out of the uterus even after activation.[30] This is likely to be important to restrict cytotoxic/inflammatory T cell responses against pregnancy. Uterine dendritic cells are also thought to contribute to pregnancy success by influencing NK cell function and the cytokine profile at the maternal-fetal interface.[29] Depletion of uterine dendritic cells in mice results in a severe impairment of implantation and embryo resorptions highlighting their importance[31] (see **Fig. 1**).

MECHANISMS OF MATERNAL IMMUNE TOLERANCE AND ADAPTATION

Extravillous trophoblast invading into the decidua and villous syncytiotrophoblast in direct contact with maternal blood evade maternal immune recognition and promote either immune inertia or immunotolerance. This is demonstrated by the presence of fetal cells and placenta-derived fragments in the maternal circulation and organs, sometimes identified decades after pregnancy.[32,33] These fetal cells may differentiate into other functional cell types, depending on the microenvironment, which may play a role in tissue repair.[32] We will describe the key strategies used by the placenta to promote such maternal immune adaptation.

Human Leukocyte Antigen Expression

Major histocompatibility complex (MHC) class I antigens, also known as human leukocyte antigens (HLA), are expressed on the surface of most nucleated cells and interact with receptors on NK and T cells to allow the immune system to distinguish invading nonself cells from self.[10] Classic HLA class Ia (HLA-A, -B, and -C) are highly polymorphic to allow fine tuning of the immune system. In contrast, Class Ib HLAs (HLA-E, -F, and -G) are "non-classical" and exhibit restricted polymorphisms. To avoid maternal immune rejection, the human placenta lacks polymorphic HLA-A and HLA-B but express HLA-C, as well as the non-classical HLA-E, HLA-F, and HLA-G.[34] Although the fetus exhibits normal MHC expression patterns, the human syncytiotrophoblast that is in contact with maternal blood throughout gestation does not express any HLA, enabling the placenta to avoid peripheral maternal immune recognition. In contrast, the extravillous trophoblast that invades into the maternal decidua is positive for HLA-C, HLA-E, HLA-G, and HLA-F.[35] These HLAs act to dampen or modulate maternal immune responses by interacting with killer immunoglobulin-like receptors (KIRs) on dNK cells, macrophages, and a subset of T cells and with the T cell receptor on CD8+ T cells.[36] Specifically, HLA-E and HLA-G expressed by extravillous trophoblasts can inhibit the cytotoxic activity of NK and T cells and instead modulate immune cell function to promote trophoblast migration and placentation[37] (see **Fig. 1**). HLA-G mRNA can be alternatively spliced to yield membrane-bound and soluble variants, and soluble HLA-G is also associated with immunomodulatory functions and promotion of placentation.[36] HLA-G can also be released from the placenta via exosomes to modulate NK and T cell function distant from the placenta.[38] A novel mechanism by which HLA-G influences dNK cell and T cell function is through trogocytosis, where NK and T cells that have acquired HLA-G are immunosuppressive.[37]

Mechanisms to Inactivate T Cells

Several mechanisms are used by the placenta to kill, inactivate, or starve T cells at the maternal-fetal interface in order to limit T cell activation and cytotoxicity.[20]

B7 family members

B7 proteins are a family of costimulatory signals that determine the response of T cells after their activation by antigen-presenting cells. B7 proteins are usually expressed by antigen-presenting cells, although trophoblasts also express these, especially the syncytiotrophoblast and extravillous trophoblasts, with levels increasing during gestation.[39] B7 family members can be either stimulatory or inhibitory for T cell activation, and B7 may play an important role in maintaining maternal tolerance. For example, villous and extravillous trophoblasts express B7H1 (also known as CD274 and PD-L1) that can interact with PD-1 on maternal T cells to promote the development and function of Tregs while inhibiting Th17 cell activation[39] (see **Fig. 1**).

Galectin-1

Galectins are part of a phylogenetically conserved family of lectins that have a wide range of subcellular localizations and functions. Galectins can recognize carbohydrate-modified residues common to many glycoproteins and can modulate cell growth, differentiation, and function.[40] Galectin-1 is expressed by the endometrium, and levels are regulated by estrogen and progesterone.[40] During pregnancy, galectin-1 is also expressed by trophoblasts, and levels have been reported to be affected by stress.[41] A deficiency in galectin-1 increases fetal loss in mouse allogeneic, but not syngeneic, pregnancies, supporting an immunomodulatory role of this protein.[41] Furthermore, supplementation with recombinant galectin-1 in stress-challenged mice prevented fetal rejection by inducing tolerogenic dendritic cells that promoted the expansion of IL-10–producing Tregs.[41]

Indoleamine 2,3-dioxygenase

Indoleamine 2,3-dioxygenase (IDO) is an enzyme that metabolizes the essential amino acid tryptophan to kynurenine.[42] Although first trimester placental expression of IDO is still controversial, multiple studies have reported that IDO is expressed by trophoblasts from the second trimester of pregnancy onwards and by decidual macrophages.[42,43] Because T cells rely on tryptophan for proliferation, depletion of tryptophan by IDO blocks cell cycle progression in activated T cells and induces their apoptosis.[1,44] Furthermore, kynurenine may also play a role in promoting the differentiation of activated T cells to Tregs.[45] Interestingly, IDO-deficient mice have uncomplicated pregnancies,[44] which may indicate redundancies between mechanisms.

TUMOR NECROSIS FACTOR–RELATED APOPTOSIS-INDUCING FAMILY

The TNF-related apoptosis-inducing superfamily describes proteins that induce apoptosis of activated immune cells, including Fas ligand (FasL) and TNF-related apoptosis-inducing ligand (TRAIL). FasL is expressed by the placental trophoblast and by secreted placental microvesicles and exosomes.[46,47] Thus, placental FasL can act on Fas-receptor expressing maternal T cells even at locations away from the implantation site to promote death and clearance of these cells.[46,47] TRAIL exhibits high homology with FasL and uses similar pathways to induce apoptosis of activated T cells.[48] TRAIL is expressed by the syncytiotrophoblast from the first trimester of pregnancy as well as by resident Hofbauer cells[48] and can also be released via placental exosomes.[47]

Diseases Associated with Dysregulation of Maternal Tolerance

Dysregulation of maternal immune tolerance or the appropriate immune regulation by the placenta can lead to a range of obstetric complications, from early pregnancy loss to preeclampsia and intrauterine growth restriction that manifest later in gestation.

Pregnancy Loss

Spontaneous abortion or miscarriage is defined as loss of a fetus before 20 weeks of gestation. Even for women with normal fertility, 1 in 3 pregnancies end in spontaneous abortion and only around 50% can be accounted for fetal chromosomal abnormalities. Immunologic alterations have been reported in the decidua of women with spontaneous and recurrent pregnancy loss (RPL). The most well-described immunologic dysregulation in these women is changes in NK cell numbers and function. Excessive dNK cell recruitment and/or expansion, as well as elevated cytotoxic activity, associate with implantation failure and RPL.[49] An imbalance in proinflammatory and antiinflammatory T-cell responses play a role in pregnancy loss, such as alterations in the Th17/Treg ratio both locally and systemically.[49] Furthermore, there may be reduced expression of the key Treg transcription factor, Foxp3, in endometrial tissues from women with RPL.[50] Increased dendritic cell numbers have also been associated with pregnancy loss.[51,52] Disrupted immunoregulatory mechanisms have also been associated with pregnancy loss. Certain combinations of maternal KIRs and fetal HLA-C variants can negatively affect NK cell function and correlate with pregnancy loss,[53] as does reduced HLA-G expression.[37] Alterations in the expression of B7 costimulatory pathways and apoptosis-inducing TNF superfamily members are associated with pregnancy losses,[54,55] and the levels of IDO expression in RPL have been reported to be reduced.[43]

Preeclampsia

Preeclampsia is clinically diagnosed by new-onset hypertension (>140/90 mm Hg) and the presence of another clinical phenotype including proteinuria, low platelet count, impaired liver or kidney function, pulmonary edema, or new-onset headaches or visual disturbances after 20 weeks of gestation. Preeclampsia affects 3% to 7% of otherwise healthy pregnant women, and currently the only definitive treatment available is delivery of the placenta and consequently, the fetus. Several lines of evidence support that preeclampsia may result from insufficient maternal immune adaptation or tolerance to paternal alloantigens. Women are at increased risk of preeclampsia during their first pregnancy, and a short interval between coitus and first conception with the same partner increases the risk of preeclampsia. Furthermore, pregnancy confers protection to preeclampsia in later pregnancies with the same partner.[34] Mechanistically, it has been shown that seminal plasma contains paternal type I and type II MHC antigens and high concentrations of TGF-β that can stimulate expansion of Tregs. In mice, exposure to seminal fluid at mating induces maternal tolerance to paternal alloantigens and an accumulation of uterine Tregs, which may facilitate implantation.[56]

Although the pathogenesis of preeclampsia remains incompletely understood, the placenta plays a central role, and there is accumulating evidence that there are early gestational alterations in the immune cells present at the maternal-fetal interface that could lead to maternal immune and vascular dysfunction later in gestation. Several studies have reported changes in decidual and circulating immune cell numbers, phenotypes, and function in women with preeclampsia. For example, alterations in dNK cell numbers and activation have been associated with preeclampsia.[57] Most studies reported higher numbers of activated decidual macrophages[58] and impaired uterine macrophage function.[59] Preeclampsia has also been associated with the recruitment of uterine dendritic cells[60] and changes in T cell ratios and function. Preeclampsia is associated with increased Th17 cells, reduced circulating and decidual Tregs, and thus, an increase in the Th17/Treg ratio.[61]

Many of the molecular mechanisms of maternal tolerance have also been reported to be altered in preeclampsia, including reduced circulating soluble HLA-G,[62] reduced placental IDO and FasL expression,[63,64] reduced circulating TRAIL levels,[65] and reduced expression of immunosuppressive B7-H1 by dendritic cells.[66] In addition, there is evidence for KIR/HLA mismatch in preeclampsia. Epidemiologic data suggest that women with KIR AA subtype carrying HLA-C2 fetuses are at increased risk for preeclampsia by affecting the cytokine and chemokines secreted by dNK cells.[67] In mice, it has been shown that this KIR/HLA combination reduces placentation.[68]

Together, these early immunologic changes at the maternal-fetal interface could manifest into systemic symptoms later in the mother because an aberrant maternal immune response against the trophoblast could result in reduced invasion, placentation, and vascular remodeling. This could lead to placental dysfunction and the release of elevated proinflammatory cytokines, placental debris, and extracellular vesicles into the maternal circulation that can trigger systemic inflammation and endothelial dysfunction. Indeed, systemic inflammation is often observed in women with preeclampsia.[34]

INNATE IMMUNE PROPERTIES OF THE PLACENTA

An infection gaining access to the maternal-fetal interface can pose a significant threat to pregnancy. Consequently, the placental trophoblast is able to sense and respond to pathogens and non-infectious danger signals through the expression of pattern recognition receptors (PRRs), and this is thought to provide a protective response against pathogens that helps to maintain and promote a healthy pregnancy[69,70] (see **Fig. 1**). However, these same placental innate immune pathways if inappropriate or inadequately controlled may play a pivotal role in infection-associated pregnancy complications by disrupting the normal distribution, phenotype, and function of decidual immune cells and/or affecting the function of the placenta itself.

Pattern Recognition Receptors

Pattern recognition receptors such as the Toll-like receptors (TLRs) and Nod-like receptors (NLRs) are activated by conserved sequences known as pathogen-associated molecular patterns (PAMPs) that are expressed by invading microorganisms or host-derived damage-associated molecular patterns (DAMPs).[69,70]

TLRs are transmembrane receptors that are present on the cell surface or in endosomes. There are 10 human and 12 murine TLRs. Each TLR has a unique ligand-binding domain that senses a specific infectious PAMP or host-derived DAMP.[71] TLR2, in cooperation with its coreceptors TLR1, TLR6, or TLR10, recognizes gram-positive bacterial peptidoglycan and lipoproteins. TLR3 senses viral dsRNA, TLR4 senses gram-negative bacterial lipopolysaccharide (LPS), TLR5 senses bacterial flagellin, TLR7 and TLR8 sense viral ssRNA, and TLR9 senses bacterial DNA.[71] Once activated, TLRs typically mediate an inflammatory response characterized by the production of cytokines/chemokines and antimicrobial/antiviral factors. However, the specificity of response generated is governed by the TLR activated and its specific signaling pathway.

NLRs are cytoplasmic PRRs that detect microbial components or DAMPs.[72] The NLRs, Nod1 and Nod2, recognize peptides derived from the degradation of bacterial peptidoglycan that occurs during normal bacterial growth or destruction. Nod1 recognizes D-glutamyl-meso-diaminopimelic acid (iE-DAP), which is only found in gram-negative bacteria, whereas Nod2 recognizes muramyl dipeptide (MDP), which is released by all bacteria. Both Nod1 and Nod2 trigger an inflammatory cytokine and chemokine response after activation.[72] Another group of NLRs are involved in mediating the production of the inflammatory cytokine IL-1β through activation of the inflammasome. The NLRs, NLRP1, NLRP3, and NLRC4 can sense infectious PAMPs, whereas NLRP3 can also be activated by danger signals such as uric acid or adenosine triphosphate.[72] On activation of these NLRs, assembly of the inflammasome occurs; a protein complex consisting of the NLR, the adapter protein, apoptosis-associated speck-like protein containing a CARD, and caspase-1. Once assembled, caspase-1 is activated and processes pro-IL-1β into its secreted form.[72] Adding to the complexity, the inflammasome requires 2 signals for activation. The first signal is usually a microbial product that activates a TLR, leading to an upregulation of pro-IL-1β expression. This is then followed by a second PAMP or DAMP signal that directly activates the NLR for inflammasome formation.[72]

Trophoblast Sensing of Pathogen-Associated Molecular Patterns and Damage-Associated Molecular Patterns

High doses of bacterial PAMPs such as LPS, iE-DAP, and MDP trigger the placental trophoblast to generate a mild proinflammatory cytokine/chemokine response through TLR4, Nod1, and Nod2, respectively, whereas lower, more physiologic doses are unable to induce this inflammation.[73–75] Instead, low-dose LPS triggers a more immunoregulatory type I interferon-β, RANTES, and IP-10 response.[76] The TLR2 trigger, gram-positive bacterial peptidoglycan, induces first trimester trophoblast apoptosis, whereas at term it is able to trigger an inflammatory response in these cells.[77] This differential response to peptidoglycan may be due to differential expression of the TLR2 coreceptor, TLR6, across gestation.[78] In contrast, the viral PAMPs dsRNA and ssRNA through TLR3 and TLR8, respectively, trigger a strong trophoblast chemokine/cytokine, type I interferon, and antiviral response.[79,80] The placenta is also able to sense and respond to DAMPs through NLRs. Uric acid activates trophoblast NLRP3 to drive inflammasome activation and IL-1β production,[81] whereas another DAMP, high-mobility group box 1 protein (HMGB-1), through activation of TLR4 induces a broad inflammatory cytokine/chemokine response.[82] In addition to inducing inflammation via TLRs and NLRs, infectious triggers may limit trophoblast migration and invasion[83–85] and induce an antiangiogenic response.[86] Although these studies demonstrate the ability of the trophoblast to sense and respond to a wide range of infectious and noninfectious triggers, they also highlight the complexity of placental TLR and NLR signaling.

Toll-like Receptor and Nod-like Receptor Activation in Pregnancy Complications

A role for infection in preterm birth is well established.[87] Although the pathways leading from infection to preterm birth are still not completely understood, there is increasing evidence suggesting that placental TLRs and NLRs may play an important role.[69,70] One of the most studied mouse model of infection-associated preterm birth uses high-dose bacterial LPS that triggers placental and uterine inflammation; and TLR4$^{-/-}$ mice are protected against this.[88] Bacterial iE-DAP, bacterial peptidoglycan, and viral dsRNA can also induce preterm birth.[89,90] Interestingly and in keeping with in vitro studies, in vivo low-dose LPS only triggers preterm birth in mice on a pathologic background, such as an active viral infection,[91] or IL-10 deficiency.[92] Thus, although TLR activation can mediate preterm birth, in normal pregnancy there seems to be some tolerance toward certain bacterial components, such as LPS, and it may take an additional signal, such as a virus, to change the way the maternal-fetal interface reacts to these bacterial signals.[91] Despite the strong role for infection in prematurity, a significant proportion of preterm deliveries show no evidence of infection,[87] suggesting that regardless of the trigger it is the inflammatory intermediaries and downstream events that cause tissue injury and the pathologic outcome. Indeed, the DAMP uric acid triggers placental inflammation and growth restriction in vivo,[93] whereas HMGB1 induces preterm birth.[94] Infections have also been associated with preeclampsia,[95] and, although studies are limited, in vivo delivery of viral components targeting TLRs have been reported to induce preeclampsia-like symptoms.[96]

Dysregulation of Placental-Immune Crosstalk

The trophoblast constantly interacts with maternal immune cells from implantation through to parturition. As discussed, this trophoblast-immune cell crosstalk is likely essential for normal maternal adaptations to pregnancy. However, placental PRR activation may alter this normal interaction. In this way, trophoblast inflammatory responses to PAMPS or DAMPs may affect the resident and recruited maternal immune cell milieu and change them from a supportive phenotype to an overactive or dangerous phenotype that may be detrimental for pregnancy success. Indeed, clinical studies and experimental models of preterm birth have reported a shift in immune cell numbers, populations, or activation status at the maternal-fetal interface, and targeting specific immune cells has highlighted their critical role in pregnancy outcome.[97] Thus, placental innate immune responses to PAMPs or DAMPs may shift in the immunologic balance.[69,97]

SUMMARY AND FUTURE DIRECTIONS

This review aims to provide an overview of our current understanding of the immunology of the placenta and mechanisms of maternal immune regulation during normal and pathologic pregnancy. However, many questions remain to be answered. What signals from the placenta trigger the specialization of maternal immune cells once they have entered the maternal-fetal interface? What are the functions of the maternal immune cell types at the decidua throughout gestation? Why is immune rejection triggered in some pregnancies but not others? Compounding this, it is clear that multiple layers of crosstalk exist between the decidua, maternal immune cells, and the placenta; and high throughput technologies have enabled the identification of new immune cell populations and dNK cell subpopulations in the human decidua.[98,99] Thus, more research is needed to better characterize the crosstalk and interactions between these cell types. Furthermore, although we know that infections can increase the risk of obstetric diseases, more clinical and in vivo studies are needed to clarify theses mechanisms involved so that we can identify predictive and therapeutic strategies in the future. Despite our efforts, the immunology of normal human pregnancy remains enigmatic and more work is needed in order to advance our understanding of the immunology of pathologic pregnancies.

DISCLOSURE

The authors have nothing to disclose.

REFERENCES

1. Mor G, Abrahams VM. The immunology of pregnancy. In: Creasy R, Resnik R, Iams J, et al, editors. Maternal-fetal medicine. 7 edition. Elsevier; 2017.
2. Bulmer JN, Pace D, Ritson A. Immunoregulatory cells in human decidua: morphology, immunohistochemistry and function. Reprod Nutr Dev 1988; 28(6B):1599–613.
3. Trundley A, Moffett A. Human uterine leukocytes and pregnancy. Tissue Antigens 2004;63(1):1–12.
4. Vacca P, Montaldo E, Croxatto D, et al. Identification of diverse innate lymphoid cells in human decidua. Mucosal Immunol 2015;8(2):254–64.
5. Tilburgs T, Schonkeren D, Eikmans M, et al. Human decidual tissue contains differentiated CD8+ effector-memory T cells with unique properties. J Immunol 2010;185(7):4470–7.
6. Moffett-King A. Natural killer cells and pregnancy. Nat Rev Immunol 2002;2(9): 656–63.
7. Keskin DB, Allan DS, Rybalov B, et al. TGFbeta promotes conversion of CD16+ peripheral blood NK cells into CD16- NK cells with similarities to decidual NK cells. Proc Natl Acad Sci U S A 2007;104(9):3378–83.
8. Manaster I, Mizrahi S, Goldman-Wohl D, et al. Endometrial NK cells are special immature cells that await pregnancy. J Immunol 2008;181(3):1869–76.
9. Gamliel M, Goldman-Wohl D, Isaacson B, et al. Trained memory of human uterine NK cells enhances their function in subsequent pregnancies. Immunity 2018; 48(5):951–962 e5.
10. Kopcow HD, Allan DS, Chen X, et al. Human decidual NK cells form immature activating synapses and are not cytotoxic. Proc Natl Acad Sci U S A 2005; 102(43):15563–8.

11. Hanna J, Goldman-Wohl D, Hamani Y, et al. Decidual NK cells regulate key developmental processes at the human fetal-maternal interface. Nat Med 2006;12(9): 1065–74.

12. Ashkar AA, Di Santo JP, Croy BA. Interferon gamma contributes to initiation of uterine vascular modification, decidual integrity, and uterine natural killer cell maturation during normal murine pregnancy. J Exp Med 2000;192(2):259–70.

13. Fraser R, Whitley GS, Johnstone AP, et al. Impaired decidual natural killer cell regulation of vascular remodelling in early human pregnancies with high uterine artery resistance. J Pathol 2012;228(3):322–32.

14. Guimond MJ, Luross JA, Wang B, et al. Absence of natural killer cells during murine pregnancy is associated with reproductive compromise in TgE26 mice. Biol Reprod 1997;56(1):169–79.

15. Ning F, Liu H, Lash GE. The role of decidual macrophages during normal and pathological pregnancy. Am J Reprod Immunol 2016;75(3):298–309.

16. Tang Z, Abrahams VM, Mor G, et al. Placental Hofbauer cells and complications of pregnancy. Ann N Y Acad Sci 2011;1221:103–8.

17. Young OM, Tang Z, Niven-Fairchild T, et al. Toll-like receptor-mediated responses by placental Hofbauer cells (HBCs): a potential pro-inflammatory role for fetal M2 macrophages. Am J Reprod Immunol 2015;73(1):22–35.

18. Houser BL, Tilburgs T, Hill J, et al. Two unique human decidual macrophage populations. J Immunol 2011;186(4):2633–42.

19. Nagamatsu T, Schust DJ. The contribution of macrophages to normal and pathological pregnancies. Am J Reprod Immunol 2010;63(6):460–71.

20. Nancy P, Erlebacher A. T cell behavior at the maternal-fetal interface. Int J Dev Biol 2014;58(2–4):189–98.

21. Mjosberg J, Berg G, Jenmalm MC, et al. FOXP3+ regulatory T cells and T helper 1, T helper 2, and T helper 17 cells in human early pregnancy decidua. Biol Reprod 2010;82(4):698–705.

22. Erlebacher A. Mechanisms of T cell tolerance towards the allogeneic fetus. Nat Rev Immunol 2013;13(1):23–33.

23. Fu B, Li X, Sun R, et al. Natural killer cells promote immune tolerance by regulating inflammatory TH17 cells at the human maternal-fetal interface. Proc Natl Acad Sci U S A 2013;110(3):E231–40.

24. Saito S, Nakashima A, Shima T, et al. Th1/Th2/Th17 and regulatory T-cell paradigm in pregnancy. Am J Reprod Immunol 2010;63(6):601–10.

25. Aluvihare VR, Kallikourdis M, Betz AG. Regulatory T cells mediate maternal tolerance to the fetus. Nat Immunol 2004;5(3):266–71.

26. Schumacher A, Zenclussen AC. Regulatory T cells: regulators of life. Am J Reprod Immunol 2014;72(2):158–70.

27. Du MR, Guo PF, Piao HL, et al. Embryonic trophoblasts induce decidual regulatory T cell differentiation and maternal-fetal tolerance through thymic stromal lymphopoietin instructing dendritic cells. J Immunol 2014;192(4):1502–11.

28. Rowe JH, Ertelt JM, Xin L, et al. Pregnancy imprints regulatory memory that sustains anergy to fetal antigen. Nature 2012;490(7418):102–6.

29. Tagliani E, Erlebacher A. Dendritic cell function at the maternal-fetal interface. Expert Rev Clin Immunol 2011;7(5):593–602.

30. Collins MK, Tay CS, Erlebacher A. Dendritic cell entrapment within the pregnant uterus inhibits immune surveillance of the maternal/fetal interface in mice. J Clin Invest 2009;119(7):2062–73.

31. Plaks V, Birnberg T, Berkutzki T, et al. Uterine DCs are crucial for decidua formation during embryo implantation in mice. J Clin Invest 2008;118(12):3954–65.

32. Bianchi DW, Zickwolf GK, Weil GJ, et al. Male fetal progenitor cells persist in maternal blood for as long as 27 years postpartum. Proc Natl Acad Sci U S A 1996;93(2):705–8.

33. Tannetta D, Collett G, Vatish M, et al. Syncytiotrophoblast extracellular vesicles - Circulating biopsies reflecting placental health. Placenta 2017;52:134–8.

34. Redman CW, Sargent IL. Immunology of pre-eclampsia. Am J Reprod Immunol 2010;63(6):534–43.

35. Hackmon R, Pinnaduwage L, Zhang J, et al. Definitive class I human leukocyte antigen expression in gestational placentation: HLA-F, HLA-E, HLA-C, and HLA-G in extravillous trophoblast invasion on placentation, pregnancy, and parturition. Am J Reprod Immunol 2017;77(6):1–11.

36. Hunt JS, Langat DK, McIntire RH, et al. The role of HLA-G in human pregnancy. Reprod Biol Endocrinol 2006;4(Suppl 1):S10.

37. Ferreira LMR, Meissner TB, Tilburgs T, et al. HLA-G: at the interface of maternal-fetal tolerance. Trends Immunol 2017;38(4):272–86.

38. Kshirsagar SK, Alam SM, Jasti S, et al. Immunomodulatory molecules are released from the first trimester and term placenta via exosomes. Placenta 2012;33(12):982–90.

39. Petroff MG, Perchellet A. B7 family molecules as regulators of the maternal immune system in pregnancy. Am J Reprod Immunol 2010;63(6):506–19.

40. Barrientos G, Freitag N, Tirado-Gonzalez I, et al. Involvement of galectin-1 in reproduction: past, present and future. Hum Reprod Update 2014;20(2):175–93.

41. Blois SM, Ilarregui JM, Tometten M, et al. A pivotal role for galectin-1 in fetomaternal tolerance. Nat Med 2007;13(12):1450–7.

42. Chang RQ, Li DJ, Li MQ. The role of indoleamine-2,3-dioxygenase in normal and pathological pregnancies. Am J Reprod Immunol 2018;79(4):e12786.

43. Ban Y, Chang Y, Dong B, et al. Indoleamine 2,3-dioxygenase levels at the normal and recurrent spontaneous abortion fetal-maternal interface. J Int Med Res 2013; 41(4):1135–49.

44. Munn DH, Zhou M, Attwood JT, et al. Prevention of allogeneic fetal rejection by tryptophan catabolism. Science 1998;281(5380):1191–3.

45. Mezrich JD, Fechner JH, Zhang X, et al. An interaction between kynurenine and the aryl hydrocarbon receptor can generate regulatory T cells. J Immunol 2010; 185(6):3190–8.

46. Abrahams VM, Straszewski-Chavez SL, Guller S, et al. First trimester trophoblast cells secrete Fas ligand which induces immune cell apoptosis. Mol Hum Reprod 2004;10(1):55–63.

47. Stenqvist AC, Nagaeva O, Baranov V, et al. Exosomes secreted by human placenta carry functional Fas ligand and TRAIL molecules and convey apoptosis in activated immune cells, suggesting exosome-mediated immune privilege of the fetus. J Immunol 2013;191(11):5515–23.

48. Phillips TA, Ni J, Pan G, et al. TRAIL (Apo-2L) and TRAIL receptors in human placentas: implications for immune privilege. J Immunol 1999;162(10):6053–9.

49. Kwak-Kim J, Bao S, Lee SK, et al. Immunological modes of pregnancy loss: inflammation, immune effectors, and stress. Am J Reprod Immunol 2014;72(2): 129–40.

50. Jasper MJ, Tremellen KP, Robertson SA. Primary unexplained infertility is associated with reduced expression of the T-regulatory cell transcription factor Foxp3 in endometrial tissue. Mol Hum Reprod 2006;12(5):301–8.

51. Askelund K, Liddell HS, Zanderigo AM, et al. CD83(+)dendritic cells in the decidua of women with recurrent miscarriage and normal pregnancy. Placenta 2004;25(2–3):140–5.
52. Huang C, Zhang H, Chen X, et al. Association of peripheral blood dendritic cells with recurrent pregnancy loss: a case-controlled study. Am J Reprod Immunol 2016;76(4):326–32.
53. Chazara O, Xiong S, Moffett A. Maternal KIR and fetal HLA-C: a fine balance. J Leukoc Biol 2011;90(4):703–16.
54. Jin LP, Fan DX, Zhang T, et al. The costimulatory signal upregulation is associated with Th1 bias at the maternal-fetal interface in human miscarriage. Am J Reprod Immunol 2011;66(4):270–8.
55. Banzato PC, Daher S, Traina E, et al. FAS and FAS-L genotype and expression in patients with recurrent pregnancy loss. Reprod Sci 2013;20(9):1111–5.
56. Robertson SA, Guerin LR, Bromfield JJ, et al. Seminal fluid drives expansion of the CD4+CD25+ T regulatory cell pool and induces tolerance to paternal alloantigens in mice. Biol Reprod 2009;80(5):1036–45.
57. Moffett A, Hiby SE. How Does the maternal immune system contribute to the development of pre-eclampsia? Placenta 2007;28(Suppl A):S51–6.
58. Schonkeren D, van der Hoorn ML, Khedoe P, et al. Differential distribution and phenotype of decidual macrophages in preeclamptic versus control pregnancies. Am J Pathol 2011;178(2):709–17.
59. Przybyl L, Haase N, Golic M, et al. CD74-downregulation of placental macrophage-trophoblastic interactions in preeclampsia. Circ Res 2016;119(1):55–68.
60. Huang SJ, Chen CP, Schatz F, et al. Pre-eclampsia is associated with dendritic cell recruitment into the uterine decidua. J Pathol 2008;214(3):328–36.
61. Saito S. Th17 cells and regulatory T cells: new light on pathophysiology of pre-eclampsia. Immunol Cell Biol 2010;88(6):615–7.
62. Yie SM, Taylor RN, Librach C. Low plasma HLA-G protein concentrations in early gestation indicate the development of preeclampsia later in pregnancy. Am J Obstet Gynecol 2005;193(1):204–8.
63. Kudo Y, Boyd CA, Sargent IL, et al. Decreased tryptophan catabolism by placental indoleamine 2,3-dioxygenase in preeclampsia. Am J Obstet Gynecol 2003;188(3):719–26.
64. Prusac IK, Zekic Tomas S, Roje D. Apoptosis, proliferation and Fas ligand expression in placental trophoblast from pregnancies complicated by HELLP syndrome or pre-eclampsia. Acta Obstet Gynecol Scand 2011;90(10):1157–63.
65. Chaemsaithong P, Chaiworapongsa T, Romero R, et al. Maternal plasma soluble TRAIL is decreased in preeclampsia. J Matern Fetal Neonatal Med 2014;27(3):217–27.
66. Darmochwal-Kolarz D, Kludka-Sternik M, Kolarz B, et al. The expression of B7-H1 and B7-H4 co-stimulatory molecules on myeloid and plasmacytoid dendritic cells in pre-eclampsia and normal pregnancy. J Reprod Immunol 2013;99(1–2):33–8.
67. Hiby SE, Walker JJ, O'Shaughnessy KM, et al. Combinations of maternal KIR and fetal HLA-C genes influence the risk of preeclampsia and reproductive success. J Exp Med 2004;200(8):957–65.
68. Kieckbusch J, Gaynor LM, Moffett A, et al. MHC-dependent inhibition of uterine NK cells impedes fetal growth and decidual vascular remodelling. Nat Commun 2014;5:3359.
69. Abrahams VM. Pattern recognition at the maternal-fetal interface. Immunol Invest 2008;37(5):427–47.

70. Abrahams VM. The role of the Nod-like receptor family in trophoblast innate immune responses. J Reprod Immunol 2011;88(2):112–7.
71. Kawai T, Akira S. The role of pattern-recognition receptors in innate immunity: update on Toll-like receptors. Nat Immunol 2010;11(5):373–84.
72. Franchi L, Warner N, Viani K, et al. Function of Nod-like receptors in microbial recognition and host defense. Immunol Rev 2009;227(1):106–28.
73. Abrahams VM, Bole-Aldo P, Kim YM, et al. Divergent trophoblast responses to bacterial products mediated by TLRs. J Immunol 2004;173(7):4286–96.
74. Costello MJ, Joyce SK, Abrahams VM. NOD protein expression and function in first trimester trophoblast cells. Am J Reprod Immunol 2007;57(1):67–80.
75. Mulla MJ, Yu AG, Cardenas I, et al. Regulation of Nod1 and Nod2 in first trimester trophoblast cells. Am J Reprod Immunol 2009;61(4):294–302.
76. Racicot K, Kwon JY, Aldo P, et al. Type I interferon regulates the placental inflammatory response to bacteria and is targeted by virus: mechanism of polymicrobial infection-induced preterm birth. Am J Reprod Immunol 2016;75(4):451–60.
77. Ma Y, Krikun G, Abrahams VM, et al. Cell type-specific expression and function of toll-like receptors 2 and 4 in human placenta: implications in fetal infection. Placenta 2007;28(10):1024–31.
78. Abrahams VM, Aldo PB, Murphy SP, et al. TLR6 modulates first trimester trophoblast responses to peptidoglycan. J Immunol 2008;180(9):6035–43.
79. Abrahams VM, Schaefer TM, Fahey JV, et al. Expression and secretion of antiviral factors by trophoblast cells following stimulation by the TLR-3 agonist, Poly(I:C). Hum Reprod 2006;21:2432–9.
80. Potter JA, Garg M, Girard S, et al. Viral single stranded RNA induces a trophoblast pro-inflammatory and antiviral response in a TLR8-dependent and -independent manner. Biol Reprod 2015;92(1):17.
81. Mulla MJ, Myrtolli K, Potter J, et al. Uric acid induces trophoblast IL-1beta production via the inflammasome: implications for the pathogenesis of preeclampsia. Am J Reprod Immunol 2011;65(6):542–8.
82. Shirasuna K, Seno K, Ohtsu A, et al. AGEs and HMGB1 increase inflammatory cytokine production from human placental cells, resulting in an enhancement of monocyte migration. Am J Reprod Immunol 2016;75(5):557–68.
83. Yamamoto-Tabata T, McDonagh S, Chang HT, et al. Human cytomegalovirus interleukin-10 downregulates metalloproteinase activity and impairs endothelial cell migration and placental cytotrophoblast invasiveness in vitro. J Virol 2004; 78(6):2831–40.
84. Arechavaleta-Velasco F, Ma Y, Zhang J, et al. Adeno-associated virus-2 (AAV-2) causes trophoblast dysfunction, and placental AAV-2 infection is associated with preeclampsia. Am J Pathol 2006;168(6):1951–9.
85. Kim YM, Romero R, Oh SY, et al. Toll-like receptor 4: a potential link between "danger signals," the innate immune system, and preeclampsia? Am J Obstet Gynecol 2005;193(3 Pt 2):921–7.
86. Nakada E, Walley KR, Nakada T, et al. Toll-like receptor-3 stimulation upregulates sFLT-1 production by trophoblast cells. Placenta 2009;30(9):774–9.
87. Goldenberg RL, Culhane JF, Iams JD, et al. Epidemiology and causes of preterm birth. Lancet 2008;371(9606):75–84.
88. Elovitz MA, Mrinalini C. Animal models of preterm birth. Trends Endocrinol Metab 2004;15(10):479–87.
89. Cardenas I, Mulla MJ, Myrtolli K, et al. Nod1 activation by bacterial iE-DAP induces maternal-fetal inflammation and preterm labor. J Immunol 2011;187(2): 980–6.

90. Koga K, Cardenas I, Aldo P, et al. Activation of TLR3 in the trophoblast is associated with preterm delivery. Am J Reprod Immunol 2009;61(3):196–212.
91. Cardenas I, Mor G, Aldo P, et al. Placental viral infection sensitizes to endotoxin-induced pre-term labor: a double hit hypothesis. Am J Reprod Immunol 2011; 65(2):110–7.
92. Murphy SP, Fast LD, Hanna NN, et al. Uterine NK cells mediate inflammation-induced fetal demise in IL-10-null mice. J Immunol 2005;175(6):4084–90.
93. Brien ME, Duval C, Palacios J, et al. Uric acid crystals induce placental inflammation and alter trophoblast function via an IL-1-dependent pathway: implications for fetal growth restriction. J Immunol 2017;198(1):443–51.
94. Gomez-Lopez N, Romero R, Plazyo O, et al. Intra-amniotic administration of HMGB1 induces spontaneous preterm labor and birth. Am J Reprod Immunol 2016;75(1):3–7.
95. Racicot K, Mor G. Risks associated with viral infections during pregnancy. J Clin Invest 2017;127(5):1591–9.
96. Chatterjee P, Weaver LE, Doersch KM, et al. Placental Toll-like receptor 3 and Toll-like receptor 7/8 activation contributes to preeclampsia in humans and mice. PLoS One 2012;7(7):e41884.
97. Gomez-Lopez N, StLouis D, Lehr MA, et al. Immune cells in term and preterm labor. Cell Mol Immunol 2014;11(6):571–81.
98. Vento-Tormo R, Efremova M, Botting RA, et al. Single-cell reconstruction of the early maternal-fetal interface in humans. Nature 2018;563(7731):347–53.
99. Vazquez J, Chavarria M, Li Y, et al. Computational flow cytometry analysis reveals a unique immune signature of the human maternal-fetal interface. Am J Reprod Immunol 2018;79(1):1–9.

Diabetes Mellitus, Obesity, and the Placenta

Gernot Desoye, PhD*, Mila Cervar-Zivkovic, MD, PhD

KEYWORDS

- Insulin • Glucose • Placental development • Fetal phenotype • Sexual dimorphism
- Stress

KEY POINTS

- Maternal metabolic and inflammatory changes in first trimester may alter placental development and determine placental trajectories ultimately contributing to fetal and neonatal phenotype.
- Placental phenotype in diabetes and obesity and molecular responses to environmental perturbation are sexually dimorphic with more plasticity in the placenta of a female fetus.
- The consequences of the manifold placental changes, observed at the end of pregnancy, associated with diabetes and/or obesity on fetal development are unclear. Indeed, they may constitute adaptive responses to the altered maternal-fetal milieu to maintain a homeostatic environment for the fetus.

THE HEALTH PROBLEM—IS THE PLACENTA INVOLVED?

Obesity and type 2 diabetes mellitus (T2DM) have become escalating global health problems. In 2016 worldwide obesity, defined by a body mass index ≥ 30 kg/m^2, had a prevalence of 13.1% among the age group 18+ years compared with 5.3% in 1980.[1] Importantly obesity is a major risk factor for T2DM, hence the number of people with diabetes mellitus, about 90% of whom are T2DM, has risen from 108 million in 1980 to 422 million in 2014. This represents an 8.5% global prevalence of diabetes mellitus among adults over 18 years in 2014.[2] Projections of the International Diabetes Federation expect this number to increase to about 500 million in 2045.[3]

Derangements of the maternal glucose-insulin axis as in pregestational (type 1 diabetes mellitus [T1DM] and T2DM) and gestational diabetes mellitus (GDM) and maternal obesity increase the risk of both mother and offspring to develop obesity and T2DM later in life. Thus, an obese pregnant woman or a woman with T1DM, T2DM, or GDM confers a risk for the offspring to become obese and also to later develop T2DM. Female offspring born to such a pregnancy may themselves become pregnant when already overweight or obese, which in turn increases the risks for the

Department of Obstetrics and Gynaecology, Medical University of Graz, Auenbruggerplatz 14, Graz 8036, Austria
* Corresponding author.
E-mail address: gernot.desoye@medunigraz.at

Obstet Gynecol Clin N Am 47 (2020) 65–79
https://doi.org/10.1016/j.ogc.2019.11.001
0889-8545/20/© 2019 Elsevier Inc. All rights reserved.

next generation. This sequence constitutes a self-perpetuating cycle that contributes to the obesity and T2DM epidemic that we are seeing.[4,5]

For this reason obesity in the youth is especially alarming. In Europe more than 20% of children are overweight or obese by the age of 10 years.[6] Epidemiologic evidence demonstrates that being born with excessive adiposity (often described as "macrosomic" or large for gestational age at birth) strongly associates with overweight or obesity in youth, commonly with features of the metabolic syndrome. These associations are independent of ethnicity and genetics and are likely mediated through epigenetic changes,[7–10] which may be induced by fetal hyperglycemia, hyperinsulinemia, or other metabolic disturbances in fetal development. For example, offspring born to obese women not only store more triglycerides, but also have a greater number of adipocytes by the age of 2 years.[11] Hence, the evidence suggests that excessive fat deposition in utero resulting in offspring being born with excess capacity for adipose storage contributes to the epidemic of obesity and T2DM. This raises the question of how the placenta, as the nutrient gatekeeper between mother and fetus, contributes to excessive neonatal adiposity.

EARLY PREGNANCY EVENTS

Although screening for GDM commonly occurs at gestational weeks 24 to 28, women who are subsequently diagnosed with GDM may be hyperglycemic earlier at weeks 9 to 10.[12] Moreover, women with pregestational diabetes, especially those with T1DM, are hyperglycemic very early in pregnancy despite marked improvement in the management of glycemia in nonpregnant adults. This distinguishes diabetes from obesity early in pregnancy, because obese pregnant women are normoglycemic and hyperinsulinemic.[13]

The rate of growth of the placenta is most rapid in the first trimester[14] and during this period placental tissues are most sensitive to environmental perturbation. Both hyperglycemia and hyperinsulinemia likely contribute to alterations in placental growth.[15,16] Notably, the early placenta exhibits more plasticity than later in pregnancy, secondary to lower average DNA methylation.[17] Placental volume (a marker of growth) at around week 11 to 13 is associated with neonatal birth weight category. At the end of the first trimester placentas of neonates born large for gestational age have a greater volume than placentas of neonates born appropriate for gestational age.[18] Although higher birthweight is a poor indicator of neonatal adiposity, a proportion of large for gestational age neonates may have accumulated excess fat during intrauterine growth. Furthermore, placental volume at week 14 and volume changes between gestational weeks 14 and 17 each correlate with fetal anthropometric parameters, including abdominal circumference, at week 36[19] (**Fig. 1**).

Because, in the first trimester, insulin receptors are primarily located at the syncytiotrophoblast surface, elevated insulin levels may directly signal to affect placental growth and metabolism. Interestingly, the area under the insulin curve after an intravenous glucose tolerance test (GTT) performed at 12 to 14 weeks' gestation, is associated with placental weight at the end of gestation, whereas the area under the insulin curve of a GTT performed before conception or at around week 34 to 36 is not.[16] This indicates that metabolic events in early gestation influence placental formation, program placental growth, and development, and suggests a role for maternal insulin in these processes. In line with this reasoning, fetal growth, which is related to placental growth and function, is determined by events in early pregnancy.[20]

We recently proposed a model linking early placental growth and maternal metabolic changes, primarily of the glucose-insulin axis, with excessive fat accumulation

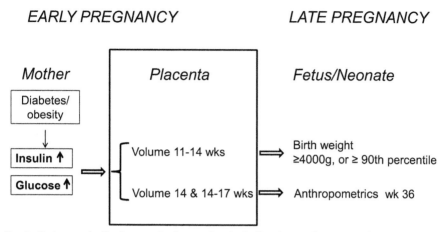

Fig. 1. Early metabolic changes in the mother including hyperglycemia and/or hyperinsulinemia may affect early placental growth, which in turn associates with fetal and neonatal phenotype. Hence, lifestyle and other interventions in the mother have to commence as early as possible in or even before pregnancy. This does not exclude early effects of other maternal metabolites, such as palmitate or inflammatory mediators, but evidence is missing.

in the fetus and neonate.[21,22] The mechanism by which glucose/insulin may stimulate early placental growth has remained elusive. It may involve stimulating fusion of cytotrophoblast with syncytiotrophoblast, thereby expanding the trophoblast compartment responsible for nutrient transport to the fetus. Insulin, through activation of syncytiotrophoblast protein kinase B, induces matrix-metalloproteinase 14 (MMP14), an enzyme located on the surface of cytotrophoblasts. MMP14 contributes to the trophoblast fusion process. MMP14 is also upregulated in pregnancies with T1DM, likely induced by maternal insulin levels, as MMP14 levels correlate with the average daily insulin dose, a proxy measure for circulating insulin levels, in the first trimester of these women.[23]

Similar mechanisms expanding the trophoblast compartment may be operative in obese women in whom tumor necrosis factor α (TNF-α) enhances MMP14 levels.[23] Conversely, insulin seems to play a lesser role in obese versus lean women because of trophoblast insulin resistance, which is inferred from a reduced insulin effect on trophoblast gene expression.[13] Hence, exposure to elevated insulin levels in early pregnancy desensitizes insulin signaling pathways in obese women.

Extracellular hyperglycemia activates mitochondrial activity in various cell types and this enhances generation of reactive oxygen species (ROS), therefore, mitochondria and their dysfunction may contribute to placental maladaptation in diabetes and obesity. Several genes regulating mitochondrial metabolism are downregulated in the first trimester trophoblast of obese compared with nonobese women.[24] However, in vitro studies commonly use 21% oxygen, which creates a state of hyperoxia that likely overwhelms cellular antioxidative defense mechanisms. Notably, when first trimester trophoblasts were incubated at lower physiologic oxygen tension, hyperglycemia increased ROS levels, but independent of mitochondrial activity, suggesting nonmitochondrial generation of ROS.[15]

Changes in oxygen tension in the intervillous space are a physiologic response to remodeling of the spiral arteries in decidua and a key driver of early placental development. Any changes in spiral artery remodeling associated with maternal diabetes, obesity, or both, will affect oxygen concentration delivered to the intervillous space, which in turn induces placental adaptive responses.[22] In pregnancies complicated with T1DM the placenta shows signs of enhanced oxidative stress attributed to altered oxygen tension in the intervillous space. Support for this notion comes from in vitro experiments with isolated primary trophoblasts in which increasing oxygen tension, but not hyperglycemia or TNF-α increased oxidative stress, are markers.[25] However, TNF-α may be harmful by enhancing inflammatory cytokines and chemokines in trophoblasts from early gestation.[26,27]

The consequences of these early placental changes for fetal growth are unclear. Historically, T1DM was accompanied by an early growth delay of the placenta and fetus[28,29] associated with small for gestational age neonates, owing to problems with implantation and remodeling of the decidual arteries.[30] In recent years, improvement in preconceptional and maternal glycemic control have alleviated these problems. However, neonates born to T1DM pregnancies are still at risk for complications, but not for overgrowth or large for gestational age.[31] An attractive hypothesis that needs testing is that maternal insulin contributes to overgrowth of the fetus resulting in neonates with excessive adiposity.

LATER IN PREGNANCY

The fetus is generally exposed to metabolic alterations before the time of GDM testing.[32] Fetal fat depots are present from week 14 onward,[33] and increased fetal adiposity can be detected as early as gestational weeks 17 to 20, well before the usual time of screening for diagnosis of GDM.[34,35] This fact emphasizes the important role of the first half of pregnancy (cf. above), and early fetal hyperinsulinemia, as a key driver of lipogenesis, which contributes to large for gestational age neonates.[36]

Fetal hyperglycemia early in gestation, but also elevated fetal concentrations of other insulin secretagogues, such as leucine and arginine, may contribute to stimulating the fetal pancreas at this time. The resulting fetal hyperinsulinemia steepens the maternal-fetal glucose concentration gradient with subsequent increased glucose flux to the fetus, the so-called "fetal glucose steal."[37] Enhanced transplacental transfer of glucose or insulin secretagogues early in gestation may associate with diabetes, obesity, or both.

AT THE END OF PREGNANCY

Multiple placental changes associated with maternal diabetes, obesity, or both, have been described at the end of pregnancy and extensively reviewed.[38–48] Some of them are listed in **Table 1**), which provides a summary of well-established findings.

At present, no framework has been conceptualized describing how any or all of these changes contribute to the excessive fetal fat accumulation characteristic of these pregnancies. We have recently proposed that, alternatively, the placental changes reflect adaptive responses to ultimately protect the fetus from the adverse intrauterine environment.[14] This paradigm shift then assigns the placenta, at least late in pregnancy, the role of an innocent bystander in determining the fetal/neonatal phenotype in pregnancies complicated by pregestational, gestational diabetes, and/ or maternal obesity. This concept is supported by data demonstrating that *maternal*-to-fetal transfer of glucose and fatty acids are not increased in such complicated pregnancies,[49–51] whereas previously this critical placental function has been regarded as unfavorably altered in conditions of maternal overnutrition, therefore, contributing to neonatal adiposity.

The concept discussed above firmly places the fetal glucose-insulin axis at the center of fetal fat accumulation, which leads to the neonatal phenotype seen in pregnancies

Table 1 Key placental changes in diabetes and/or obesity	References
Fetal hypoxia can occur in GDM and pregestational diabetes. Placental exchange area is increased in diabetes as a result of enhanced angiogenesis. Fetal insulin is one of the proangiogenic factors but also others are overproduced and/or antiangiogenic factors secreted in reduced amounts (**Fig. 2**).	83–90
Placenta is heavier in diabetes and obesity. It contains more DNA, and stores more glycogen around feto-placental vessels and more triglycerides in the syncytiotrophoblast.	53,91–95
Obesity is associated with villous inflammation and thrombosis. T1DM is associated with fibrinoid necrosis and atherosis in the spiral arteries.	30,96,97
Inflammatory cytokines (IL-1b, IL-8, CXCR2, and MCP-1) are overexpressed in placenta particularly in obesity.	98
Genes involved in the regulation of growth, cytoskeletal structure, oxidative stress, inflammation, coagulation, and apoptosis are altered in diabetic placentas.	98–100
Gene expression in diabetic placentas is sexually dimorphic with more changes in placentas from female than male placentas.	101
Placental genes related to lipid metabolism are altered in obesity, GDM, and pregestational diabetes. Transplacental transfer of fatty acids is low and unchanged or reduced in GDM and obesity.	50,51,53,77,102–105
GDM is associated only with small changes of the proteome, likely because of adequate glycemic control.	106
Total placental levels of glucose transporters is unchanged in diabetes resulting in unchanged or reduced transplacental glucose transfer in GDM.	49,107,108
Changes in amino acid transporters in diabetes and obesity are inconclusive, with no information available about transplacental transfer.	109–111
Mitochondrial respiration in placenta in diabetes and obesity is associated with overproduction of superoxide, oxidative stress, and mitochondrial damage.	112–114
Placental DNA methylation is globally increased in either diabetes or obesity with locus-specific changes. Also miRNA profiles are modified in a sex-specific manner.	115–121

with maternal diabetes mellitus, obesity, or both. However, there has been an ongoing debate about the potential contribution of maternal lipids in particular fatty acids to the process. Maternal triglycerides are hydrolyzed on the surface of the syncytiotrophoblast by endothelial lipase to release free fatty acids.[52] An increased maternal triglyceride concentration is often associated with diabetes and obesity leading to elevated free fatty acid concentrations on the maternal side of the placenta. These fatty acids are taken up by the syncytiotrophoblast and, after re-esterification, stored as lipid droplets.[53,54] When there are excessive maternal fatty acids trophoblast storage capacity may be overwhelmed and fatty acids spill over to reach the fetal circulation. The proportion of maternally derived fatty acids in the total fetal fatty acid pool is unknown, but overall transplacental transfer is notably low (2%–3%).[55]

EFFECTS OF PREVENTIVE MEASURES ON THE PLACENTA

The conclusion from the evidence presented above is that, in late gestation, the placenta contributes little to determining the neonatal phenotype associated with

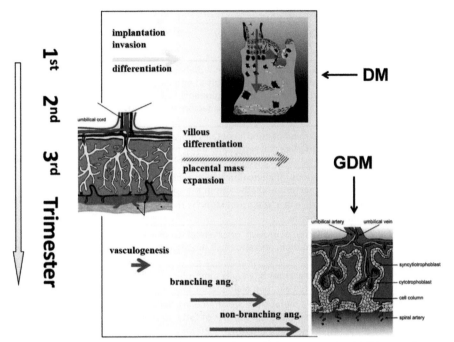

Fig. 2. Hypervascularization of the placenta at the end of pregnancy is a well-known feature in many pregnancies complicated by diabetes and presumably also by obesity of the women. It may originate early in pregnancy. Pregestational diabetes (DM) could have a negative impact on trophoblast invasion in the first trimester of gestation, resulting in impaired vasculogenesis and blood supply in the second trimester of pregnancy, leading to inadequate fetal oxygenation and eventually to adverse pregnancy outcome. Metabolic derangements in gestational diabetes (GDM) primarily, but not exclusively, target placental villi in the second and third trimester. Stimulation of fetal metabolism by insulin enhances oxygen demand, which requires an increase in placental area for oxygen exchange. This is achieved by enhanced angiogenesis of the feto-placental vasculature, mainly induced by fetal signals, such as insulin. (*Modified from* Rampersad R, Cervar-Zivkovic M, Nelson DM. Development and Anatomy of the Human Placenta. In: Kay HH, Neslon DM, Wang Y, editors. The Placenta, From Development to Disease. West Sussex: Blackwell Publishing Ltd; 2011; with permission.)

pregnancies complicated by maternal diabetes, obesity, or both. Following on from this interventions to prevent the development of this phenotype will have to concentrate on the mother and have to begin before or as early as possible in pregnancy.[33]

Dietary supplementation of mothers with n-3 long-chain polyunsaturated fatty acids did not alter offspring fat at up to 1 year. However, it affected the placental transcriptome in a sexually dimorphic manner with a greater number of transcripts altered by the intervention in placentas of female compared with male fetuses.[56]

Many women with GDM are vitamin D deficient, which confers some risk for developing GDM.[57] This has led to intervention studies using vitamin D supplementation to prevent GDM and, hopefully, also reduce the accompanying adiposity in the offspring. These trials have, however, not been successful, but may have altered placental function in several ways given the broad range of vitamin D effects on the placenta.[58–62] Analysis of placental samples from women undergoing this intervention may provide useful information about potential compensatory mechanisms, which may have precluded a beneficial intervention effect on the fetus and neonate.

A lifestyle intervention that reduced sedentary behavior in pregnant obese women has been shown to successfully reduce neonatal adiposity.[63] Although the effects of physical activity on the placenta have been documented,[64,65] the role of reducing sedentary behavior for placental development and function has not yet been studied.

AREAS FOR FUTURE RESEARCH

Despite enormous research efforts, a large number of gaps still limit our understanding of the effects of maternal metabolic derangements on placental development and function and the consequences for the growing fetus. Therefore, future research should focus on closing some of these gaps to improve our understanding to ultimately allow establishment of conceptualized frameworks for the dialog between mother, placenta, and fetus in these pregnancies. Listed below are some areas of research priorities we have identified. They agree with published suggestions in this field,[22,66,67] but the selection is of course biased.[68]

- How is first trimester placental development and function affected by metabolic changes and the inflammatory environment associated with maternal adiposity/obesity, pregestational diabetes, or hyperglycemia short of a GDM diagnosis?
- How do these placental changes track throughout pregnancy and how do they determine fetal growth and development and neonatal outcome?
- GDM is a heterogeneous condition characterized not only by changes in insulin resistance, insulin secretory defects, or a combination of the 2,[69] but also by other metabolic changes.[70] Likewise, obesity is not a homogeneous entity, because a subgroup of obese women is regarded metabolically healthy, that is with normal metabolism.[71] Future research will have to use a more detailed phenotypic characterization of women to define subtypes of placental responses to these conditions.
- Sexual dimorphism in the placental transcriptome has been well established at the whole tissue and cellular level and may explain some of the sex dependency of changes in maternal diabetes and obesity.[72–74] However, much less is known about the structural and functional consequences of these differences in gene expression. Their further characterization will help understand (1) how evolutionary pressure has facilitated development of placental phenotypes and (2) how the placenta may contribute to programming offspring phenotype and subsequent sex-dependent developmental changes in childhood.
- Although much research has focused on studying placental response to maternal changes, little efforts have been made to describe the placental contribution to the maternal metabolic and inflammatory responses.[75] We proposed a bidirectional interaction with maternal signals affecting placental development and function, especially in early pregnancy, and that these placental changes then feed back to the maternal system through placental-specific signals.[76] These signals may include hormones, such as placenta-specific growth hormone, chorionic gonadotropin, placental lactogens, and others, as well as placentally derived microvesicles, which may all contribute to maternal adaptation to pregnancy.
- Enhanced fat accretion in the fetus may result from increased transplacental fatty acid transfer. However, the fetus is capable of de novo fatty acid synthesis using glucose as precursor and indeed an overabundance of fetal glucose is present in pregnancies with maternal diabetes, obesity, or both. The contribution of maternally derived fatty acids to fetal fat accretion is unclear, but is thought to be small based on its limited transfer and the further reduction of free fatty acid transfer in

GDM and obesity.[50,51] Although oxidative stress and mitochondrial function in the placenta has been well studied, endoplasmic reticulum stress has not received the same attention. Lipotoxicity was demonstrated in the placenta in maternal obesity,[77,78] but its consequences for placental function remain unknown.[79]

- The fetus in diabetic pregnancy is often low in oxygen, as reflected by increased red blood cell count and cord blood erythropoietin. How metabolic changes in the placenta affect partitioning of oxygen is unclear. In addition, transplacental iron transfer may be altered to facilitate fetal generation of the various fetal hemoglobins, but details and regulatory mechanisms are unknown.
- Placental microvesicles are secreted into the fetal circulation, but their role is unknown.[80,81] They may constitute important signals targeting various fetal organs and thus contribute to phenotypic and functional changes, which may emerge only in the neonatal period and thereafter.
- A further important area of future research will include deciphering the role of the placenta, if any, in determining offspring phenotype in childhood. The association of placenta alkaline phosphatase with adiposity in children at the age of 4 and 6 to 7 years[82] suggests such a role, but future efforts will need to demonstrate causality and unravel underlying mechanisms.

Collectively, while an enormous amount of data has been accumulated over the past 70 years related to the placenta and fetus in the setting of maternal diabetes mellitus and obesity, we are far from understanding the role of the placenta in determining the immediate, but even more so the long-term consequences of these conditions for the mother and, predominantly, for the offspring.

DISCLOSURE

The authors have nothing to disclose. Work of the authors was funded by grants of the Austrian Science Fund (FWF), Vienna, and the Jubilee Fund of the Austrian National Bank (OENB), Vienna, as well as by the European Commission (Brussels).

REFERENCES

1. WHO. Available at: https://www.who.int/gho/ncd/risk_factors/overweight_obesity/obesity_adults/en/.
2. Emerging Risk Factors Collaboration, Sarwar N, Gao P, Seshasai SR, et al. Diabetes mellitus, fasting blood glucose concentration, and risk of vascular disease: a collaborative meta-analysis of 102 prospective studies. Lancet 2010; 375(9733):2215–22.
3. Cho NH, Shaw JE, Karuranga S, et al. IDF diabetes atlas: global estimates of diabetes prevalence for 2017 and projections for 2045. Diabetes Res Clin Pract 2018;138:271–81.
4. Catalano PM. Obesity and pregnancy—the propagation of a viscous cycle? J Clin Endocrinol Metab 2003;88(8):3505–6.
5. Dabelea D, Harrod CS. Role of developmental overnutrition in pediatric obesity and type 2 diabetes. Nutr Rev 2013;71(Suppl 1):S62–7.
6. Ahrens W, Pigeot I, Pohlabeln H, et al. Prevalence of overweight and obesity in European children below the age of 10. Int J Obes 2014;38(Suppl 2):S99–107.
7. Gu S, An X, Fang L, et al. Risk factors and long-term health consequences of macrosomia: a prospective study in Jiangsu Province, China. J Biomed Res 2012;26(4):235–40.

8. Boney CM, Verma A, Tucker R, et al. Metabolic syndrome in childhood: association with birth weight, maternal obesity, and gestational diabetes mellitus. Pediatrics 2005;115(3):e290–6.

9. Raghavan S, Zhang W, Yang IV, et al. Association between gestational diabetes mellitus exposure and childhood adiposity is not substantially explained by offspring genetic risk of obesity. Diabet Med 2017;34(12):1696–700.

10. Hjort L, Novakovic B, Grunnet LG, et al. Diabetes in pregnancy and epigenetic mechanisms—how the first 9 months from conception might affect the child's epigenome and later risk of disease. Lancet Diabetes Endocrinol 2019;7(10): 796–806.

11. Spalding KL, Arner E, Westermark PO, et al. Dynamics of fat cell turnover in humans. Nature 2008;453(7196):783–7.

12. Riskin-Mashiah S, Damti A, Younes G, et al. First trimester fasting hyperglycemia as a predictor for the development of gestational diabetes mellitus. Eur J Obstet Gynecol Reprod Biol 2010;152(2):163–7.

13. Lassance L, Haghiac M, Leahy P, et al. Identification of early transcriptome signatures in placenta exposed to insulin and obesity. Am J Obstet Gynecol 2015; 212(5):647.e1-11.

14. Desoye G. The human placenta in diabetes and obesity: friend or foe? The 2017 Norbert Freinkel Award Lecture. Diabetes care 2018;41(7):1362–9.

15. Frohlich JD, Huppertz B, Abuja PM, et al. Oxygen modulates the response of first-trimester trophoblasts to hyperglycemia. Am J Pathol 2012;180(1):153–64.

16. O'Tierney-Ginn P, Presley L, Myers S, et al. Placental growth response to maternal insulin in early pregnancy. J Clin Endocrinol Metab 2015;100(1): 159–65.

17. Novakovic B, Yuen RK, Gordon L, et al. Evidence for widespread changes in promoter methylation profile in human placenta in response to increasing gestational age and environmental/stochastic factors. BMC Genomics 2011;12:529.

18. Effendi M, Demers S, Giguere Y, et al. Association between first-trimester placental volume and birth weight. Placenta 2014;35(2):99–102.

19. Thame M, Osmond C, Bennett F, et al. Fetal growth is directly related to maternal anthropometry and placental volume. Eur J Clin Nutr 2004;58(6):894–900.

20. Smith GC. First-trimester determination of complications of late pregnancy. Jama 2010;303(6):561–2.

21. Desoye G, van Poppel M. The feto-placental dialogue and diabesity. Best Pract Res Clin Obstet Gynaecol 2015;29(1):15–23.

22. Hoch D, Gauster M, Hauguel-de Mouzon S, et al. Diabesity-associated oxidative and inflammatory stress signalling in the early human placenta. Mol Aspects Med 2019;66:21–30.

23. Hiden U, Glitzner E, Ivanisevic M, et al. MT1-MMP expression in first-trimester placental tissue is upregulated in type 1 diabetes as a result of elevated insulin and tumor necrosis factor-alpha levels. Diabetes 2008;57(1):150–7.

24. Lassance L, Haghiac M, Minium J, et al. Obesity-induced down-regulation of the mitochondrial translocator protein (TSPO) impairs placental steroid production. J Clin Endocrinol Metab 2015;100(1):E11–8.

25. Gauster M, Majali-Martinez A, Maninger S, et al. Maternal type 1 diabetes activates stress response in early placenta. Placenta 2017;50:110–6.

26. Siwetz M, Blaschitz A, El-Heliebi A, et al. TNF-alpha alters the inflammatory secretion profile of human first trimester placenta. Lab Invest 2016;96(4): 428–38.

27. Lewis RM, Demmelmair H, Gaillard R, et al. The placental exposome: placental determinants of fetal adiposity and postnatal body composition. Ann Nutr Metab 2013;63(3):208–15.

28. Brown ZA, Mills JL, Metzger BE, et al. Early sonographic evaluation for fetal growth delay and congenital malformations in pregnancies complicated by insulin-requiring diabetes. National Institute of Child Health and Human Development Diabetes in Early Pregnancy Study. Diabetes care 1992;15(5):613–9.

29. Pedersen JF, Sorensen S, Molsted-Pedersen L. Serum levels of human placental lactogen, pregnancy-associated plasma protein A and endometrial secretory protein PP14 in first trimester of diabetic pregnancy. Acta Obstet Gynecol Scand 1998;77(2):155–8.

30. Barth WH Jr, Genest DR, Riley LE, et al. Uterine arcuate artery Doppler and decidual microvascular pathology in pregnancies complicated by type I diabetes mellitus. Ultrasound Obstet Gynecol 1996;8(2):98–103.

31. Mackin ST, Nelson SM, Kerssens JJ, et al. Diabetes and pregnancy: national trends over a 15 year period. Diabetologia 2018;61(5):1081–8.

32. Tisi DK, Burns DH, Luskey GW, et al. Fetal exposure to altered amniotic fluid glucose, insulin, and insulin-like growth factor-binding protein 1 occurs before screening for gestational diabetes mellitus. Diabetes Care 2011;34(1):139–44.

33. Poissonnet CM, Burdi AR, Garn SM. The chronology of adipose tissue appearance and distribution in the human fetus. Early Hum Dev 1984;10(1–2):1–11.

34. Macaulay S, Munthali RJ, Dunger DB, et al. The effects of gestational diabetes mellitus on fetal growth and neonatal birth measures in an African cohort. Diabet Med 2018;35(10):1425–33.

35. Sovio U, Murphy HR, Smith GC. Accelerated fetal growth prior to diagnosis of gestational diabetes mellitus: a prospective cohort study of nulliparous women. Diabetes care 2016;39(6):982–7.

36. Carpenter MW, Canick JA, Hogan JW, et al. Amniotic fluid insulin at 14-20 weeks' gestation: association with later maternal glucose intolerance and birth macrosomia. Diabetes care 2001;24(7):1259–63.

37. Desoye G, Nolan CJ. The fetal glucose steal: an underappreciated phenomenon in diabetic pregnancy. Diabetologia 2016;59(6):1089–94.

38. Desoye G, Hauguel-de Mouzon S. The human placenta in gestational diabetes mellitus. The insulin and cytokine network. Diabetes care 2007;30(Suppl 2):S120–6.

39. Hauguel-de Mouzon S, Shafrir E. Carbohydrate and fat metabolism and related hormonal regulation in normal and diabetic placenta. Placenta 2001;22(7):619–27.

40. Herrera E, Desoye G. Maternal and fetal lipid metabolism under normal and gestational diabetic conditions. Horm Mol Biol Clin Investig 2016;26(2):109–27.

41. Gauster M, Desoye G, Totsch M, et al. The placenta and gestational diabetes mellitus. Curr Diab Rep 2012;12(1):16–23.

42. Desoye G, Gauster M, Wadsack C. Placental transport in pregnancy pathologies. Am J Clin Nutr 2011;94(6 Suppl):1896S–902S.

43. Hiden U, Lang I, Ghaffari-Tabrizi N, et al. Insulin action on the human placental endothelium in normal and diabetic pregnancy. Curr Vasc Pharmacol 2009;7(4):460–6.

44. Hiden U, Glitzner E, Hartmann M, et al. Insulin and the IGF system in the human placenta of normal and diabetic pregnancies. J Anat 2009;215(1):60–8.

45. Desoye G, Shafrir E. Placental metabolism and its regulation in health and diabetes. Mol Aspects Med 1994;15(6):505–682.

46. Jiang S, Teague AM, Tryggestad JB, et al. Effects of maternal diabetes and fetal sex on human placenta mitochondrial biogenesis. Placenta 2017;57:26–32.
47. Subiabre M, Villalobos-Labra R, Silva L, et al. Role of insulin, adenosine, and adipokine receptors in the foetoplacental vascular dysfunction in gestational diabetes mellitus. Biochim Biophys Acta Mol Basis Dis 2019. [Epub ahead of print].
48. Jayabalan N, Nair S, Nuzhat Z, et al. Cross talk between adipose tissue and placenta in obese and gestational diabetes mellitus pregnancies via exosomes. Front Endocrinol (Lausanne) 2017;8:239.
49. Osmond DT, Nolan CJ, King RG, et al. Effects of gestational diabetes on human placental glucose uptake, transfer, and utilisation. Diabetologia 2000;43(5): 576–82.
50. Pagan A, Prieto-Sanchez MT, Blanco-Carnero JE, et al. Materno-fetal transfer of docosahexaenoic acid is impaired by gestational diabetes mellitus. Am J Physiol Endocrinol Metab 2013;305(7):E826–33.
51. Gazquez A, Prieto-Sanchez MT, Blanco-Carnero JE, et al. Altered materno-fetal transfer of ^{13}C-polyunsaturated fatty acids in obese pregnant women. Clin Nutr 2019 [pii:S0261-5614(19)30187-6].
52. Gauster M, Hiden U, van Poppel M, et al. Dysregulation of placental endothelial lipase in obese women with gestational diabetes mellitus. Diabetes 2011;60(10): 2457–64.
53. Hirschmugl B, Desoye G, Catalano P, et al. Maternal obesity modulates intracellular lipid turnover in the human term placenta. Int J Obes 2017;41(2):317–23.
54. Stirm L, Kovarova M, Perschbacher S, et al. BMI-independent effects of gestational diabetes on human placenta. J Clin Endocrinol Metab 2018;103(9): 3299–309.
55. Dancis J, Jansen V, Kayden HJ, et al. Transfer across perfused human placenta. II. Free fatty acids. Pediatr Res 1973;7(4):192–7.
56. Sedlmeier EM, Brunner S, Much D, et al. Human placental transcriptome shows sexually dimorphic gene expression and responsiveness to maternal dietary n-3 long-chain polyunsaturated fatty acid intervention during pregnancy. BMC Genomics 2014;15:941.
57. Xia J, Song Y, Rawal S, et al. Vitamin D status during pregnancy and the risk of gestational diabetes mellitus: a longitudinal study in a multiracial cohort. Diabetes Obes Metab 2019;21(8):1895–905.
58. Knabl J, Huttenbrenner R, Hutter S, et al. Gestational diabetes mellitus upregulates vitamin D receptor in extravillous trophoblasts and fetoplacental endothelial cells. Reprod Sci 2015;22(3):358–66.
59. Shin JS, Choi MY, Longtine MS, et al. Vitamin D effects on pregnancy and the placenta. Placenta 2010;31(12):1027–34.
60. Corcoy R, Mendoza LC, Simmons D, et al. The DALI vitamin D randomized controlled trial for gestational diabetes mellitus prevention: no major benefit shown besides vitamin D sufficiency. Clin Nutr 2019 [pii:S0261-5614(19) 30161-X].
61. Longtine MS, Cvitic S, Colvin BN, et al. Calcitriol regulates immune genes CD14 and CD180 to modulate LPS responses in human trophoblasts. Reproduction 2017;154(6):735–44.
62. Hepp P, Hutter S, Knabl J, et al. Histone H3 lysine 9 acetylation is downregulated in GDM placentas and calcitriol supplementation enhanced this effect. Int J Mol Sci 2018;19(12) [pii:E4061].

63. van Poppel MNM, Simmons D, Devlieger R, et al. A reduction in sedentary behaviour in obese women during pregnancy reduces neonatal adiposity: the DALI randomised controlled trial. Diabetologia 2019;62(6):915–25.

64. Brett KE, Ferraro ZM, Holcik M, et al. Prenatal physical activity and diet composition affect the expression of nutrient transporters and mTOR signaling molecules in the human placenta. Placenta 2015;36(2):204–12.

65. Bergmann A, Zygmunt M, Clapp JF 3rd. Running throughout pregnancy: effect on placental villous vascular volume and cell proliferation. Placenta 2004; 25(8–9):694–8.

66. Schaefer-Graf U, Napoli A, Nolan CJ, et al. Diabetes in pregnancy: a new decade of challenges ahead. Diabetologia 2018;61(5):1012–21.

67. McIntyre D, Desoye G, Dunne F, et al. FIGO analysis of research priorities in hyperglycemia in pregnancy. Diabetes Res Clin Pract 2018;145:5–14.

68. McIntyre D, Catalano P, Zhang C, et al. Gestational diabetes mellitus. Nat Rev Dis Primers 2019;5(1):47.

69. Powe CE, Allard C, Battista MC, et al. Heterogeneous contribution of insulin sensitivity and secretion defects to gestational diabetes mellitus. Diabetes care 2016;39(6):1052–5.

70. Layton J, Powe C, Allard C, et al. Maternal lipid profile differs by gestational diabetes physiologic subtype. Metabolism 2019;91:39–42.

71. Stefan N, Haring HU, Hu FB, et al. Metabolically healthy obesity: epidemiology, mechanisms, and clinical implications. Lancet Diabetes Endocrinol 2013;1(2): 152–62.

72. Cvitic S, Longtine MS, Hackl H, et al. The human placental sexome differs between trophoblast epithelium and villous vessel endothelium. PLoS One 2013; 8(10):e79233.

73. Gonzalez TL, Sun T, Koeppel AF, et al. Sex differences in the late first trimester human placenta transcriptome. Biol Sex Differ 2018;9(1):4.

74. Cvitic S, Novakovic B, Gordon L, et al. Human fetoplacental arterial and venous endothelial cells are differentially programmed by gestational diabetes mellitus, resulting in cell-specific barrier function changes. Diabetologia 2018;61(11): 2398–411.

75. Napso T, Yong HEJ, Lopez-Tello J, et al. The role of placental hormones in mediating maternal adaptations to support pregnancy and lactation. Front Physiol 2018;9:1091.

76. Hiden U, Maier A, Bilban M, et al. Insulin control of placental gene expression shifts from mother to foetus over the course of pregnancy. Diabetologia 2006; 49(1):123–31.

77. Saben J, Lindsey F, Zhong Y, et al. Maternal obesity is associated with a lipotoxic placental environment. Placenta 2014;35(3):171–7.

78. Saben J, Zhong Y, Gomez-Acevedo H, et al. Early growth response protein-1 mediates lipotoxicity-associated placental inflammation: role in maternal obesity. Am J Physiol Endocrinol Metab 2013;305(1):E1–14.

79. Jarvie E, Hauguel-de-Mouzon S, Nelson SM, et al. Lipotoxicity in obese pregnancy and its potential role in adverse pregnancy outcome and obesity in the offspring. Clin Sci 2010;119(3):123–9.

80. Saez T, de Vos P, Sobrevia L, et al. Is there a role for exosomes in foetoplacental endothelial dysfunction in gestational diabetes mellitus? Placenta 2018;61: 48–54.

81. Miranda J, Paules C, Nair S, et al. Placental exosomes profile in maternal and fetal circulation in intrauterine growth restriction—liquid biopsies to monitoring fetal growth. Placenta 2018;64:34–43.
82. Hirschmugl B, Crozier S, Matthews N, et al. Relation of placental alkaline phosphatase expression in human term placenta with maternal and offspring fat mass. Int J Obes 2018;42(6):1202–10.
83. Teasdale F. Histomorphometry of the placenta of the diabetic women: class A diabetes mellitus. Placenta 1981;2(3):241–51.
84. Teasdale F. Histomorphometry of the human placenta in class B diabetes mellitus. Placenta 1983;4(1):1–12.
85. Teasdale F. Histomorphometry of the human placenta in class C diabetes mellitus. Placenta 1985;6(1):69–81.
86. Arany E, Hill DJ. Fibroblast growth factor-2 and fibroblast growth factor receptor-1 mRNA expression and peptide localization in placentae from normal and diabetic pregnancies. Placenta 1998;19(2–3):133–42.
87. Cvitic S, Desoye G, Hiden U. Glucose, insulin, and oxygen interplay in placental hypervascularisation in diabetes mellitus. Biomed Res Int 2014;2014:145846.
88. Mayhew TM. Enhanced fetoplacental angiogenesis in pre-gestational diabetes mellitus: the extra growth is exclusively longitudinal and not accompanied by microvascular remodelling. Diabetologia 2002;45(10):1434–9.
89. Babawale MO, Lovat S, Mayhew TM, et al. Effects of gestational diabetes on junctional adhesion molecules in human term placental vasculature. Diabetologia 2000;43(9):1185–96.
90. Loegl J, Nussbaumer E, Cvitic S, et al. GDM alters paracrine regulation of fetoplacental angiogenesis via the trophoblast. Lab Invest 2017;97(4):409–18.
91. Desoye G, Hofmann HH, Weiss PA. Insulin binding to trophoblast plasma membranes and placental glycogen content in well-controlled gestational diabetic women treated with diet or insulin, in well-controlled overt diabetic patients and in healthy control subjects. Diabetologia 1992;35(1):45–55.
92. Makhseed M, Musini VM, Ahmed MA, et al. Placental pathology in relation to the White's classification of diabetes mellitus. Arch Gynecol Obstet 2002;266(3):136–40.
93. Robb SA, Hytten FE. Placental glycogen. Br J Obstet Gynaecol 1976;83(1):43–53.
94. Jones CJ, Desoye G. Glycogen distribution in the capillaries of the placental villus in normal, overt and gestational diabetic pregnancy. Placenta 1993;14(5):505–17.
95. Diamant YZ, Metzger BE, Freinkel N, et al. Placental lipid and glycogen content in human and experimental diabetes mellitus. Am J Obstet Gynecol 1982;144(1):5–11.
96. Staff AC, Redman CW, Williams D, et al. Pregnancy and long-term maternal cardiovascular health: progress through harmonization of research cohorts and biobanks. Hypertension 2016;67(2):251–60.
97. Leon-Garcia SM, Roeder HA, Nelson KK, et al. Maternal obesity and sex-specific differences in placental pathology. Placenta 2016;38:33–40.
98. Roberts KA, Riley SC, Reynolds RM, et al. Placental structure and inflammation in pregnancies associated with obesity. Placenta 2011;32(3):247–54.
99. Oliva K, Barker G, Riley C, et al. The effect of pre-existing maternal obesity on the placental proteome: two-dimensional difference gel electrophoresis coupled with mass spectrometry. J Mol Endocrinol 2012;48(2):139–49.

100. Radaelli T, Varastehpour A, Catalano P, et al. Gestational diabetes induces placental genes for chronic stress and inflammatory pathways. Diabetes 2003;52(12):2951–8.

101. Mao J, Zhang X, Sieli PT, et al. Contrasting effects of different maternal diets on sexually dimorphic gene expression in the murine placenta. Proc Natl Acad Sci U S A 2010;107(12):5557–62.

102. Dube E, Gravel A, Martin C, et al. Modulation of fatty acid transport and metabolism by maternal obesity in the human full-term placenta. Biol Reprod 2012; 87(1):14, 11-11.

103. Brass E, Hanson E, O'Tierney-Ginn PF. Placental oleic acid uptake is lower in male offspring of obese women. Placenta 2013;34(6):503–9.

104. Radaelli T, Lepercq J, Varastehpour A, et al. Differential regulation of genes for fetoplacental lipid pathways in pregnancy with gestational and type 1 diabetes mellitus. Am J Obstet Gynecol 2009;201(2):209.e1-10.

105. Lepercq J, Cauzac M, Lahlou N, et al. Overexpression of placental leptin in diabetic pregnancy: a critical role for insulin. Diabetes 1998;47(5):847–50.

106. Lapolla A, Porcu S, Roverso M, et al. A preliminary investigation on placenta protein profile reveals only modest changes in well controlled gestational diabetes mellitus. Eur J Mass Spectrom (Chichester) 2013;19(3):211–23.

107. Jansson T, Ekstrand Y, Wennergren M, et al. Placental glucose transport in gestational diabetes mellitus. Am J Obstet Gynecol 2001;184(2):111–6.

108. Sciullo E, Cardellini G, Baroni M, et al. Glucose transporters (GLUT 1, GLUT 3) mRNA in human placenta of diabetic and non-diabetic pregnancies. Ann Ist Super Sanita 1997;33(3):361–5.

109. Gallo LA, Barrett HL, Dekker Nitert M. Review: placental transport and metabolism of energy substrates in maternal obesity and diabetes. Placenta 2017; 54:59–67.

110. Vaughan OR, Rosario FJ, Powell TL, et al. Regulation of placental amino acid transport and fetal growth. Prog Mol Biol Transl Sci 2017;145:217–51.

111. San Martin R, Sobrevia L. Gestational diabetes and the adenosine/L-arginine/ nitric oxide (ALANO) pathway in human umbilical vein endothelium. Placenta 2006;27(1):1–10.

112. Coughlan MT, Vervaart PP, Permezel M, et al. Altered placental oxidative stress status in gestational diabetes mellitus. Placenta 2004;25(1):78–84.

113. Myatt L. Review: reactive oxygen and nitrogen species and functional adaptation of the placenta. Placenta 2010;31(Suppl):S66–9.

114. Myatt L, Cui X. Oxidative stress in the placenta. Histochem Cell Biol 2004; 122(4):369–82.

115. Armstrong DA, Lesseur C, Conradt E, et al. Global and gene-specific DNA methylation across multiple tissues in early infancy: implications for children's health research. FASEB J 2014;28(5):2088–97.

116. Reichetzeder C, Dwi Putra SE, Pfab T, et al. Increased global placental DNA methylation levels are associated with gestational diabetes. Clin Epigenetics 2016;8:82.

117. Finer S, Mathews C, Lowe R, et al. Maternal gestational diabetes is associated with genome-wide DNA methylation variation in placenta and cord blood of exposed offspring. Hum Mol Genet 2015;24(11):3021–9.

118. Cardenas A, Gagne-Ouellet V, Allard C, et al. Placental DNA methylation adaptation to maternal glycemic response in pregnancy. Diabetes 2018;67(8): 1673–83.

119. Gagne-Ouellet V, Houde AA, Guay SP, et al. Placental lipoprotein lipase DNA methylation alterations are associated with gestational diabetes and body composition at 5 years of age. Epigenetics 2017;12(8):616–25.
120. Nomura Y, Lambertini L, Rialdi A, et al. Global methylation in the placenta and umbilical cord blood from pregnancies with maternal gestational diabetes, pre-eclampsia, and obesity. Reprod Sci 2014;21(1):131–7.
121. Strutz J, Cvitic S, Hackl H, et al. Gestational diabetes alters microRNA signatures in human feto-placental endothelial cells depending on fetal sex. Clin Sci 2018;132(22):2437–49.

The Placental Basis of Fetal Growth Restriction

Rebecca L. Zur, MD[a], John C. Kingdom, MD[a],*, W. Tony Parks, MD[b], Sebastian R. Hobson, MD, PhD, MPH[a]

KEYWORDS

- Fetal growth restriction (FGR) • Intrauterine growth restriction (IUGR)
- Placental dysfunction • Placental insufficiency
- Maternal vascular malperfusion (MVM) • Fetal vascular malperfusion (FVM)
- Placental pathology • Placental growth factor (PlGF)

KEY POINTS

- Placental dysfunction is a major contributing factor to fetal growth restriction. Although definitions vary, a common definition is an estimated fetal weight of less than the 10th centile for gestational age.
- Placental-mediated fetal growth restriction occurs through chronic fetal hypoxia owing to poor placental perfusion.
- Maternal vascular malperfusion may present with signs of chorion regression or uteroplacental vascular insufficiency on ultrasound examination.
- Circulating angiogenic growth factors are frequently abnormal in pregnancies with placental fetal growth restriction and can be used in to identify and manage these.
- Because a range of placental diseases may be associated with fetal growth restriction and have varying recurrence risks, histopathologic examination of the placenta after delivery can guide future care.

INTRODUCTION

The past decade has seen a substantial advancement in our understanding of placental diseases that are associated with fetal growth restriction (FGR).[1] This increased understanding of placental pathophysiology has been achieved largely through the application of contemporary imaging methods, combined with biomarker and molecular testing. Much of the recent stimulus for these advances is credited to the Human Placenta Project, funded by the National Institutes of Health, with new

[a] Placenta Program, Maternal-Fetal Medicine Division, Department of Obstetrics & Gynaecology, Mount Sinai Hospital, University of Toronto, 600 University Avenue, Toronto, Ontario M5G 1X5, Canada; [b] Department of Pathology and Laboratory Medicine, Mount Sinai Hospital, University of Toronto, 600 University Avenue, Toronto, Ontario M5G 1X5, Canada
* Corresponding author. Department of Obstetrics & Gynaecology, Mount Sinai Hospital, Room 3-904, 600 University Avenue, Toronto, Ontario M5G 1X5, Canada.
E-mail address: john.kingdom@sinaihealthsystem.ca

knowledge regarding disease pathogenesis being translated into the delivery of improved patient outcomes. In developed countries with equitable access to maternity care, FGR remains the most common underlying cause of "preventable stillbirth." The risk of stillbirth remains unacceptably high, averaging 1 in 300 births,[2] despite adequate access to ultrasound examinations.[3] Because most cases are associated with clinically silent placental disease and only postnatal evidence of FGR,[4] the challenge for clinician-researchers is to now test the clinical effectiveness of screening strategies that demonstrate high test precision.[5]

Definitions of fetal growth restriction

The definition of FGR currently used in clinical research varies worldwide[6] and is largely constrained by limitations of ultrasound test precision. In Canada, FGR is defined as an estimated fetal weight of less that the 10th centile accompanied by evidence of a pathologic process,[7] although in many countries, FGR is defined more simply by an estimated fetal weight or fetal abdominal circumference of less than the 10th centile.[6] In Spain, recognition of the common association between FGR and placental disease has resulted in a definition of either extreme growth impairment alone (estimated fetal weight of less than the third centile), or growth less than the 10th centile accompanied by abnormal umbilical and/or fetal Doppler waveforms, in addition to timing of onset (early vs late).[8] However, FGR-related stillbirth or severe morbidity is ultimately the most important outcome measure. In this context, Sovio and colleagues[9] from the United Kingdom demonstrated that routine third trimester ultrasound considerably improved the sensitivity for this functional outcome in comparison with selective ultrasound examination, capturing relevant adverse events with birthweights above the 10th centile.[10]

Fetal Pathophysiology of Placenta-Mediated Fetal Growth Restriction

The underlying basis of antepartum stillbirth in FGR is asphyxia, based on autopsy data in critically affected organs, especially the brain.[11] The vulnerable FGR fetus exists in a chronically hypoxic state, which has been demonstrated using fetal blood sampling[12] and correlated with abnormal umbilical artery Doppler waveforms. In placenta-mediated FGR, the fetus adapts for survival through reduced growth velocity. More recently, this adaptive state has been characterized further using T2* MRI.[13] The adaptive circulatory changes are designed to protect the vulnerable fetal brain, given the brain's relatively high oxygen consumption, and are characterized by a substantial increase in cerebral blood flow at the expense of blood flow to the lower body. These changes can be demonstrated by middle cerebral artery Doppler[8] along with largely preserved head growth and brain development at the expense of abdominal growth, thereby resulting in asymmetric FGR.[14]

The clinical and ultrasound presentation of placental FGR is strikingly variable and consequently the detection of this condition, especially in the late-onset form, remains a major challenge in clinical practice. This variability is largely caused by the heterogeneity in type, severity, and progression of the underlying placental disease and is combined with the intrinsic variability of the fetus to adapt and conserve cerebral oxygenation. Finally, placental dysfunction may affect the mother, causing hypertension, which may remain mild and treatable for some time, or alternatively may progress rapidly to severe forms of preeclampsia, including hemolysis, elevated liver enzymes, low platelets syndrome, or acute abruption. A more in-depth understanding of placental disease type and severity in the context of FGR may greatly aid clinical decision making.

Key Steps in Placental Development

After implantation, the embryo is surrounded by an outer trophoblastic shell that penetrates into the endometrial stroma. Here, the extravillous cytotrophoblast (EVT) cells proliferate to occlude nearby maternal blood vessels, which allows the embryo to form in a hypoxic environment free of oxidative stress signals, sustained by endometrial glandular secretions.[15] Primitive chorionic villi form all around the embryo and grow into the definitive placenta (chorion frondosum) in the most hypoxic regions of the uterine wall that are effectively occluded by the EVT.[16] The remainder of the chorion surrounding the embryo is deficient in EVT and therefore well-oxygenated and thins out to form the definitive fetal membranes (chorion leave). By the time of the 11- to 13-week nuchal translucency ultrasound examination, the spiral arterioles feeding the base of the placenta are transformed and dilated,[17] with established distinction between the placenta and membranes (**Fig. 1**). Indeed, first trimester development is critical to the future success of placental function. The extent of transformation of the spiral arteries by EVT largely dictates placental size. Clinical evidence of disruption of this process includes persistent vaginal bleeding[18] along with abnormal maternal serum levels of alpha-fetoprotein and/or pregnancy-associated plasma protein-A in early pregnancy, which in combination are important biochemical risk factors for subsequent complications attributable to placental dysfunction.[19–21]

Types of Placental Disease Associated with Fetal Growth Restriction

Maternal vascular malperfusion

The most commonly observed placental disease in association with FGR is maternal vascular malperfusion (MVM) (for a recent review see[22]). Based on a composite of the opinions of recent publications,[23,24] including our own work,[25] we present our working diagnostic criteria to define MVM in **Table 1**. Apart from small placental size and/or weight for gestation at delivery, 1 or more of a variety of macroscopic and histologic features are required to establish the diagnosis of MVM. Gross lesions include multifocal infarction or hemorrhage, whereas histologic lesions are found in the decidual vessels and/or the placental villi. An illustrative example of an MVM placenta with several diagnostic criteria is illustrated in **Fig. 2**. A typical case scenario of severe MVM disease resulting in preterm Cesarean delivery owing to evolving chronic abruption is illustrated in **Fig. 3**. The histologic features of MVM pathology are shown in **Fig. 4**.

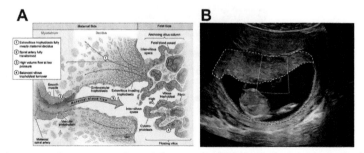

Fig. 1. Diagrammatic representation of the maternal-fetal interface at the end of the first trimester. (*A*) The spiral arteries in the placental bed are transformed to perfuse the developing placental villi. (*B*) Ultrasound demonstration of the distinction between the definitive placenta (*white dashed line*) and membranes (*red dashed line*) at 13 weeks gestation. (*Adapted from* Kingdom JC, Drewlo S. Is heparin a placental anticoagulant in high-risk pregnancies? Blood 2011;118(18):4781; with permission.)

Table 1
Diagnostic features of MVM on placental pathology

Type	Definition
Gross findings	
Placental hypoplasia	Placental weight at less than the 10th centile for gestational age and/or umbilical cord at less than the 10th centile in diameter
Placental infarction	Any infarction in a preterm placenta, or nonperipheral infarction of >5% at any gestational age. Chronicity of infarction and/or infarcts of multiple ages should be noted.
Retroplacental hemorrhage	Blood accumulation on maternal placental surface, with congestion and/or compression of the overlying parenchyma
Microscopic findings	
DVH	Decrease in villi relative to the surrounding stem villi. Villi are often elongated and thin in appearance. May be focal or diffuse.
Accelerated villous maturation	Presence of small, short villi relative to gestational age.
Syncytial knots	Aggregation of syncytiotrophoblast nuclei along villi. A feature of both DVH and accelerated villous maturation.
Decidual vasculopathy	Vascular lesions of the basal plate, membrane roll, or both. Features include: acute atherosis, fibrinoid necrosis, mural hypertrophy, chronic perivasculitis, and arterial thrombosis

Abbreviation: DVH, distal villous hypoplasia.
  Data from Refs.[24–26,85]

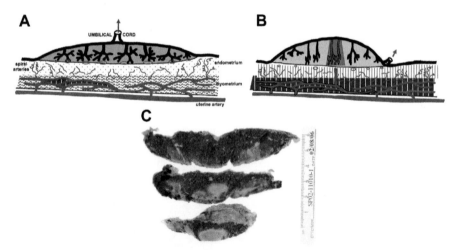

Fig. 2. Diagrammatic representation of the development of MVM pathology of the placenta. (*A*) In normal circumstances, the spiral arteries are transformed by the EVT over a larger area, occupying up to 25% of the uterine surface area. Note, the spiral arteries are maximally transformed in the center of the placental bed and the villi branch normally. (*B*) In MVM disease, EVT fail to interact normally with the spiral arteries, especially in the center of the placental bed. The placenta regresses in surface area and the umbilical cord may be marginal and have only one umbilical artery. (*B*) Diseased central spiral arteries may occlude and cause central wedge-shaped areas of infarction that are identified on (*C*) gross inspection of serial fixed placental sections.

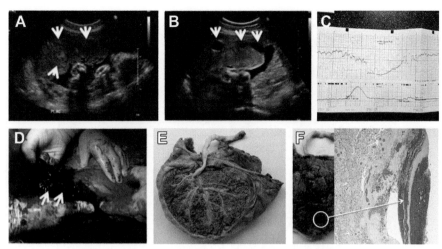

Fig. 3. Severe MVM presenting with preeclampsia and FGR at 33 weeks of gestation. Ultrasound examination on admission revealed asymmetric FGR with abnormal uterine and umbilical artery Dopplers. (*A*) A small fundal placenta was suspicious for several infarcts (*arrowheads*). Fetal Dopplers and heart rate tracing were normal. Steroids were given for fetal lung maturation. (*B*) Two days later, ultrasound examination was repeated for vague abdominal pain, demonstrating several black spaces suspicious for retroplacental hemorrhages (*arrowheads*). (*C*) Fetal heart rate tracing demonstrated a large late deceleration in response to a Braxton-Hicks contraction. (*D*) Old retroplacental hemorrhages (*arrowheads*) were found at emergency Cesarean delivery. (*E*) Fetal surface of the placenta weighing 225g (third to fifth centiles) with peripheral cord insertion (1.7 cm from the margin). (*F*) Focal black area of consolidated retroplacental hemorrhage (*circle*) confirmed by hematoxylin and eosin staining (*arrow*). ([*A–D*] *Adapted from* Kingdom JC, Audette MC, Hobson SR, et al. A placenta clinic approach to the diagnosis and management of fetal growth restriction. Am J Obstet Gynecol 2018;218(2S):S803-S817; with permission; and [*E, F*] *Courtesy of* E.K. Morgen, MD, MPH, FRCPC, Richmond, CA.)

From a clinical perspective, the current diagnostic criteria for MVM are very broad and, with some exceptions,[26,27] generally do not take disease impact into account. Small placental size reflects disease severity[21,28] and is a prerequisite in some publications,[24,25] although multiple gross and histologic features of MVM may be found in placentas greater than the 10th centile. In deliveries at less than 32 weeks of gestation, the majority of MVM placentas are less than the 10th centile for weight.[29,30] At later gestational ages, placentas from FGR deliveries may meet MVM criteria, although the phenotype is much less striking and the overall association between FGR and placental MVM disease is weaker.[31] The most severe form of MVM disease may present as so-called preventable stillbirth[4,32] owing to MVM's association with FGR.[10,33,34]

As an illustration of the wide definition of MVM disease, our recent prospective study of placental diseases in a low-risk cohort of nulliparous women found MVM pathology in 12%, yet one-half were asymptomatic.[25] The wide spectrum of placental abnormalities that constitute MVM disease in theory present challenges for the development of effective screening programs.[35] This was illustrated in the DIGITAT trial, where a high proportion of subjects in each arm of the study had no postnatal evidence of FGR.[36] Strongly associated with FGR, screening for early-onset preeclampsia has a much higher sensitivity than for disease near term[37] and collectively these studies illustrate a strong gestational age–dependent correlation of severity between FGR and MVM disease.

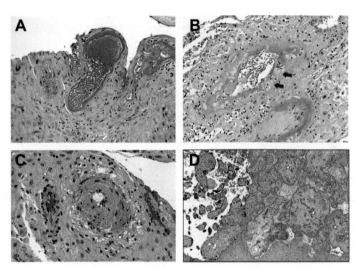

Fig. 4. Maternal vascular malperfusion. (*A*) Fibrinoid necrosis. The wall of this spiral has been replaced by dense, brightly eosinophilic fibrinoid. (H&E stain, 20x magnification). (*B*) Fibrinoid necrosis with atherosis. The walls of these 2 spiral artery cross-sections have been replaced by dense, eosinophilic fibrinoid. Scattered foamy macrophages are also present in the vessel on the left, highlighted by the *arrows*. (H&E stain, 20x magnification). (*C*) Mural hypertrophy. The spiral artery on the right shows marked thickening of the vessel's smooth muscle wall. (H&E stain, 20x magnification). (*D*) Remote infarct. The right half of this image shows old infarction of the placental parenchyma, identified by asterisks. Damaged but still viable villi are present along the left side of the image. (H&E stain, 10x magnification).

The diagnosis of MVM can be broadly divided into 2 components, the first comprising poor elaboration of the definitive placenta (which we have termed "chorion regression") and the second reflecting features of impaired uteroplacental blood flow owing to abnormal spiral arteries (which we have termed "uteroplacental vascular insufficiency"). Both components result in small placentas with weights of less than the 10th centile for gestational age.[25]

Chorion regression Fig. 5 illustrates the features of chorion regression, which can include a 2-vessel cord as an early developmental feature of the disease. Low pregnancy-associated plasma protein-A at first trimester screening may precede this type of FGR-associated disease,[20] which reflects reduced placental size.[21] The more obvious examples of chorion regression may be identified at the 11 to 13 week ultrasound using 3-dimensional methods,[38] and as pregnancy advances, reduced placental size may be identified using conventional 2-dimensional ultrasound methods[39–41] or 3-dimensional imaging.[42] Sometimes, these placental types may transform into an expanded ball, largely comprising maternal blood, owing to progressive rupture of the deficient anchoring villi. This phenomenon has been described as placental hyperinflation and is pathognomonic of severe MVM disease.[43] The typical histologic appearances of the placental villi in this context are described as distal villous hypoplasia,[44] which is characterized by poor formation of gas-exchanging villi.[45] The syncytiotrophoblast layer covering villi with distal villous hypoplasia is typically very thin, and is characterized by wave-like knotting and loss of underlying cytotrophoblasts, implying an arrest of new syncytiotrophoblast formation.[46] Chorion

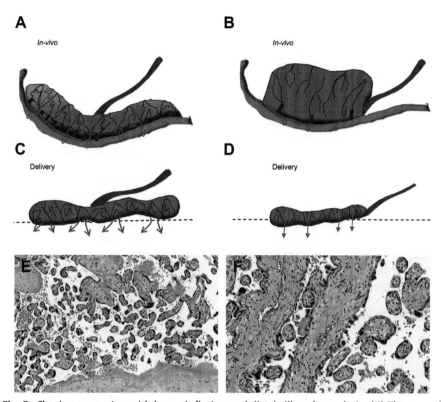

Fig. 5. Chorion regression with hyper-inflation and distal villous hypoplasia. (*A*) The normal placenta is inflated by the pressure of maternal blood in the intervillous space, and (*B*) deflates after delivery as maternal blood leaks out of the basal plate veins. In severe chorion regression, anchoring villi that normally keep the placental surfaces parallel are lost, such that (*C*) the placenta expands into a ball-like structure, (*D*) which collapses after delivery. (*E*) In distal villous hypoplasia, the villi are very long and thin with little branching. (H&E Stain, 4x magnification). (*F*) Wave-like syncytial knots in a midtrimester placenta show increased syncytial knots, which line up focally, line up along the surfaces of stem villi. (H&E Stain, 20x magnification). ([*A–D*] *Adapted from* Kingdom JC, Audette MC, Hobson SR, et al. A placenta clinic approach to the diagnosis and management of fetal growth restriction. Am J Obstet Gynecol 2018;218(2S):S811; with permission.)

regression alone may cause severe FGR, but in this context uterine artery Doppler is often normal, and the risk of coexistent preeclampsia is low.[21,43] The fetus can become hypoxic when chorion regression is present with normal uterine artery Dopplers because the impairment in transplacental gas transfer occurs distally at the level of the gas-exchanging placental villi.[47]

Uteroplacental vascular insufficiency In contrast, ischemic pathologic features largely arise from defective implantation biology, whereby the EVT are unable to transform the distal uteroplacental spiral arteries.[48] Under normal circumstances, the funneling distal spiral arterioles create a Venturi effect, which sprays maternal blood at low pressure into the intervillous space surrounding the placental villi, while the more proximal arterioles are dilated by estrogen and denervated. Uteroplacental blood flow is therefore perfusion dependent and stable in the absence of hypotension. The histopathologic term "decidual vasculopathy" (for a review see[49]) refers to a constellation of observations in spiral artery segments resulting from failed extravillous trophoblast invasion,[17,50] which leads to untransformed vessels that may be damaged by fibrinoid necrosis, narrowed by atherosis, and develop occlusive thrombosis. These diseased vessels create unstable high-velocity blood flow, which leads to ischemia-reperfusion injury, disruption of the placental architecture, and focal infarction of villous segments. Normal placentas may exhibit minor areas of peripheral placental infarction, because peripheral spiral arteries are small. However, multiple infarcts, especially if centrally located or of varying ages, imply significant uteroplacental vascular disease (see **Fig. 2C**). Diseased spiral arteries are also at risk of dissection,[51] leading to hemorrhage and potentially abruption along the normal placental cleavage plane.[52] Hemorrhage in various parenchymal sites is a diagnostic feature of MVM.

Chronic ischemia of the developing placental villi is associated with structural alterations in their development, especially in their overlying villous trophoblast compartment. They are described as accelerated in their development (accelerated villous maturation), with areas of syncytial knot formation known as Tenney-Parker changes.[53] The villous trophoblast layer shows several alterations as illustrated in **Fig. 6**. First, there are decreased numbers of proliferating cytotrophoblasts[46] owing to premature loss via cell death.[54] These cells divide asymmetrically with the daughter postmitotic cells fusing into the outer syncytiotrophoblast layer, thereby retaining the progenitor cytotrophoblast cell. The transcription factor Glial Cell Missing-1 (GCM-1) mediates this asymmetrical division,[55] whereas GCM-1's downstream partner, Syncytin, enables syncytial fusion. Placental expression of GCM-1 and Syncytin are deficient in placentas with severe preeclampsia or FGR.[56] The clinical relevance of a deficient GCM-1–mediated fusion pathway is that under normal circumstances GCM-1 promotes the synthesis and release of placenta growth factor (PlGF) into maternal blood.[57] PlGF has now emerged as a key diagnostic marker for severe FGR, preeclampsia, or both.

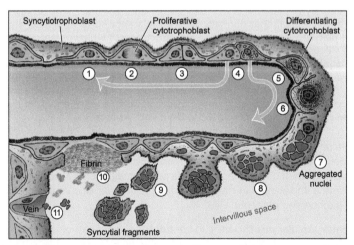

Fig. 6. Diagrammatic representation of normal villous trophoblast turnover (upper portion, 1–4) and abnormal villous trophoblast surface in MVM with excess syncytial knot formation (lower portion). In severe MVM disease, syncytial fusion events are reduced (5–6) and syncytial knots (7–8) form containing dense nuclei. These may detach as knots or as smaller fragments into the maternal circulation (9–11). (*Adapted from* Kingdom JC, Drewlo S. Is heparin a placental anticoagulant in high-risk pregnancies? Blood 2011;118(18):4784; with permission.)

Angiogenic growth factors and the fetal growth restriction placenta PlGF originates principally from the placental villi. This protein is detectable in maternal blood when the uteroplacental circulation is established between 11 and 13 weeks of gestation and thereafter blood levels rise throughout the second trimester[37] to reach a peak (median 240 pg/mL) at 28 weeks of gestation. Blood levels then decline by 36 weeks of gestation to a median of 100 pg/mL.[5] PlGF levels are low (<100 pg/mL) in FGR pregnancies,[58] with concentrations related to placental disease severity.[59] A recent retrospective cohort study of 274 women with suspected pre-eclampsia explored the diagnostic potential of PlGF to detect FGR in a blinded manner.[60] All 6 stillbirths had evidence of FGR, 5 of which had PlGF levels of less that the fifth centile. These low levels of PlGF preceded stillbirth by at least 10 days, which suggests a potential window of opportunity to prevent this outcome.

Placental villi globally suppress protein transcription and translation in response to hypoxia or hypoxia-reoxygenation injury[61] and this response has been specifically demonstrated in the context of PlGF production.[57] Explanted placental villi from pregnancies with preeclampsia with severe features and FGR demonstrate substantially impaired PlGF secretion.[62] The severe MVM placenta is also known to secrete excess amounts of the antiangiogenic protein soluble fms-like tyrosine kinase-1,[63,64] with intense production demonstrated from areas of placental villi arranged as syncytial knots.[65] Soluble fms-like tyrosine kinase-1 has been combined as a ratio test with PlGF to augment diagnostic precision for FGR[5] and to identify pregnancies with more severe MVM pathology.[26] The relationship between altered villous morphology and aberrant angiogenic growth factor expression and secretion is demonstrated in **Fig. 7.**

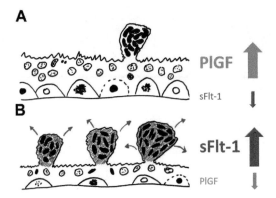

Fig. 7. Diagrammatic representation of the villous trophoblast surface at the beginning of the third trimester (*A*) in normal pregnancy and (*B*) in a pregnancy with MVM of the placenta expressed as early-onset preeclampsia with FGR and an elevated maternal serum sFlt-1/PlGF ratio. (*A*) Villous cytotrophoblast cells undergo asymmetrical divisions, producing daughter cells expressing glial cell missing-1 (GCM-1) in the nucleus (nucleus represented by a *black circle*) that enables syncytial fusion (*dashed cell border*). Fused syncytial nuclei eventually aggregate in syncytial knots and may even shed into maternal blood, where they remain functionally active. (*B*) Note the decreased numbers of cytotrophoblasts, implying less syncytial fusion and a reduced syncytiotrophoblast volume. Despite reduced syncytial turnover, this layer is characterized by increased syncytial knot formation where soluble fms-like tyrosine kinase-1 synthesis is found. Explanted placental villi in this disease context secrete less PlGF and more soluble fms-like tyrosine kinase-1.[62]

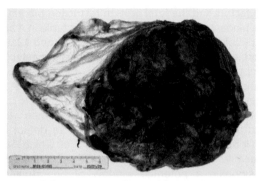

Fig. 8. Gross appearance of the placenta infiltrated by MPVFD.

Massive Perivillous Fibrin Deposition, Chronic Histiocytic Intervillositis, and Villitis of Unknown Etiology

Massive perivillous fibrin deposition (MPVFD) and chronic histiocytic intervillositis (CHIV) are much rarer placental diseases than MVM. They may coexist, are strongly associated with severe FGR, and may present as stillbirth with no prior clinical risk factors. MPVFD and CHIV are each noted for their high (>30%) risk of recurrence.[66,67] MPVFD is recognizable at delivery as a rigid yellow-colored placenta, as shown in **Fig. 8**. The typical ultrasound features of MPVFD, in the context of early-onset FGR, is a markedly heterogeneous abnormal placental texture with normal uterine artery Doppler, as shown in **Fig. 9**.[30]

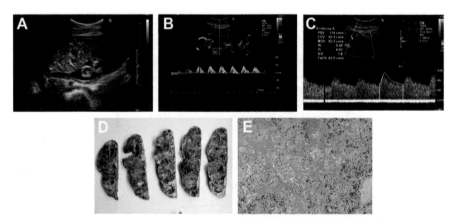

Fig. 9. Normotensive woman referred at 28 weeks with suspected FGR and previous 22-week stillbirth. Ultrasound examination demonstrates asymmetric FGR, (*A*) accompanied by thick placenta with diffusely abnormal texture, (*B*) with absent end-diastolic flow velocity waveforms in umbilical arteries, (*C*) yet bilateral normal uterine artery Doppler waveforms. Gross findings in (*D*) serial sections of fixed placenta demonstrate extensive replacement of villous tissue with lacelike pale fibrinoid material consistent with massive perivillous fibrinoid deposition of placenta (maternal floor infarction) accompanied by CHIV. (*E*) Massive perivillous fibrin deposition. This section shows a broad swathe of perivillous fibrin entrapping multiple villi and filling the entirety of the image. (H&E stain, 10x magnification). ([*A*–*D*] *From* Kingdom JC, Audette MC, Hobson SR, et al. A placenta clinic approach to the diagnosis and management of fetal growth restriction. Am J Obstet Gynecol 2018;218(2S):S812; with permission.)

Villitis of unknown etiology (VUE) is another inflammatory placental disease that is typically associated with late-onset FGR when VUE diffusely affects the organ.[68] In 1 study, VUE affected 5% of placentas submitted for pathology at greater than 37 weeks of gestation for suspected FGR at birth.[69] Representative histologic images of VUE and CHIV are shown in **Fig. 10**.

Fetal Thrombotic Vasculopathy

Several studies reporting the association between MVM placental pathology and FGR show a mixed pattern of disease and, although MVM dominates, coexistent histologic features of fetal vascular malperfusion may be present.[29,30,70,71] In a related study of 435 preeclamptic placentas, MVM disease was 2- to 3-fold

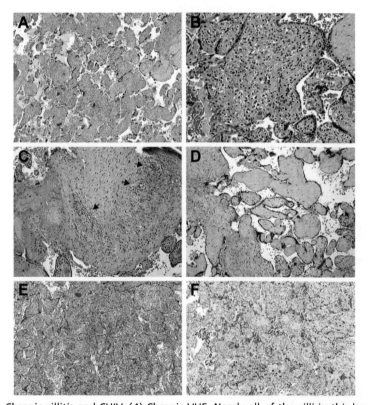

Fig. 10. Chronic villitis and CHIV. (*A*) Chronic VUE. Nearly all of the villi in this low-power image are infiltrated by numerous chronic inflammatory cells. (H&E, 4x magnification). (*B*) Chronic VUE. The villi in this high-power image show diffuse infiltration by chronic inflammatory cells. All of the villous vessels have been obliterated. (H&E, 20x magnification). (*C*) Stem vessel obliteration. The chronic inflammatory cells in this image selectively involve and destroy the stem villous vessels. *Arrows* point to involved stem villous vessels. (H&E, 10x magnification). (*D*) Avascular villi resulting from chronic villitis. With the frequent destruction of vessels by chronic villitis, the downstream villi often become avascular. (H&E, 10x magnification). (*E*) CHIV. The intervillous space in this placenta is clogged by large numbers of histiocytes. The villi appear largely unremarkable, with no evidence of chronic villitis. (H&E, 10x magnification). (*F*) CHIV—CD68 immunostain. CD68 immunostaining confirms that the cells in the intervillous space are macrophages. Modest numbers of macrophages are also present in the villi. (CD68 stain, 10x magnification).

more common than fetal vascular malperfusion. Using the more stringent diagnosis of fetal thrombotic vasculopathy,[24] a single-center study of 132 demonstrated an association with both FGR and with neurologic injury that was compounded by abnormal umbilical artery Doppler.[72] A typical example is shown in **Fig. 11**.

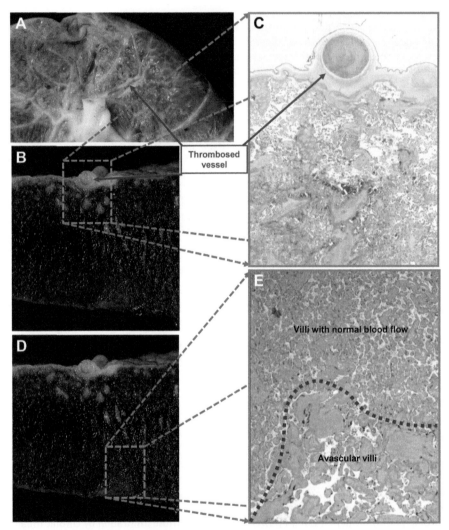

Fig. 11. Fetal vascular malperfusion. (*A*) At an elective Cesarean delivery at term, distal arm skin necrosis was evident and inspection of the fetal surface revealed chorionic plate surface vessels suspicious for thrombosis. (*B*) Placental cross-section with (*C*) corresponding hematoxylin and eosin (H&E) histology showing thrombosis within chorionic plate vessel. (*D*) Slightly pale basal region of same placental cross-section (note that central red band is fixation artifact) suggests distal vascular disease induced by proximal vascular thrombosis. (*E*) Corresponding H&E histology of the basal region demonstrating avascular villi in portions of the villous tree that were perfused by the now occluded chorionic plate vessel. (*From* Kingdom JC, Audette MC, Hobson SR, et al. A placenta clinic approach to the diagnosis and management of fetal growth restriction. Am J Obstet Gynecol 2018;218(2S):S813; with permission.)

Prenatal Diagnosis of Placental Diseases Causing Fetal Growth Restriction

Uterine artery Doppler

MVM pathology is strongly associated with abnormal bilateral uterine artery Doppler. In a cohort of 196 singleton severe FGR pregnancies delivering at less than 32 weeks of gestation with abnormal umbilical artery Doppler waveforms, 80% of placentas with this disease were from women with bilateral high-resistance uterine artery waveforms.[30] Other groups have made similar observations.[73–76] The incorporation of uterine artery Doppler into first trimester[77] and early second trimester[37] screening programs for early-onset preeclampsia likely reflects this association.

Placental morphologic imaging The logic of visualizing placental size, shape and gross anatomy is based on the macroscopic findings of the MVM placenta following delivery. Two-dimensional ultrasound measurements of maximum placental length and thickness, together with cord insertion, may recognize MVM as a placental basis for FGR, especially in early-onset FGR with abnormal uterine artery Doppler[21,39,43](for further review see[1]). Some of these sonographic abnormalities are virtually diagnostic of MVM disease in the context of early-onset FGR; yet, when incorporated into a screening program for low-risk women in the second trimester, they are of limited usefulness.[25] In addition to MPVFD and CHIV, other rare placental diseases associated with FGR, which may be recognized using ultrasound morphology, include Breus' mole,[78] triploidy,[79] and mesenchymal dysplasia.[80] Three-dimensional placental assessment is technically easier at 11 to 13 weeks of gestation than at later gestational ages, and can define the chorionic plate surface.[38] Information from first trimester 3-dimensional ultrasound examination has been incorporated into screening algorithms,[81,82] but these methods have not yet been incorporated into clinical practice.

Role of MRI in the Diagnosis of Placenta-Mediated Fetal Growth Restriction

MRI methods are increasingly used in high-risk pregnancy settings to improve both prenatal diagnosis and the functional significance of placental pathologies in the context of FGR. Placental volume growth in normal pregnancy was recently reported.[83] In comparing normal and FGR pregnancies, differences in regional blood flow rates, oxygen delivery and consumption have been observed.[13] A study of 59 pregnancies with postnatally confirmed MVM pathology demonstrated an 82% positive predictive value,[84] which is much higher than was previously reported using 2-dimensional ultrasound examination.[39]

SUMMARY

Placental dysfunction is a major contributor to FGR. Although the definition of FGR varies worldwide, the most accepted diagnostic criteria include an estimated fetal weight of less than the 10th centile for gestational age, with or without signs of pathology. Placental-mediated FGR results from chronic fetal hypoxia owing to poor placental perfusion through a variety of mechanisms. MVM is the most common placental disorder contributing to FGR, but the role of rare placental disorders, such as MPVFD, CHIV, and VUE, should not be overlooked. Although macroscopic and microscopic characteristics of MVM are identifiable on placental pathology, antepartum diagnostic methods are still evolving. Placental imaging and uterine artery Doppler, used in conjunction with angiogenic growth factors (specifically PlGF and sFlt-1), play an increasingly important role in the identification and management of pregnancies at risk of placental mediated FGR.

REFERENCES

1. Kingdom JC, Audette MC, Hobson SR, et al. A placenta clinic approach to the diagnosis and management of fetal growth restriction. Am J Obstet Gynecol 2017;1–15. https://doi.org/10.1016/j.ajog.2017.11.575.
2. Flenady V, Wojcieszek A, Middleton P, et al. Series ending preventable stillbirths 4 stillbirths: recall to action in high-income countries. Lancet 2016;1–12. https://doi.org/10.1016/S0140-6736(15)01020-X.
3. You JJ, Alter DA, Stukel TA, et al. Proliferation of prenatal ultrasonography. CMAJ 2010;182(2):143–51.
4. Ptacek I, Sebire NJ, Man JA, et al. Systematic review of placental pathology reported in association with stillbirth. Placenta 2014;35(8):552–62.
5. Gaccioli F, Sovio U, Cook E, et al. Screening for fetal growth restriction using ultrasound and the sFLT1/PlGF ratio in nulliparous women: a prospective cohort study. Lancet Child Adolesc Health 2018;2(8):569–81.
6. McCowan LM, Figueras F, Anderson NH. Evidence-based national guidelines for the management of suspected fetal growth restriction: comparison, consensus, and controversy. Am J Obstet Gynecol 2018;218(2S):S855–68.
7. Lausman A, Kingdom J. Intrauterine growth restriction: screening, diagnosis, and management. J Obstet Gynaecol Can 2013;35(8):741–8.
8. Figueras F, Caradeux J, Crispi F, et al. Diagnosis and surveillance of late-onset fetal growth restriction. Am J Obstet Gynecol 2018;218(2S):790–802.e1.
9. Sovio U, white IR, Dacey A, et al. Articles Screening for fetal growth restriction with universal third trimester ultrasonography in nulliparous women in the Pregnancy Outcome Prediction (POP) study: a prospective cohort study. Lancet 2015;1–9. https://doi.org/10.1016/S0140-6736(15)00131-2.
10. Iliodromiti S, Mackay DF, Smith GC, et al. Customised and noncustomised birth weight centiles and prediction of stillbirth and infant mortality and morbidity: a cohort study of 979,912 term singleton pregnancies in Scotland. PLoS Med 2017;14(1). e1002228.
11. Chang KTE, Keating S, Costa S, et al. Third-trimester stillbirths: correlative neuropathology and placental pathology. Pediatr Dev Pathol 2011;14(5):345–52.
12. Pardi G, Cetin I, Marconi AM, et al. Diagnostic value of blood sampling in fetuses with growth retardation. N Engl J Med 1993;328(10):692–6.
13. Zhu MY, Milligan N, Keating S, et al. The hemodynamics of late-onset intrauterine growth restriction by MRI. Am J Obstet Gynecol 2016;214(3):367.e1-17.
14. Riyami NA, Walker MG, Proctor LK, et al. Utility of head/abdomen circumference ratio in the evaluation of severe early-onset intrauterine growth restriction. J Obstet Gynaecol Can 2011;33(7):715–9.
15. Burton GJ, Hempstock J, Jauniaux E. Nutrition of the human fetus during the first trimester—a review. Placenta 2001;22:S70–7.
16. Jauniaux E, Hempstock J, Greenwold N, et al. Trophoblastic oxidative stress in relation to temporal and regional differences in maternal placental blood flow in normal and abnormal early pregnancies. Am J Pathol 2003;162(1):115–25.
17. Robson SC, Simpson H, Ball E, et al. Punch biopsy of the human placental bed. Am J Obstet Gynecol 2002;187(5):1349–55.
18. Saraswat L, Maheshwari A, Bhattacharya S. Maternal and perinatal outcome in women with threatened miscarriage in the first trimester: a systematic review. BJOG 2010;117(3):245–57.

19. Smith GC, Shah I, Crossley JA, et al. Pregnancy-associated plasma protein A and alpha-fetoprotein and prediction of adverse perinatal outcome. Obstet Gynecol 2006;107(1):161–6.
20. Hughes AE, Sovio U, Gaccioli F, et al. The association between first trimester AFP to PAPP-A ratio and placentally-related adverse pregnancy outcome. Placenta 2019;81:25–31.
21. Proctor LK, Toal M, Keating S, et al. Placental size and the prediction of severe early-onset intrauterine growth restriction in women with low pregnancy-associated plasma protein-A. Ultrasound Obstet Gynecol 2009;34(3):274–82.
22. Ernst LM. Maternal vascular malperfusion of the placental bed. APMIS 2018; 126(7):551–60.
23. Redline RW. Classification of placental lesions. Am J Obstet Gynecol 2015;213(4 Suppl):S21–8.
24. Khong TY, Mooney EE, Ariel I, et al. Sampling and definitions of placental lesions: Amsterdam placental workshop group consensus statement. Arch Pathol Lab Med 2016;140(7):698–713.
25. Wright E, Audette MC, Ye XY, et al. Maternal vascular malperfusion and adverse perinatal outcomes in low-risk nulliparous women. Obstet Gynecol 2017;130(5): 1112–20.
26. Korzeniewski SJ, Romero R, Chaiworapongsa T, et al. Maternal plasma angiogenic index-1 (placental growth factor/soluble vascular endothelial growth factor receptor-1) is a biomarker for the burden of placental lesions consistent with uteroplacental underperfusion: a longitudinal case-cohort study. Am J Obstet Gynecol 2016;214(5):629.e1-17.
27. Parra-Saavedra M, Simeone S, Triunfo S, et al. Correlation between histological signs of placental underperfusion and perinatal morbidity in late-onset small-for-gestational-age fetuses. Ultrasound Obstet Gynecol 2015;45(2):149–55.
28. Toal M, Chan C, Fallah S, et al. Usefulness of a placental profile in high-risk pregnancies. Am J Obstet Gynecol 2007;196(4):363.e1-7.
29. Walker MG, Fitzgerald B, Keating S, et al. Sex-specific basis of severe placental dysfunction leading to extreme preterm delivery. Placenta 2012;33(7):568–71.
30. Levytska K, Higgins M, Keating S, et al. Placental pathology in relation to uterine artery doppler findings in pregnancies with severe intrauterine growth restriction and abnormal umbilical artery doppler changes. Am J Perinatol 2017;34(05): 451–7.
31. Parra-Saavedra M, Crovetto F, Triunfo S, et al. Placental findings in late-onset SGA births without Doppler signs of placental insufficiency. Placenta 2013. https://doi.org/10.1016/j.placenta.2013.09.018.
32. Man J, Hutchinson JC, Heazell AE, et al. Stillbirth and intrauterine fetal death: role of routine histopathological placental findings to determine cause of death. Ultrasound Obstet Gynecol 2016;48(5):579–84.
33. Reinebrant HE, Leisher SH, Coory M, et al. Making stillbirths visible: a systematic review of globally reported causes of stillbirth. BJOG 2018;125(2):212–24.
34. Francis A, Hugh O, Gardosi J. Customized vs INTERGROWTH-21st standards for the assessment of birthweight and stillbirth risk at term. Am J Obstet Gynecol 2018;218(2S):S692–9.
35. Smith GC. Best practice & research clinical obstetrics and gynaecology. Best Pract Res Clin Obstet Gynaecol 2016;38(C):71–82.
36. Boers KE, Vijgen SMC, Bijlenga D, et al. Induction versus expectant monitoring for intrauterine growth restriction at term: randomised equivalence trial (DIGITAT). BMJ 2010;341:c7087.

37. Myers JE, Kenny LC, McCowan LME, et al. Angiogenic factors combined with clinical risk factors to predict preterm pre-eclampsia in nulliparous women: a predictive test accuracy study. BJOG 2013;120(10):1215–23.

38. Schwartz N, Mandel D, Shlakhter O, et al. Placental morphologic features and chorionic surface vasculature at term are highly correlated with sonographic measurements at 11 to 14 weeks. J Ultrasound Med 2011;30(9):1171–8.

39. Toal M, Keating S, Machin G, et al. Determinants of adverse perinatal outcome in high-risk women with abnormal uterine artery Doppler images. Am J Obstet Gynecol 2008;198(3):330.e1-7.

40. Costantini D, Walker M, Milligan N, et al. Pathologic basis of improving the screening utility of 2-dimensional placental morphology ultrasound. Placenta 2012;33(10):845–9.

41. Schwartz N, Wang E, Parry S. Two-dimensional sonographic placental measurements in the prediction of small-for-gestational-age infants. Ultrasound Obstet Gynecol 2012;40(6):674–9.

42. Quant HS, Sammel MD, Parry S, et al. Second-trimester 3-dimensional placental sonography as a predictor of small-for-gestational-age birth weight. J Ultrasound Med 2016;35(8):1693–702.

43. Porat S, Fitzgerald B, Wright E, et al. Placental hyperinflation and the risk of adverse perinatal outcome. Ultrasound Obstet Gynecol 2013;42(3):315–21.

44. Mukherjee A, Chan ADC, Keating S, et al. The placental distal villous hypoplasia pattern: interobserver agreement and automated fractal dimension as an objective metric. Pediatr Dev Pathol 2016;19(1):31–6.

45. Krebs C, Macara LM, Leiser R, et al. Intrauterine growth restriction with absent end-diastolic flow velocity in the umbilical artery is associated with maldevelopment of the placental terminal villous tree. Am J Obstet Gynecol 1996;175(6):1534–42.

46. Fitzgerald B, LEVYTSKA K, Kingdom J, et al. Villous trophoblast abnormalities in extremely preterm deliveries with elevated second trimester maternal serum hCG or inhibin-A. Placenta 2011;32(4):339–45.

47. Kingdom JC, Kaufmann P. Oxygen and placental villous development: origins of fetal hypoxia. Placenta 1997;18(8):613–21 [discussion: 623–6].

48. Burton GJ, Woods AW, Jauniaux E, et al. Rheological and physiological consequences of conversion of the maternal spiral arteries for uteroplacental blood flow during human pregnancy. Placenta 2009;30(6):473–82.

49. Staff AC, Dechend R, Redman CWG. Review: preeclampsia, acute atherosis of the spiral arteries and future cardiovascular disease: two new hypotheses. Placenta 2013;34(Suppl):S73–8.

50. Reister F, Frank HG, Kingdom JC, et al. Macrophage-induced apoptosis limits endovascular trophoblast invasion in the uterine wall of preeclamptic women. Lab Invest 2001;81(8):1143–52.

51. Fitzgerald B, Shannon P, Kingdom J, et al. Basal plate plaque: a novel organising placental thrombotic process. J Clin Pathol 2011;64(8):725–8.

52. Neville G, Russell N, O'Donoghue K, et al. Rounded intraplacental hematoma - A high risk placental lesion as illustrated by a prospective study of 26 consecutive cases. Placenta 2019;81:18–24.

53. Fogarty NME, Ferguson-Smith AC, Burton GJ. Syncytial knots (Tenney-Parker changes) in the human placenta: evidence of loss of transcriptional activity and oxidative damage. Am J Pathol 2013;183(1):144–52.

54. Longtine MS, Chen B, Odibo AO, et al. Villous trophoblast apoptosis is elevated and restricted to cytotrophoblasts in pregnancies complicated by preeclampsia, IUGR, or preeclampsia with IUGR. Placenta 2012;33(5):352–9.
55. Baczyk D, Drewlo S, Proctor L, et al. Glial cell missing-1 transcription factor is required for the differentiation of the human trophoblast. Cell Death Differ 2009; 16(5):719–27.
56. Langbein M, Strick R, Strissel PL, et al. Impaired cytotrophoblast cell-cell fusion is associated with reduced Syncytin and increased apoptosis in patients with placental dysfunction. Mol Reprod Dev 2008;75(1):175–83.
57. Chiu Y-H, Yang M-R, Wang L-J, et al. New insights into the regulation of placental growth factor gene expression by the transcription factors GCM1 and DLX3 in human placenta. J Biol Chem 2018;293(25):9801–11.
58. Benton SJ, Hu Y, Xie F, et al. Can placental growth factor in maternal circulation identify fetuses with placental intrauterine growth restriction? Am J Obstet Gynecol 2012. https://doi.org/10.1016/j.ajog.2011.09.019.
59. Benton SJ, McCowan LM, Heazell AEP, et al. Placental growth factor as a marker of fetal growth restriction caused by placental dysfunction. Placenta 2016; 42(C):1–8.
60. Griffin M, Seed PT, Duckworth S, et al. Predicting delivery of a small-for-gestational-age infant and adverse perinatal outcome in women with suspected pre-eclampsia. Ultrasound Obstet Gynecol 2018;51(3):387–95.
61. Hung T-H, Burton GJ. Hypoxia and reoxygenation: a possible mechanism for placental oxidative stress in preeclampsia. Taiwanese J Obstet Gynecol 2006; 45(3):189–200.
62. O'Brien M, Baczyk D, Kingdom JC. Endothelial dysfunction in severe preeclampsia is mediated by soluble factors, rather than extracellular vesicles. Sci Rep 2017;7(1):5887.
63. Ahmad S, Ahmed A. Elevated placental soluble vascular endothelial growth factor receptor-1 inhibits angiogenesis in preeclampsia. Circ Res 2004;95(9): 884–91.
64. Drewlo S, Levytska K, Sobel M, et al. Heparin promotes soluble VEGF receptor expression in human placental villi to impair endothelial VEGF signaling. J Thromb Haemost 2011;9(12):2486–97.
65. Taché V, LaCoursiere DY, Saleemuddin A, et al. Placental expression of vascular endothelial growth factor receptor-1/soluble vascular endothelial growth factor receptor-1 correlates with severity of clinical preeclampsia and villous hypermaturity. Hum Pathol 2011;42(9):1283–8.
66. Contro E, deSouza R, Bhide A. Chronic intervillositis of the placenta: a systematic review. Placenta 2010;31(12):1106–10.
67. Chen A, Roberts DJ. Placental pathologic lesions with a significant recurrence risk - what not to miss! APMIS 2018;126(7):589–601.
68. Derricott H, Jones RL, Greenwood SL, et al. Characterizing villitis of unknown etiology and Inflammation in Stillbirth. Am J Pathol 2016;186(4):952–61.
69. Kovo M, Ganer Herman H, Gold E, et al. Villitis of unknown etiology - prevalence and clinical associations. J Matern Fetal Neonatal Med 2016;29(19):3110–4.
70. Ravikumar G, Crasta J. Do Doppler Changes reflect pathology of placental vascular lesions in IUGR pregnancies? Pediatr Dev Pathol 2019;204. 1093526619837790.
71. Gluck O, Schreiber L, Marciano A, et al. Pregnancy outcome and placental pathology in small for gestational age neonates in relation to the severity of their growth restriction. J Matern Fetal Neonatal Med 2019;32(9):1468–73.

72. Chisholm KM, Heerema-McKenney A. Fetal thrombotic vasculopathy: significance in liveborn children using proposed society for pediatric pathology diagnostic criteria. Am J Surg Pathol 2015;39(2):274–80.
73. Ferrazzi E, Bulfamante G, Mezzopane R, et al. Uterine Doppler velocimetry and placental hypoxic-ischemic lesion in pregnancies with fetal intrauterine growth restriction. Placenta 1999;20(5–6):389–94.
74. Aardema MW, Oosterhof H, Timmer A, et al. Uterine artery Doppler flow and uteroplacental vascular pathology in normal pregnancies and pregnancies complicated by pre-eclampsia and small for gestational age fetuses. Placenta 2001; 22(5):405–11.
75. Parra-Saavedra M, Crovetto F, Triunfo S, et al. Association of Doppler parameters with placental signs of underperfusion in late-onset small-for-gestational-age pregnancies. Ultrasound Obstet Gynecol 2014;44(3):330–7.
76. Orabona R, Donzelli CM, Falchetti M, et al. Placental histological patterns and uterine artery Doppler velocimetry in pregnancies complicated by early or late pre-eclampsia. Ultrasound Obstet Gynecol 2016;47(5):580–5.
77. Rolnik DL, Wright D, Poon LC, et al. Aspirin versus placebo in pregnancies at high risk for preterm preeclampsia. N Engl J Med 2017;377(7):613–22.
78. Alanjari A, Wright E, Keating S, et al. Prenatal diagnosis, clinical outcomes, and associated pathology in pregnancies complicated by massive subchorionic thrombohematoma (Breus' mole). Prenat Diagn 2013;33(10):973–8.
79. Massalska D, Bijok J, Ilnicka A, et al. Triploidy - variability of sonographic phenotypes. Prenat Diagn 2017;37(8):774–80.
80. Guenot C, Kingdom J, De Rham M, et al. Placental mesenchymal dysplasia: an underdiagnosed placental pathology with various clinical outcomes. Eur J Obstet Gynecol Reprod Biol 2019;234:155–64.
81. Schwartz N, Sammel MD, Leite R, et al. First-trimester placental ultrasound and maternal serum markers as predictors of small-for-gestational-age infants. Am J Obstet Gynecol 2014;211(3):253.e1-8.
82. Papastefanou I, Chrelias C, Siristatidis C, et al. Placental volume at 11 to 14 gestational weeks in pregnancies complicated with fetal growth restriction and preeclampsia. Prenat Diagn 2018;38(12):928–35.
83. León RL, Li KT, Brown BP. A retrospective segmentation analysis of placental volume by magnetic resonance imaging from first trimester to term gestation. Pediatr Radiol 2018;48(13):1936–44.
84. Messerschmidt A, Baschat A, Linduska N, et al. Magnetic resonance imaging of the placenta identifies placental vascular abnormalities independently of Doppler ultrasound. Ultrasound Obstet Gynecol 2011;37(6):717–22.
85. Kelly R, Holzman C, Senagore P, et al. Placental vascular pathology findings and pathways to preterm delivery. Am J Epidemiol 2009;170(2):148–58.

Placental Anatomy and Function in Twin Gestations

Matthew A. Shanahan, MD, Michael W. Bebbington, MD, MHSc*

KEYWORDS

- Twin placenta • Monochorionic placenta • Twin-to-twin transfusion syndrome
- Selective intrauterine growth restriction • Twin anemia-polycythemia sequence
- Twin reversed arterial perfusion

KEY POINTS

- Monochorionic twins are susceptible to complications because of their unique placental architecture, including twin-to-twin transfusion syndrome, the twin anemia-polycythemia sequence, selective intrauterine growth restriction, and the twin reversed arterial perfusion sequence.
- Net unidirectional blood flow from 1 twin to the other via intertwin anastomoses can lead to twin-to-twin transfusion syndrome or the twin reversed arterial perfusion sequence.
- Unequal sharing of a monochorionic placenta among twins can result in 1 twin being growth restricted, termed selective intrauterine growth restriction.
- Detailed placental evaluation of twin gestations, especially monochorionic diamniotic twins, is important in understanding the various complications associated with these complex pregnancies.

INTRODUCTION

With the increasing number of pregnancies in women over 40 years, and the ever-expanding use of assisted reproductive technologies (ART), the rate of twin pregnancies is continuing to rise. In 2017, approximately 3% of all births in the United States were twin births,[1] with that number only expected to continue to rise. With an increasing incidence of twins, understanding the inherent risks associated with these pregnancies is essential to the practice of modern obstetrics. Twin pregnancies, have increased rates of prematurity, low birth weight, and congenital anomalies.[2] The twin mortality rate is approximately 5 times higher than in singletons.[1] The unique differences in placentation in twin gestations contribute to the increased risks.

Thirty percent of twin gestations have monochorionic (MC) placentas which are susceptible to complications related to the angioarchitecture of the placenta,

Department of Obstetrics & Gynecology, Division of Maternal-Fetal Medicine, Washington University in St. Louis School of Medicine, 660 South Euclid Avenue, Mailstop 8064-37-1005, St. Louis, MO 63110, USA
* Corresponding author.
E-mail address: bebbingtonm@wustl.edu

Obstet Gynecol Clin N Am 47 (2020) 99–116
https://doi.org/10.1016/j.ogc.2019.10.010
0889-8545/20/© 2019 Elsevier Inc. All rights reserved.

including twin-to-twin transfusion syndrome, twin anemia-polycythemia sequence (TAPS), selective intrauterine growth restriction (sIUGR), and the twin reversed arterial perfusion (TRAP) sequence. The incidence of MC twins is also rising, secondary to the increased use of ART. The incidence of MC twins increases 3-fold after ovulation induction or conventional in vitro fertilization and 13-fold following intracytoplasmic sperm injection.[3] Although prevention of unnecessary multiple gestations is an important goal in ART, management of MC gestations, whether twins or part of a higher order multiple gestation, is now part of routine obstetric practice. An understanding of the placental pathophysiology of these conditions is critical for understanding the natural history and ultimate clinical course of these diseases, and to guide antenatal surveillance, delivery, the role for directed fetal therapy or potential selective fetal reduction.

ZYGOSITY, CHORIONICITY, AND THEIR CLINICAL IMPLICATIONS

Twin gestations are either the result of a single zygote that splits after fertilization (monozygotic [MZ]), or of the concurrent fertilization of 2 separate ova that were ovulated simultaneously (dizygotic [DZ]).[4] DZ twin gestations result from 2 independent ovulations of 2 viable oocytes fertilized with normal sperm cells in a temporality that allows concurrent implantation within the endometrium. DZ twins are genetically different and account for approximately 70% of twin gestations. MZ twins result from the splitting of a single zygote, initially formed by 1 oocyte and 1 sperm. MZ twins are thus genetically identical and account for about 30% of spontaneously conceived twins. MZ twins are estimated at 0.4% of nonstimulated *in vivo* conceptions.[5]

Because DZ gestations result from 2 distinct fertilization events, each zygote has a distinct chorion, amnion, and placental mass, referred to as dichorionic, diamniotic placentas. Dichorionic placentas may either be 2 separate placental masses or a single fused placental mass, depending on the proximity of the implantation sites of the blastocyts.[4] Fused placental masses function independently as discrete fetoplacental circulations, no different from 2 geographically discrete placental masses.

The chorionicity of MZ twin gestations is determined by the timing of the division of the zygote.[4,6] Overall, 25% to 30% of MZ twins are dichorionic, diamniotic resulting from a zygote split within 3 days after fertilization, before embryonic cell differentiation (**Fig. 1**). The remaining 70% to 75% of MZ twins are monochorionic diamniotic (MCDA), where the inner cell mass divides during the preimplantation blastocyst stage between days 4 and 8 after fertilization. If the division takes place in the after implantation blastocyst phase, usually days 8 to 12 after fertilization, then monochorionic monoamniotic (MCMA) twins occur. Notably, only 1% to 2% of MZ twins are MCMA. If division takes place beyond 12 days after fertilization, conjoined MCMA twins develop, occurring about 1 in 100,000.[4]

The perinatal outcome of DZ twins and dichorionic MZ twins is the same. Monochorionic twins, however, are susceptible to additional complications because of their unique placental architecture (**Fig. 2**). Given the higher risks of perinatal morbidity and mortality in MC gestations, early, accurate determination of chorionicity is essential. This determination is best performed in the first trimester by ultrasound.[7] It is an oft repeated aphorism that there is no diagnosis of twins. There are only MC twins or dichorionic twins.[8] All MC placentas are characterized by the presence of vascular connections between the circulations of the fetuses. These can be between pairs of arteries, pairs of veins, or arteries connected to veins. The number and type of vessels involved are unique to each pregnancy. The net effect is dynamic bidirectional blood

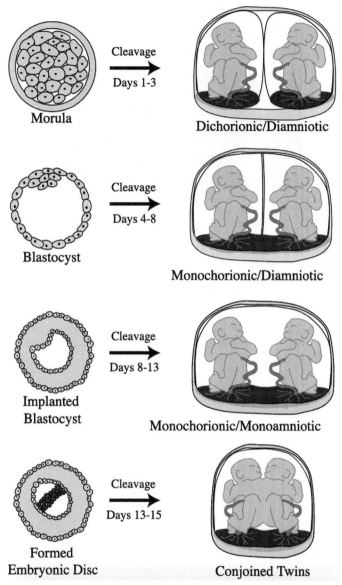

Fig. 1. Timing of embryonal division and the subsequent chorionicity that results. (*Courtesy of* K.R. Dufendach, MD, MS, FAAP, Cincinnati, OH.)

flow between the cotwins. Abnormalities in the nature of the connections or in the balance of blood flow between the fetuses create clinical problems unique to MCDA pregnancies. These include twin-to-twin transfusion syndrome (TTTS), TAPS, sIUGR, and TRAP sequence. The vascular connections also link the fetuses in terms of outcomes. Intrauterine death of 1 fetus increases the risk of death or cerebral damage in the cotwin likely due to acute transfusion from the normal twin into the lower pressure circulation of the dying twin through the placental anastomoses.[9–11] This risk has been reported to be as high as 30% to 50%.

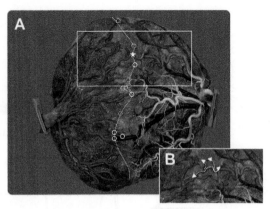

Fig. 2. Vascular anastomoses in monochorionic twin pregnancies. Healthy monochorionic diamniotic placenta delivered at 35 weeks without any antenatal complications. (*A*) Each twin has its own individual placental territory (veins colored blue for twin 1 and veins colored brown for twin 2) defined by venous chorionic plate vessels of each twin (*dotted line*). There is 1 artery-to-artery anastomosis (*star*); 5 arteriovenous anastomoses (from twin 1 to 2) (open circles); and 6 oppositely directed venoarterial anastomoses (*dotted circles*). (*B*) Magnification of artery-to-artery anastomosis. Each artery-to-artery anastomosis functions as flexible arteriovenous anastomosis. Depending on direction of flow, it can act as arteriovenous anastomosis from twin 1 to 2 (*solid arrow*), or as venoarterial anastomosis from twin 2 to 1 (*dotted arrows*). (*From* Lewi L, Deprest J, Hecher K. The vascular anastomoses in monochorionic twin pregnancies and their clinical consequences. Am J Obstet Gynecol 2013;208(1):21; with permission.)

After a spontaneous demise of 1 twin, the rate of demise in the cotwin is twice as high in MC twins compared with dichorionic twins (**Table 1**).[12] Even if the cotwin survives there is a significant risk of neurologic sequelae. Hypotension and hypoxia then lead to under perfusion of the cotwin causing tissue damage. These significant risks illustrate why in a MC twin gestation where 1 fetus demonstrates abnormalities that may be associated with intrauterine fetal demise (IUFD), selective termination can be advocated to optimize the chances for intact survival of the cotwin and as an alternative to termination of the entire pregnancy.[13]

PLACENTAL EVALUATION AND INJECTION STUDIES

Placental injection studies performed on a fresh MC placenta after delivery can demonstrate the underlying angioarchitecture responsible for clinical syndromes seen in MC twin gestations. The technique is well described in the literature.[14] This can describe the placental distribution and the number, size, and type of vascular anastomoses that underlie complications associated with MC twins. However, there is a time-sensitive window to perform the staining before tissue breakdown, and often demise of either or both twins an MC yields a placenta not amenable to injection limiting the ability to outline the causative angioarchitecture.[15]

TWIN-TO-TWIN TRANSFUSION SYNDROME

TTTS is only observed in MC twin gestations and has a spectrum of severity. Approximately 10% to 15% of MC gestations will develop TTTS,[16] although this may be an

Table 1
Perinatal outcomes in monochorionic twins compared with dichorionic twins

Adverse Outcome in Cotwin	Monochorionic Event Rate	Dichorionic Event Rate	Odds Ratio [95% CI] Comparing MC vs. DC
Cotwin intrauterine fetal death	41.0% [95% CI, 33.7, 49.9] I^2 = 44.2%, 32 studies, 379 pregnancies	22.4% [95% CI, 16.2, 30.9] I^2 = 21.7%, 20 studies, 255 pregnancies	**2.06 [95% CI, 1.14, 3.71] P = .016, I^2 = 0.0%, 19 studies, 441 pregnancies**
Preterm birth	58.5% [95% CI, 48.2, 70.9] I^2 = 11.7%, 20 studies, 202 pregnancies	53.7% [95% CI, 40.8, 70.6] I^2 = 0.0%, 12 studies, 107 pregnancies	1.42 [95% CI, 0.67, 2.99] P = .356, I^2 = 1.5%, 10 studies, 167 pregnancies
Abnormal antenatal brain fMRI	20.0% [95% CI, 12.8, 31.1] I^2 = 21.9%, 6 studies, 116 pregnancies	NP	NP
Abnormal postnatal brain imaging	43.0% [95% CI, 32.8, 56.3] I^2 = 12.4%, 12 studies, 140 pregnancies	21.2% [95% CI, 10.6, 42.4] I^2 = 0.7%, 7 studies, 75 pregnancies	**5.41 [95% CI, 1.03, 28.58] P = .047, I^2 = 45.8%, 7 studies, 142 pregnancies**
Neuro-developmental comorbidity	28.5% [95% CI, 19.0, 42.7] I^2 = 0.0%, 13 studies, 103 pregnancies	10% [95% CI, 3.9, 27.7] I^2 = 0.0%, 8 studies, 62 pregnancies	3.06 [95% CI, 0.88, 10.61] P = .08, I^2 = 0.0%, 8 studies, 129 pregnancies
Neonatal death	27.9% [95% CI, 21.1, 36.9] I^2 = 0.0%, 18 studies, 206 pregnancies	21.2% [95% CI, 14.5, 31.2] I^2 = 0.0%, 12 studies, 130 pregnancies	1.95 [95% CI, 1.00, 3.79] P = .051, I^2 = 0.0%, 11 studies, 232 pregnancies

Bold denotes statistically significant results.

P value in the odds ratio (OR) column denotes the significance of OR = 1.

Abbreviations: DC, dichorionic; fMRI, fetal magnetic resonance imaging; MC, monochorionic; NP, not possible to calculate.

From Mackie FL, Rigby A, Morris RK, et al. Prognosis of the co-twin following spontaneous single intrauterine fetal death in twin pregnancies: a systematic review and meta-analysis. BJOG 2019;126(5):569-578; with permission.

underestimation, as early demises may occur before diagnosing TTTS. TTTS is typically staged by the criteria published by Quintero (**Table 2**).[17] The typical presentation is a MC pregnancy with 1 twin developing oligohydramnios and the other twin showing concurrent polyhydramnios. TTTS can develop at any gestational age, with different degrees of severity and with dynamic findings from 1 evaluation to the next. Indeed, some cases demonstrate rapid progression whereas others follow an indolent course. The reasons for the degree of clinical variations are poorly understood and clinicians cannot predict TTTS development, and if a case will demonstrate stable TTTS, or show rapid clinical progression.[18] Although the Quintero staging is helpful for prognostication and for distinguishing mild cases from severe cases, TTTS often does not progress in a linear, stepwise fashion.

Table 2
Staging system for twin-to-twin transfusion syndrome

TTTS Stage	Diagnostic Criteria
1	Donor with <2 cm MVP & recipient with >8 cm MVP
2	Stage 1 criteria plus absent bladder in donor twin
3	Stage 1 or 2 criteria, with any of the following: absent or reversed end-diastolic flow in umbilical artery, pulsatile flow in umbilical vein, or reversed flow in ductus venosus
4	Hydrops fetalis of 1 or both twins
5	Intrauterine demise of 1 or both twins

Abbreviation: MVP, maximum vertical pocket of amniotic fluid.
From Quintero RA, Morales WJ, Allen MH, et al. Staging of twin-twin transfusion syndrome. J Perinatol 1999;19(8 Pt 1):550-555; with permission.

The presence of arteriovenous (AV) anastomoses without compensatory arterioarterial (AA) anastomoses is associated with a higher risk for the development of TTTS (**Fig. 3**),[19] but severe AV imbalance without AA anastomoses is present in 14% of TTTS placentas.[20] The transfusion between fetuses is likely influenced not only by the underlying angioarchitecture but also by the diameter of the vessels involved and the intrinsic placental resistance. About half of TTTS pregnancies have a marginal or velamentous cord insertion,[20] and the smaller twin usually commands a smaller placental area.[4]

If the shift of blood flow becomes hemodynamically significant, the donor becomes hypovolemic and oliguric and the recipient becomes hypervolemic and polyuric. In the donor, the decreased circulating volume activates the renin-angiotensin system (RAS), increasing the tubular reabsorption and the production of angiotensin-2, which causes vasoconstriction to maintain circulating volume. This produces hypertension

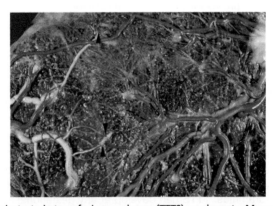

Fig. 3. Effect of twin-to-twin transfusion syndrome (TTTS) on placenta. Monochorionic, diamniotic placenta affected with TTTS with intrauterine demise of both twins. (*Left*) Placental share of the donor twin. (*Right*) Placental share of the recipient twin. The donor twin's arteries are in red and the donor's veins are in yellow. The recipient's arteries are in red and the recipient's veins are in green. (*Black arrows*) Arteriovenous (AV) anastomoses between the recipient on the right and the donor on the left. (*From* De Paepe ME, Shapiro S, Greco D, et al. Placental markers of twin-to-twin transfusion syndrome in diamniotic-monochorionic twins: A morphometric analysis of deep artery-to-vein anastomoses. Placenta 2010;31(4):272; with permission.)

within the donor and may also have the paradoxic effect of decreasing renal and placental perfusion, worsening oliguria and resulting in growth restriction. The observation of decreased or absent diastolic flow in the umbilical artery (UA) of the donor would implicate the effect of the above endocrine products on the vascular tone of the placental bed. In the recipient twin, a variety of mediators may be involved in response to increased blood volume. The increased atrial pressure mediates an increase in cardiac atrial natriuretic peptide synthesis. This increases glomerular filtration rate and decreases tubular reabsorption in the kidney.[21] Suppression of antidiuretic hormone also increases the recipient's production of urine. Downregulation of the RAS is the expected response to the recipient hypervolemia, and study of the recipient kidneys has revealed changes consistent with hypertensive microangiopathy owing to high levels of circulating RAS effectors.[22] These effectors may be transferred from the donor to the recipient through the placental anastomoses. The recipient placenta may also play a role as a source for RAS activation in the recipient twin.[23] Cardiovascular findings in the recipient, such as ventricular hypertrophy, atrioventricular valve regurgitation, and increased pulmonary outflow and aortic outflow velocities can be attributed to volume overload. However, if the changes within the recipient only occur in response to volume loading, there should be an increase in the combined cardiac output. This has not been observed. The observed cardiomegaly appears to result from myocardial hypertrophy rather than cardiac dilation.[24,25] The development of pulmonic stenosis and obstruction of the right ventricular outflow tract would not be expected strictly from volume loading, suggesting an increase in cardiac afterload secondary to the development of systemic hypertension.[26]

Thus, the imbalance of blood volume due to vascular anastomoses initiates a cascade of events in both fetuses that would be adaptive, were they not confined to an intrauterine environment. However, occurring in utero, they lead to the significant morbidity and mortality, which is associated with untreated TTTS. Indeed, outcomes of untreated TTTS are poor in part because TTTS usually appears before fetal viability. Outcomes are improved in TTTS pregnancies treated via laser therapy to ablate the causative intertwin anastomoses. Indeed, 86% of these pregnancies will have survival of 1 twin, and 74% of pregnancies will have survival of both cotwins,[27] although some data suggest a lower survival rate of the smaller, donor twin.[27,28] Notably, 5% of surviving twins will have cerebral palsy, and up to 10% will have neurocognitive impairment.[15,27] Occasionally after laser ablation of anastomoses for TTTS, residual anastomoses may persist after laser ablation (**Fig. 4**) and may lead to recurrent TTTS or twin anemia-polycythemia sequence.[29]

TWIN ANEMIA-POLYCYTHEMIA SEQUENCE

The TAPS is a complication of MC twin pregnancies characterized postnatally by a significant intertwin hemoglobin discordance, with 1 anemic twin and the other twin polycythemic.[30] TAPS can arise spontaneously in utero[31] or iatrogenically after laser treatment of TTTS.[30] The placentas in pregnancies affected by TAPS tend to have smaller and fewer intertwin anastomoses when compared with placentas of pregnancies with TTTS. This results in an overall slower net transfusion from the donor to the recipient in TAPS, compared with TTTS, leading to the donor becoming anemic and the recipient becoming polycythemic. The chronic nature of the unidirectional blood flow allows time for both fetuses to equilibrate to volume shifts. TAPS itself is primarily transfusion of red blood cells, not plasma, between the twins. Notably, either polyhydramnios nor oligohydramnios develops in neither twin, distinguishing TAPS from TTTS, where significant plasma and endocrine factors exchange between fetuses occurs.[14,15,30,32–34]

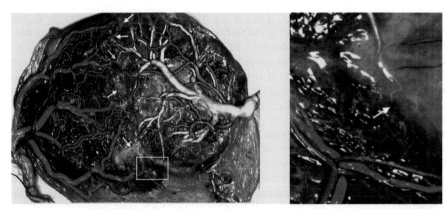

Fig. 4. Effect of laser ablation of a monochorionic, diamniotic placenta affected with TTTS. (*Left*) Monochorionic, diamniotic placenta affected with TTTS with laser ablation of inter-twin anastomoses at approximately 17 weeks' gestation. The placental share of the ex-donor is on the left side of the placenta (arteries are blue, veins are orange). The placental share of the ex-recipient is on the right side (arteries are green, veins are yellow). The white arrows indicate the successfully ablated anastomoses. The light blue arrow indicates a residual venovenous anastomosis. (*Right*) Magnification of a residual arteriovenous anastomosis (diameter <1 mm) between an artery (*blue*) from the ex-donor and a vein (*yellow*) from the ex-recipient. (*From* Lopriore E, Middeldorp JM, Oepkes D, et al. Residual anastomoses after fetoscopic laser surgery in twin-to-twin transfusion syndrome: frequency, associated risks and outcome. Placenta 2007;28(2-3):205; with permission.)

AA anastomoses are protective against development of TAPS, as they mediate bidirectional blood flow and allow equilibration of the volume shifts from the chronic interfetal transfusion (**Fig. 5**).[32,35–38] Placentas affected by TAPS have 10% to 20% AA anastomoses compared with 80% in unaffected MC placentas.[15,32,39] The AA anastomoses in TAPS placentas are smaller than the AA anastomoses in uncomplicated MC

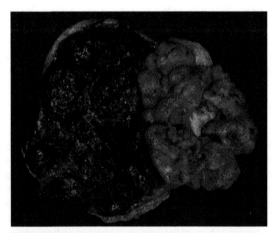

Fig. 5. Monochorionic, diamniotic placenta affected by the twin anemia-polycythemia sequence (TAPS). The left side of the basal plate of the placenta, obviously polycythemic, represents the recipient twin's placental share, and the pale right side of the placenta represents the donor (anemic) twin's placental share. (*From* Fitzgerald B. Histopathological examination of the placenta in twin pregnancies. APMIS 2018;126(7):633; with permission.)

placentas,[40] contributing to the inability of the placenta to compensate for the net unidirectional blood flow.[15,35,41] Another interesting characteristic of TAPS placentas is the placental share of the donor twin is usually greater than the placental share of the recipient, despite the donor twin commonly being the smaller twin.[42] This is opposite of the placental share and fetal growth that is observed in sIUGR (described in detail below). This pattern supports the theory that the overall net blood flow is the primary determinant of fetal growth, rather than percentage of placenta shared, in twin pregnancies complicated by TAPS.[32] A larger placental share is what allows the anemic donor twin to survive.[43] Placentas of pregnancies complicated by post-laser TAPS tend to have fewer intertwin anastomoses and a lower number of AA anastomoses when compared with the spontaneously arising TAPS.[44]

TAPS is diagnosed antenatally by intertwin differential peak systolic velocity within the middle cerebral artery (MCA-PSV) as determined by Doppler velocimetry. TAPS is defined as the donor twin with greater than 1.50 multiples of the median (MoM) in MCA-PSV and the recipient twin having less than 1.0 MoM in MCA-PSV.[45] TAPS can be staged antenatally based on the severity of the intertwin MCA-PSV differential, the presence of UA or vein Doppler changes, or hydrops or demise of either twin (**Table 3**). TAPS can also be staged postnatally based on the intertwin serum hemoglobin concentrations.[45]

Spontaneous TAPS affects ≤5% of MC pregnancies[46–49] and presents later in gestation past the threshold of viability, leading to a lower risk of perinatal morbidity and mortality than TTTS. The later development of the disease process likely is a reflection of the chronic, gradual change in blood flow between the fetuses which allows for hemodynamic compensation, unlike the rapid fluid shifts seen in TTTS.[15,50] The occasional progression of TAPS requires treatment, and can result in premature delivery or IUFD. Serial ultrasound surveillance should be performed when monitoring or surveilling for TAPS, and serial fetal MCA Doppler velocimetry every 2 weeks should be included starting at 16 to 20 weeks' gestation.[7]

TAPS resulting after incomplete laser treatment of TTTS affects 2% to 16% of MC twins after laser therapy,[31,51,52] with the wide range related to surgical technique and diagnostic criteria in the published literature.[32] TAPS evolves when anastomoses remain, despite the attempt to ablate them all. Anastomoses at the periphery may be too small to visualize. The Solomon technique decreases the number of residual

Table 3		
Antenatal staging criteria for the twin anemia-polycythemia sequence		
TAPS Stage	**Diagnostic Criteria**	
1	Donor with >1.50 MoM MCA-PSV and recipient with <1.00 MoM MCA-PSV	
2	Donor with >1.70 MoM MCA-PSV and recipient with <0.80 MoM MCA-PSV	
3	Meets stage 1 or 2 criteria, with any of the following: absent or reversed end-diastolic flow in umbilical artery, pulsatile flow in umbilical vein, or increased pulsatility index or reversed flow in the ductus venosus	
4	Hydrops fetalis of donor twin	
5	Intrauterine demise of 1 or both twins	

Abbreviations: MCA-PSV, middle cerebral artery peak systolic velocity; MoM, multiples of the median.

Adapted from Slaghekke F, Kist WJ, Oepkes D, et al. Twin Anemia-Polycythemia Sequence: Diagnostic Criteria, Classification, Perinatal Management and Outcome. Fetal Diagn Ther 2010;27(4):185; with permission.

anastomoses.[52] Post-laser TAPS typically presents 1 to 5 weeks after laser treatment,[31] and often the former donor becomes polycythemic and the former recipient becomes anemic, contrary to what may be expected.[32,53,54] The mechanism for this may be related to the former recipient twin's colloid osmotic pressure being markedly elevated before and shortly after the laser procedure, with the osmotic pressure subsequently driving fluid from the maternal circulation to the former recipient's circulation, thereby expanding blood volume.[55] This may also explain why the former recipient does not develop oligohydramnios after becoming the TAPS donor.[32] Long-term outcome data in TAPS are lacking. One small cohort study found that twins with TAPS had similar rates of perinatal mortality, cerebral injury, and severe neonatal morbidity when compared with similarly matched unaffected MC twins.[56]

SELECTIVE INTRAUTERINE GROWTH RESTRICTION

sIUGR describes MC pregnancies in which the twins have significantly different growth patterns. sIUGR is typically defined as 1 twin $\leq$10th percentile estimated fetal weight (EFW) and an EFW discordance of $\geq$ 25% between the twins.[7,57,58] Notably, sIUGR is used when the twin with the appropriate EFW has a normal amniotic fluid volume, that is, when there is no evidence of TTTS. Distinguishing sIUGR from TTTS can be challenging as they can coexist, which is associated with a worse prognosis for the growth-restricted twin.

sIUGR results from the MC placenta being unequally shared, with a larger placental territory supplying the larger fetus.[19,42,57,59–63] A marginal or velamentous cord insertion is associated with an increased risk of sIUGR.[61,62,64]

sIUGR is classified into 3 types, characterized by the UA Doppler waveforms in the growth-restricted twin,[65] reflecting different arrangements and types of intertwin vascular anastomoses within the MC placenta.[19,42,61,62] Type 1 sIUGR is characterized by constant forward (normal) flow through the UA during diastole in the growth-restricted twin (**Fig. 6**). The presence of diastolic flow is indicative that the discrepancy between the placental territories supplying each twin is mild to moderate in magnitude. Seventy percent of type 1 sIUGR pregnancies have multiple AA intertwin anastomoses,[15] which allow bidirectional intertwin blood flow, thus supplying the smaller fetus with nutrients and oxygenated blood while also mitigating the impact of the smaller placental mass available to the growth-restricted fetus. A recent meta-analysis[63] demonstrated a smaller birth weight discordance (23% vs. 44%)

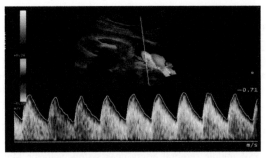

Fig. 6. Umbilical artery Doppler velocimetry of a monochorionic, diamniotic twin pregnancy affected with type 1 selective intrauterine growth restriction. Note the constant presence of forward end-diastolic flow in the umbilical artery waveform. (*Courtesy of* M.W. Bebbington, MD, MHSc, St. Louis, MO.)

and lower perinatal mortality (4% vs. 16%) when compared with type 2 sIUGR. The smaller placental territory imbalance between the twins and the AA anastomoses explain the better perinatal outcomes in type 1.

Type 2 sIUGR is characterized by persistently absent or reversed flow through the UA at the end of diastole in the growth-restricted twin (**Fig. 7**). The placental territory difference between the twins is greater than in type 1, with the smaller fetus commanding a smaller fraction of placenta. There tends to be fewer AA placental anastomoses, which are usually smaller in diameter,[15] limiting the amount of bidirectional blood flow that can be exchanged between the twins. As a result, there is a decreased overall ability to compensate the growth-restricted fetus, and the pregnancies are more likely to deteriorate earlier in gestation.[15,62,65,66] UA Doppler changes in type 2 sIUGR tend to be progressive throughout gestation. There is persistent absent end-diastolic flow, progressing to reversed end-diastolic flow, and ultimately necessitating earlier delivery. Type 2 sIUGR progresses slower than singleton or dichorionic IUGR pregnancies.[67] Perinatal outcomes are worse in type 2 compared with type 1, including a 4-fold higher risk of perinatal mortality, earlier gestational age at delivery, and more pronounced birth weight discordance.[63]

Type 3 sIUGR is characterized by intermittently absent or reversed flow through the UA at the end of diastole in the growth-restricted twin (**Fig. 8**). This pattern is only observed in MC placentas and indicates a large number and size of AA anastomoses,[68–70] with 98% of type 3 placentas having greater than 2 mm AA anastomoses.[15] The intermittent abnormal patterns represent the systolic waveform of the larger twin being transmitted through the AA anastomoses, into the UA of the smaller fetus. Both twins pump into common vessels, but from opposite directions. The balance point shifts as the intravascular pressures between the 2 fluctuate. The balance point is also affected by the synchronicity of each twin's cardiac cycle compared with the other twin's cardiac cycle, which varies with the fetal heart rate and the different blood pressure in systole compared with diastole. The constantly shifting balance point is reflected in the UA Doppler waveforms by the variable end-diastolic flow in the IUGR twin, with periods of normal flow mixed with periods of end-diastolic flow that is, absent or reversed. Importantly, the Doppler pattern in type 3 contrasts with singleton IUGR pregnancies by reflecting the total vascular resistance, rather than solely the placental resistance.

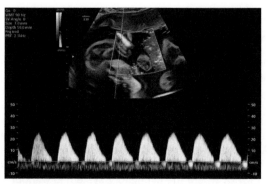

Fig. 7. Umbilical artery Doppler velocimetry of a monochorionic diamniotic twin pregnancy affected with Type 2 selective intrauterine growth restriction (sIUGR). (*Courtesy of* M.W. Bebbington, MD, MHSc, St. Louis, MO.)

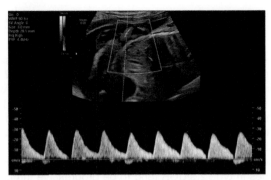

Fig. 8. Umbilical artery Doppler velocimetry of a monochorionic, diamniotic twin pregnancy affected by type 3 selective intrauterine growth restriction (sIUGR). (*Courtesy of* M.W. Bebbington, MD, MHSc, St. Louis, MO.)

The magnitude of the reversal observed in the growth-restricted fetus' UA Dopplers is affected by the growth discordance between the twins, the distance between the placental cord insertion sites (with decreasing distance increasing the magnitude of the reversal of flow), and the number and size of the AA anastomoses.[62,68,69] The placental territory discordance between the twins is unpredictable in type 3. The large AA connections allow for constant bidirectional blood flow between the twins, which can compensate for placental territory discordance. In such cases, the nongrowth-restricted fetus serves as a pump for the smaller twin through the vast AA network, which explains why the normal-sized twin shows evidence of hypertrophic cardiomyopathy-type cardiac changes in 20% of type 3 pregnancies compared with 2% of type 1 or 2.[62,71]

The large AA blood flow also has risks. Hypotensive events or episodes of bradycardia in the smaller twin can result in a larger hemodynamic pressure gradient between the 2 fetuses, causing a volume shift from the normal twin to the growth restricted twin. This rapid volume shift can lead to demise from hypovolemia or ischemic neurologic injury in the larger twin and demise of the growth-restricted fetus from acute hypervolemia.[42,65] Because these events are sudden and unpredictable, the clinical course of type 3 sIUGR is unpredictable. IUFD occurs despite recent normal Dopplers, raising challenges in the clinical management of these pregnancies.[62,63]

TWIN REVERSED ARTERIAL PERFUSION SEQUENCE

The TRAP sequence affects 2.6% of all MC pregnancies and approximately 1 in 9500 to 11,000 of all pregnancies.[72] The TRAP sequence only affects MC pregnancies and is present when a normal donor, or pump twin, provides all of the circulatory support for the second twin, which is dysmorphic and either has no heart or has a heart that is, rudimentary and nonfunctional, referred to as "acardiac."[73] There are generally 2 criteria that must be present for the TRAP sequence to develop. The first is the presence of a large AA anastomosis connecting the circulations of both fetuses within the placenta (**Fig. 9**). The second is either a malformation or agenesis of the heart in the second twin, or an IUFD, where the circulatory system is without a functional heart to maintain blood pressure within the second twin.[73–75] Fulfillment of these 2 criteria allows for blood flow directly from the UA of the normal twin into an UA of the acardiac twin in a retrograde manner, hence the description of reversed arterial perfusion.[34] Of

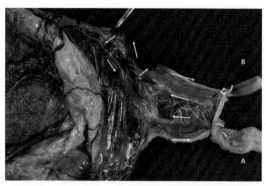

Fig. 9. Arterioarterial anastomosis in Twin Reversed Arterial Perfusion (TRAP) Sequence. Arterioarterial anastomosis between the 2 umbilical cords in a monochorionic diamniotic twin gestation affected by TRAP sequence. The white arrows point out the direction of arterial blood flow from the umbilical artery of the Pump fetus (*B*) directly into the umbilical artery of the TRAP fetus (*A*). The yellow arrows show direction of venous blood from the TRAP fetus back to the pump twin. (*Courtesy of* M.W. Bebbington, MD, MHSc, St. Louis, MO.)

note, acardiac twins typically have a single UA.[4] Because the blood flows from the UA of the normal twin, the acardiac twin is supplied with deoxygenated blood. Furthermore, because the acardiac twin receives blood via retrograde flow through the UA, a branch off the internal iliac artery, the caudal portion of the acardiac fetus receives

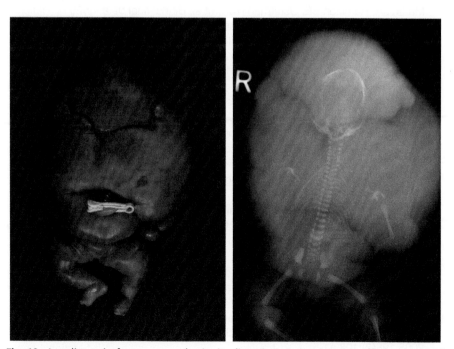

Fig. 10. Acardiac twin from a monochorionic, diamniotic twin gestation affected by TRAP sequence. (*Left*) Gross photograph of the obviously dysmorphic acardiac (recipient) twin. (*Right*) Plain radiograph of the same twin demonstrating a relatively preserved skeletal system. (*Courtesy of* M.W. Bebbington, MD, MHSc, St. Louis, MO.)

most of the bloody supply. The dysmorphic fetus commonly has preserved lower limbs but typically has upper body, cardiac, and central nervous system anomalies (**Fig. 10**).[4,15]

Blood usually returns from the acardiac twin to the normal twin via a venovenous anastomosis. The acardiac fetus is entirely dependent on the normal twin for blood supply, and the normal twin is thus at risk for high output cardiac failure,[76] development of polyhydramnios, preterm delivery, and IUFD.[15] Strikingly, the perinatal mortality of the normal twin in untreated TRAP approaches 50%.[75,77]

SUMMARY

Detailed placental evaluation of twin gestations, especially MC diamniotic twins, is important in understanding the complications associated with these complex pregnancies. Knowing the clinical correlations of placental anatomy and function in these gestations helps perinatal pathologists perform a more informed placental evaluation, which in turn provides the obstetrician and neonatologist with a more comprehensive understanding of each patient's case. This ultimately allows for better care for the mother and her children.

DISCLOSURE

The authors have no financial disclosures or conflicts of interest to report.

REFERENCES

1. Martin JA, Hamilton BE, Osterman MJK, et al. Births: final data for 2017. National vital statistics reports: from the Centers for Disease Control and Prevention, National Center for Health Statistics. Natl Vital Stat Syst 2018;67(8):1–50.
2. Chauhan SP, Scardo JA, Hayes E, et al. Twins: prevalence, problems, and preterm births. Am J Obstet Gynecol 2010;203(4):305–15.
3. Schachter M. Monozygotic twinning after assisted reproductive techniques: a phenomenon independent of micromanipulation. Hum Reprod 2001;16(6): 1264–9.
4. Paepe MED. Examination of the twin placenta. Semin Perinatol 2015;39(1):27–35.
5. Derom C, Vlietinck R, Derom R, et al. Increased monozygotic twinning rate after ovulation induction. Lancet 1987;1(8544):1236–8.
6. Hall JG. Twinning: mechanisms and genetic implications. Curr Opin Genet Dev 1996;6(3):343–7.
7. Khalil A, Rodgers M, Baschat A, et al. ISUOG practice guidelines: role of ultrasound in twin pregnancy. Ultrasound Obstet Gynecol 2016;47(2):247–63.
8. Moise KJ Jr, Johnson A. There is NO diagnosis of twins. Am J Obstet Gynecol 2010;203(1):1–2.
9. Rossi AC, D'Addario V. Umbilical cord occlusion for selective feticide in complicated monochorionic twins: a systematic review of literature. Am J Obstet Gynecol 2009;200(2):123–9.
10. Moise KJ Jr, Johnson A, Moise KY, et al. Radiofrequency ablation for selective reduction in the complicated monochorionic gestation. Am J Obstet Gynecol 2008;198(2):198.e1-5.
11. Roman A, Papanna R, Johnson A, et al. Selective reduction in complicated monochorionic pregnancies: radiofrequency ablation vs. bipolar cord coagulation. Ultrasound Obstet Gynecol 2010;36(1):37–41.

12. Mackie FL, Rigby A, Morris RK, et al. Prognosis of the co-twin following sponta-neous single intrauterine fetal death in twin pregnancies: a systematic review and meta-analysis. BJOG 2019;126(5):569–78.

13. Bebbington M. Selective reduction in complex monochorionic gestations. Am J Perinatol 2014;31(Suppl 1):S51–8.

14. Zhao D, de Villiers SF, Oepkes D, et al. Monochorionic twin placentas: injection technique and analysis. Diagnóstico Prenatal 2014;25(2):35–42.

15. Lewi L, Deprest J, Hecher K. The vascular anastomoses in monochorionic twin pregnancies and their clinical consequences. Am J Obstet Gynecol 2013; 208(1):19–30.

16. Sebire NJ, Snijders RJ, Hughes K, et al. The hidden mortality of monochorionic twin pregnancies. Br J Obstet Gynaecol 1997;104(10):1203–7.

17. Quintero RA, Morales WJ, Allen MH, et al. Staging of twin-twin transfusion syn-drome. J Perinatol 1999;19(8 Pt 1):550–5.

18. Bebbington M. Twin-to-twin transfusion syndrome: current understanding of path-ophysiology, in-utero therapy and impact for future development. Semin Fetal Neonatal Med 2010;15(1):15–20.

19. Denbow ML, Cox P, Taylor M, et al. Placental angioarchitecture in monochorionic twin pregnancies: relationship to fetal growth, fetofetal transfusion syndrome, and pregnancy outcome. Am J Obstet Gynecol 2000;182(2):417–26.

20. De Paepe ME, Shapiro S, Greco D, et al. Placental markers of twin-to-twin trans-fusion syndrome in diamniotic–monochorionic twins: a morphometric analysis of deep artery-to-vein anastomoses. Placenta 2010;31(4):269–76.

21. Bajoria R, Ward S, Sooranna SR. Atrial natriuretic peptide mediated polyuria: pathogenesis of polyhydramnios in the recipient twin of twin-twin transfusion syn-drome. Placenta 2001;22(8–9):716–24.

22. Mahieu-Caputo D, Meulemans A, Martinovic J, et al. Paradoxic activation of the renin-angiotensin system in twin-twin transfusion syndrome: an explanation for cardiovascular disturbances in the recipient. Pediatr Res 2005;58(4):685–8.

23. Galea P, Barigye O, Wee L, et al. The placenta contributes to activation of the renin angiotensin system in twin–twin transfusion syndrome. Placenta 2008; 29(8):734–42.

24. Wohlmuth C, Boudreaux D, Moise KJ Jr, et al. Cardiac pathophysiology in twin-twin transfusion syndrome: new insights into its evolution. Ultrasound Obstet Gy-necol 2018;51(3):341–8.

25. Barrea C, Alkazaleh F, Ryan G, et al. Prenatal cardiovascular manifestations in the twin-to-twin transfusion syndrome recipients and the impact of therapeutic am-nioreduction. Am J Obstet Gynecol 2005;192(3):892–902.

26. Mahieu-Caputo D, Salomon LJ, Le Bidois J, et al. Fetal hypertension: an insight into the pathogenesis of the twin-twin transfusion syndrome. Prenat Diagn 2003;23(8):640–5.

27. Snowise S, Moise KJ, Johnson A, et al. Donor death after selective fetoscopic laser surgery for twin-twin transfusion syndrome. Obstet Gynecol 2015;126(1): 74–80.

28. Rossi AC, D'Addario V. Comparison of donor and recipient outcomes following laser therapy performed for twin-twin transfusion syndrome: a meta-analysis and review of literature. Am J Perinatol 2009;26(1):27–32.

29. Lopriore E, Middeldorp JM, Oepkes D, et al. Residual anastomoses after feto-scopic laser surgery in twin-to-twin transfusion syndrome: frequency, associated risks and outcome. Placenta 2007;28(2–3):204–8.

30. Lopriore E, Middeldorp JM, Oepkes D, et al. Twin anemia–polycythemia sequence in two monochorionic twin pairs without oligo-polyhydramnios sequence. Placenta 2007;28(1):47–51.

31. Robyr R, Lewi L, Salomon LJ, et al. Prevalence and management of late fetal complications following successful selective laser coagulation of chorionic plate anastomoses in twin-to-twin transfusion syndrome. Am J Obstet Gynecol 2006; 194(3):796–803.

32. Tollenaar LSA, Slaghekke F, Middeldorp JM, et al. Twin anemia polycythemia sequence: current views on pathogenesis, diagnostic criteria, perinatal management, and outcome. Twin Res Hum Genet 2016;19(3):222–33.

33. Moaddab A, Nassr AA, Espinoza J, et al. Twin anemia polycythemia sequence: a single center experience and literature review. Eur J Obstet Gynecol Reprod Biol 2016;205:158–64.

34. Couck I, Lewi L. The placenta in twin-to-twin transfusion syndrome and twin anemia polycythemia sequence. Twin Res Hum Genet 2016;19(03):184–90.

35. De Villiers S, Slaghekke F, Middeldorp JM, et al. Arterio-arterial vascular anastomoses in monochorionic twin placentas with and without twin anemia-polycythemia sequence. Placenta 2012;33(3):227–9.

36. Lopriore E, van den Wijngaard JP, Middeldorp JM, et al. Assessment of feto-fetal transfusion flow through placental arterio-venous anastomoses in a unique case of twin-to-twin transfusion syndrome. Placenta 2007;28(2–3):209–11.

37. Suzuki S. Twin anemia-polycythemia sequence with placental arterio-arterial anastomoses. Placenta 2010;31(7):652.

38. van Meir H, Slaghekke F, Lopriore E, et al. Arterio-arterial anastomoses do not prevent the development of twin anemia-polycythemia sequence. Placenta 2010;31(2):163–5.

39. Fitzgerald B. Histopathological examination of the placenta in twin pregnancies. APMIS 2018;126(7):626–37.

40. Zhao DP, de Villiers SF, Slaghekke F, et al. Prevalence, size, number and localization of vascular anastomoses in monochorionic placentas. Placenta 2013; 34(7):589–93.

41. Lopriore E, Deprest J, Slaghekke F, et al. Placental characteristics in monochorionic twins with and without twin anemia-polycythemia sequence. Obstet Gynecol 2008;112(4):753–8.

42. Lewi L, Cannie M, Blickstein I, et al. Placental sharing, birthweight discordance, and vascular anastomoses in monochorionic diamniotic twin placentas. Am J Obstet Gynecol 2007;197(6):587.e1-8.

43. Zhao D, Slaghekke F, Middeldorp JM, et al. Placental share and hemoglobin level in relation to birth weight in twin anemia-polycythemia sequence. Placenta 2014; 35(12):1070–4.

44. De Villiers SF, Slaghekke F, Middeldorp JM, et al. Placental characteristics in monochorionic twins with spontaneous versus post-laser twin anemia-polycythemia sequence. Placenta 2013;34(5):456–9.

45. Slaghekke F, Kist WJ, Oepkes D, et al. Twin anemia-polycythemia sequence: diagnostic criteria, classification, perinatal management and outcome. Fetal Diagn Ther 2010;27(4):181–90.

46. Gucciardo L, Lewi L, Vaast P, et al. Twin anemia polycythemia sequence from a prenatal perspective. Prenat Diagn 2010;30(5):438–42.

47. Lewi L, Jani J, Blickstein I, et al. The outcome of monochorionic diamniotic twin gestations in the era of invasive fetal therapy: a prospective cohort study. Am J Obstet Gynecol 2008;199(5):514.e1-8.

48. Lopriore E, Slaghekke F, Middeldorp JM, et al. Residual anastomoses in twin-to-twin transfusion syndrome treated with selective fetoscopic laser surgery: localization, size, and consequences. Am J Obstet Gynecol 2009;201(1):66.e1-4.

49. Yokouchi T, Murakoshi T, Mishima T, et al. Incidence of spontaneous twin anemia-polycythemia sequence in monochorionic-diamniotic twin pregnancies: single-center prospective study. J Obstet Gynaecol Res 2015;41(6):857–60.

50. Tollenaar LSA, Zhao DP, Middeldorp JM, et al. Can color difference on the maternal side of the placenta distinguish between acute peripartum twin–twin transfusion syndrome and twin anemia–polycythemia sequence? Placenta 2017;57:189–93.

51. Habli M, Bombrys A, Lewis D, et al. Incidence of complications in twin-twin transfusion syndrome after selective fetoscopic laser photocoagulation: a single-center experience. Am J Obstet Gynecol 2009;201(4):417.e1-7.

52. Slaghekke F, Lewi L, Middeldorp JM, et al. Residual anastomoses in twin-twin transfusion syndrome after laser: the Solomon randomized trial. Am J Obstet Gynecol 2014;211(3):285.e1-7.

53. Lewi L, Jani J, Cannie M, et al. Intertwin anastomoses in monochorionic placentas after fetoscopic laser coagulation for twin-to-twin transfusion syndrome: is there more than meets the eye? Am J Obstet Gynecol 2006;194(3):790–5.

54. Yamamoto M, El Murr L, Robyr R, et al. Incidence and impact of perioperative complications in 175 fetoscopy-guided laser coagulations of chorionic plate anastomoses in fetofetal transfusion syndrome before 26 weeks of gestation. Am J Obstet Gynecol 2005;193(3 Pt 2):1110–6.

55. van den Wijngaard JP, Lewi L, Lopriore E, et al. Modeling severely discordant hematocrits and normal amniotic fluids after incomplete laser therapy in twin-to-twin transfusion syndrome. Placenta 2007;28(7):611–5.

56. Lopriore E, Slaghekke F, Oepkes D, et al. Clinical outcome in neonates with twin anemia-polycythemia sequence. Am J Obstet Gynecol 2010;203(1):54.e1-5.

57. Lewi L, Gucciardo L, Huber A, et al. Clinical outcome and placental characteristics of monochorionic diamniotic twin pairs with early- and late-onset discordant growth. Am J Obstet Gynecol 2008;199(5):511.e1-7.

58. Valsky DV, Eixarch E, Martinez JM, et al. Selective intrauterine growth restriction in monochorionic diamniotic twin pregnancies. Prenat Diagn 2010;30(8):719–26.

59. Fick AL, Feldstein VA, Norton ME, et al. Unequal placental sharing and birth weight discordance in monochorionic diamniotic twins. Am J Obstet Gynecol 2006;195(1):178–83.

60. Chang Y-L, Chang S-D, Chao A-S, et al. Clinical outcome and placental territory ratio of monochorionic twin pregnancies and selective intrauterine growth restriction with different types of umbilical artery Doppler. Prenat Diagn 2009;29(3):253–6.

61. Lopriore E, Pasman SA, Klumper FJ, et al. Placental characteristics in growth-discordant monochorionic twins: a matched case-control study. Placenta 2012;33(3):171–4.

62. Bennasar M, Eixarch E, Martinez JM, et al. Selective intrauterine growth restriction in monochorionic diamniotic twin pregnancies. Semin Fetal neonatal Med 2017;22(6):376–82.

63. Buca D, Pagani G, Rizzo G, et al. Outcome of monochorionic twin pregnancy with selective intrauterine growth restriction according to umbilical artery Doppler flow pattern of smaller twin: systematic review and meta-analysis. Ultrasound Obstet Gynecol 2017;50(5):559–68.

64. Machin GA. Velamentous cord insertion in monochorionic twin gestation. An added risk factor. J Reprod Med 1997;42(12):785–9.
65. Gratacós E, Lewi L, Muñoz B, et al. A classification system for selective intrauterine growth restriction in monochorionic pregnancies according to umbilical artery Doppler flow in the smaller twin. Ultrasound Obstet Gynecol 2007;30(1):28–34.
66. Ishii K, Murakoshi T, Takahashi Y, et al. Perinatal outcome of monochorionic twins with selective intrauterine growth restriction and different types of umbilical artery Doppler under expectant management. Fetal Diagn Ther 2009;26(3):157–61.
67. Vanderheyden TM, Fichera A, Pasquini L, et al. Increased latency of absent end-diastolic flow in the umbilical artery of monochorionic twin fetuses. Ultrasound Obstet Gynecol 2005;26(1):44–9.
68. Wee LY, Taylor MJ, Vanderheyden T, et al. Transmitted arterio-arterial anastomosis waveforms causing cyclically intermittent absent/reversed end-diastolic umbilical artery flow in monochorionic twins. Placenta 2003;24(7):772–8.
69. Gratacós E, Lewi L, Carreras E, et al. Incidence and characteristics of umbilical artery intermittent absent and/or reversed end-diastolic flow in complicated and uncomplicated monochorionic twin pregnancies. Ultrasound Obstet Gynecol 2004;23(5):456–60.
70. Gratacós E, Antolin E, Lewi L, et al. Monochorionic twins with selective intrauterine growth restriction and intermittent absent or reversed end-diastolic flow (type III): feasibility and perinatal outcome of fetoscopic placental laser coagulation. Ultrasound Obstet Gynecol 2008;31(6):669–75.
71. Muñoz-Abellana B, Hernandez-Andrade E, Figueroa-Diesel H, et al. Hypertrophic cardiomyopathy-like changes in monochorionic twin pregnancies with selective intrauterine growth restriction and intermittent absent/reversed end-diastolic flow in the umbilical artery. Ultrasound Obstet Gynecol 2007;30(7):977–82.
72. Van Gemert MJC, Van Den Wijngaard JPHM, Vandenbussche FPHA. Twin reversed arterial perfusion sequence is more common than generally accepted. Birth Defects Res A Clin Mol Teratol 2015;103(7):641–3.
73. Van Allen MI, Smith DW, Shepard TH. Twin reversed arterial perfusion (TRAP) sequence: a study of 14 twin pregnancies with acardius. Semin Perinatol 1983;7(4):285–93.
74. Gembruch U, Viski S, Bagamery K, et al. Twin reversed arterial perfusion sequence in twin-to-twin transfusion syndrome after the death of the donor co-twin in the second trimester. Ultrasound Obstet Gynecol 2001;17(2):153–6.
75. Moore TR, Gale S, Benirschke K. Perinatal outcome of forty-nine pregnancies complicated by acardiac twinning. Am J Obstet Gynecol 1990;163(3):907–12.
76. Van Gemert MJC, Ross MG, Nikkels PGJ, et al. Acardiac twin pregnancies part III: model simulations. Birth Defects Res A Clin Mol Teratol 2016;106(12):1008–15.
77. Healey MG. Acardia: predictive risk factors for the co-twin's survival. Teratology 1994;50(3):205–13.

Placental Implantation Disorders

Eric Jauniaux, MD, PhD, FRCOG[a],*, Ashley Moffett, MD, MRCP, MRCPath, FRCOG[b],
Graham J. Burton, MD, DSc[c]

KEYWORDS

- Placenta • Previa • Accreta • Circumvallate • Velamentous insertion
- Cesarean section • In vitro fertilization

KEY POINTS

- The main disorders of placental implantation are associated with a high maternal and fetal morbidity and possible mortality.
- Placental implantation disorders are essentially iatrogenic, with more than 90% of cases resulting from multiple cesarean deliveries and in vitro fertilization.
- In vitro fertilization has been associated with blastocyst malrotation at implantation leading to low-lying/placenta previa and velamentous insertion of the umbilical cord.
- Caesarean scars have become the leading predisposing factor for placenta previa accreta in subsequent pregnancies.

INTRODUCTION

Primary placental implantation disorders have been known to midwives and obstetricians for at least 100 years. Overall, these anomalies have only been described in human pregnancies and are associated with a high risk of antenatal and perinatal complications. Thus they cannot be considered as an evolutionary reproductive advantage. Their etiopathology is still not completely understood, but their prevalence and incidence are increased by iatrogenic factors that may have a direct or indirect impact on the functional integrity of the endometrium.

The most common of these congenital disorders, placenta previa, may have been first described by Hippocrates (460–370 BC) in "De Superfoeratione" and "De Morbis Mulierum".[1] In his apocryphal writings, he highlights the main signs: "a great flow of blood without pain occurring to the parturient before birth of the child" and "the

[a] Academic Department of Obstetrics and Gynaecology, The EGA Institute for Women's Health, University College London (UCL), 86-96 Chenies Mews, London WC1E 6HX, UK; [b] Department of Pathology, Centre for Trophoblast Research, University of Cambridge, Tennis Court Road, Cambridge CB2 1QP, UK; [c] Department of Physiology, Development and Neuroscience, The Centre for Trophoblast Research, University of Cambridge, Physiology Building, Downing Street, Cambridge CB2 3EG, UK
* Corresponding author.
E-mail address: e.jauniaux@ucl.ac.uk

Obstet Gynecol Clin N Am 47 (2020) 117–132
https://doi.org/10.1016/j.ogc.2019.10.002
0889-8545/20/© 2019 Elsevier Inc. All rights reserved.

obgyn.theclinics.com

placenta is delivered before the child", both of which have been used since in the clinical diagnosis of the condition. When undiagnosed before delivery, placenta previa is associated with high maternal and fetal mortality, and in 1878 the famous Scottish obstetrician Charles Bell described placenta previa as "the most dreaded complication in midwifery."[2] Not surprisingly, when radiology was developed one of its first uses in obstetric practice was the prenatal diagnosis of placenta previa.[3] With the development of ultrasound imaging, screening for placenta previa has become an essential part of the routine detailed mid-trimester fetal anomaly scan.

Other primary placental anomalies of implantation include placenta accreta spectrum (PAS), abnormal insertion of the umbilical cord, and abnormal placental shape. These anomalies were first described by obstetricians during the first half of the 20th century when they were still extremely rare.[4–6] Both PAS and velamentous cord insertion (VCI) have been associated with a high risk of perinatal complications, and their incidence has risen rapidly in the last 2 decades with the increased use of caesarean delivery (CD) and artificial reproduction technologies (ARTs), and in particular with in vitro fertilization (IVF). Thus, primary placental anomalies of implantation are a consequence of modern obstetric and reproductive practices, and are likely to become increasingly common as women delay childbearing, require reproductive assistance, and enter pregnancy with medical comorbidities. This article aims to describe and discuss current knowledge of the epidemiology and pathophysiology of primary intrauterine placental anomalies of implantation. Placental hematomas and placenta abruptio are secondary anomalies of placentation caused by the rupture of one or more spiral arteries. As their epidemiology is heterogeneous and etiopathology different from that of placental anomalies resulting from a primary abnormal implantation process, they have not been included in this article.

LOW-LYING PLACENTA AND PLACENTA PREVIA

Placenta previa now has a prevalence of 5 cases per 1000 (1 in 200) pregnancies and is caused by the implantation of the placenta fully or partially in the lower uterine segment.[7] The term placenta previa should only be used when the placenta lies directly over the internal os of the uterine cervix. If the placental edge is less than 2 cm from the internal os, but not covering it, at the 20-week detailed anatomy scan, the placenta should be labeled as low-lying. The increase in distance between the lower placental edge and the cervix that occurs normally with advancing gestation following the development of the lower uterine segment during the third trimester of pregnancy results in resolution of a low-lying placenta in 90% of cases before 37 weeks.[7]

Placenta previa is associated with prior CD, use of ART, and maternal smoking (**Table 1**). With CD rates ranging between 20% and 50% in most high- and medium-income countries, a prior CD is the most common risk factor for placenta previa in subsequent pregnancies. This association has been confirmed by several systematic reviews and meta-analyses with a significant dose-response pattern in women with multiple prior CDs.[9–12] A CD will result in major structural changes with formation of scar tissue in the lower uterine segment that is likely to modify the directionality of the physiologic uterine peristaltic waves and thus the flow of intrauterine endometrial secretions. Repeat CDs are also often associated with the development of large scar defects or niches,[20] which can also affect intrauterine flow, leading to more blastocysts implanting around or within the lower segment scar area.

ARTs, and in particular IVF, have also been associated with a higher incidence of placenta previa independently of the high rate of multiple pregnancies.[13–16] A large

Table 1
Clinical variables associated with placenta previa in large epidemiologic studies and systematic reviews

Variables	Author, Year/Type of Study	Risk Calculation for Placenta Previa
Prior CD	Ananth et al,[8] 1997/SR&MA of 3.7 million pregnancies including 170,640 with data on the numbers of prior CDs	Overall RR: 2.6 (95% CI 2.3–3.0) RR after 1 CD: 4.5 (95% CI 3.6–5.5) RR after 2 CDs: 7.4 (95% CI 7.1–7.7) RR after 3 CD: 6.5 (95% CI 6.6–11.6) RR after >3 CDs: 44.9 (95% CI 13.5–149.5)
	Getahun et al,[9] 2006/cohort study of 187,577 singleton pregnancies	RR after 1 CD: 1.5 (95% CI 1.3–1.8) RR after 2 CDs: 2.0 (95% CI 1.3–3.0)
	Marshall et al,[10] 2011/SR&MA of 2,282,922 deliveries	Summary OR: 1.48–3.95
	Klar et al,[11] 2014/SR&MA of prior CDs	Summary RR: 1.47 (95% CI:1.44–1.51) Summary OR: 1.62 (95% CI:1.42–1.86)
	Keag et al,[12] 2018/SR&MA of 7,101,692 prior CDs	OR: 1.74 (95% CI 1.62–1.87)
IVF	Grady et al,[13] 2012/SR&MA of 269 single embryo transfer	RR: 6.02 (95% CI 2.79–13.01)
	Ginstrom Ernstad et al,[14] 2016/ population-based study of 4819 singleton pregnancies after blastocyst transfer	aOR: 6.38 (95% CI 5.31–7.66)
	Qin et al,[15] 2016/SR&MA of 161,370 ART conceived singleton pregnancies	RR: 3.71 (95% CI 2.67–5.16)
	Karami et al,[16] 2018/SR&MA of singleton and twin ART conceived pregnancies	Singleton aOR: 2.59 (95% CI 1.70–3.48) Twins aOR: 2.91 (95% CI 1.08–4.73)
Smoking	Aliyu et al,[17] 2011/population-based study of 1,224,133 singleton pregnancies	OR: 1.34 (95% CI 1.27–1.45)
	Rombauts et al,[18] 2014/4537 ART conceived singleton pregnancies	aOR: 2.58 (95% CI 1.07–6.24)
	Shobeiri et al,[19] 2017/SR&MA of 9,094,443 participants	OR: 1.42 (95% CI 1.30–1.54) RR: 1.27 (95% CI 1.18–1.35)

Abbreviations: aOR, adjusted odds ratio; CD, cesarean delivery; MA, meta-analysis; OR, odds ratio; RR, relative risk; SR, systematic review.

Swedish population-based retrospective registry study analysis found that the risk of placenta previa is higher in pregnancies after blastocyst transfer compared with pregnancies after cleavage-stage replacements (adjusted odds ratio [aOR], 2.08; 95% confidence interval [CI], 1.70–2.55) and to spontaneous conceptions (aOR, 6.38; 95% CI, 5.31–7.66).[21] Overall, these findings suggest that the technique of transcervical embryo transfer, even if the catheter is inserted high within the uterine cavity, changes the physiologic interaction between the blastocyst and the endometrium and/or intrauterine flows. By contrast to pregnancies after CD or resulting from ART, there have been contradictory reports regarding the incidence of placenta previa in multiple gestation pregnancies (MGPs). One would assume that additional placental volume would increase the risk of abnormal placental location; however, a national retrospective cohort study of 1,172,405 twin live births and stillbirths in the United States from 1989 through 1998 found no increased risk in twins.[22] A recent retrospective cohort of 67,895 singleton and twin pregnancies found that both dichorionic and monochorionic twins had an increased risk of placenta previa (aOR 1.54, 95% CI 1.15–2.06 and RR 3.29, 95% CI 1.32–8.21, respectively) compared to singleton.[23]

Maternal smoking before and during pregnancy is an independent risk factor for placenta previa.[17–19] Smoking alters the epithelial development of many organs and tissues, and in particular of the uterine endometrium. The expression of regulatory cytokines and receptivity markers, such as the C-X-C motif chemokine ligand 12 (CXCL12) and fibroblast growth factor 2 (FGF2), is decreased in women who smoke compared with nonsmokers.[24] Smoking also inhibits recruitment of bone marrow-derived stem cells to the uterus and stem cell differentiation[25] and increases the endometrial content of cadmium and lead.[26] These findings suggest that endometrial receptivity is altered in women who smoke, and could explain previa implantation in spontaneous pregnancies in primigravidae. Other risk factors that may have an impact on the site of implantation include uterine leiomyoma (aOR 2.21; 95% CI: 1.48, 2.94)[27] and endometrial thickness.[18] Compared with women with an endometrial thickness of less than 9 mm, women with an endometrial thickness of 9 to 12 mm and women with an endometrial thickness greater than 12 mm have an aOR of 2.02 (95% CI 1.12–3.65) and of 3.74 (95% CI 1.90–7.34), of developing a placenta previa respectively. The authors have suggested that the endometrium thickness could influence fundus-to-cervix uterine peristalsis, explaining the increased risk of implantation in the lower uterine segment in women with thicker endometrium.[18]

Some authors have hypothesized that placentation in the lower segment of the uterus could be associated with suboptimal vascular development of the utero-placental and the umbilico-placental circulations.[28,29] These studies were poorly controlled for the number of active smokers and medical disorders such as thrombophilia, and the women in the placenta previa group were delivered on average 3 weeks before their nonprevia controls, making the evaluation of placental weight and fetal birthweight inaccurate. A population-based, retrospective cohort study of singleton live births in women diagnosed with placenta previa reported a higher rate of low birth weight (LBW) caused by preterm delivery, which was not significant when adjusted for gestational age at delivery.[30] A recent retrospective large cohort study of 724 women diagnosed prenatally with placenta previa found no increase in the incidence of fetal growth restriction (FGR).[31] The presence of bleeding and the type of the placenta (ie, low-lying placenta [partial previa] and placenta previa [marginal or complete]) did not impact the risk of FGR. These data and the authors' recent study showing no difference in the rate of FGR in both low-lying and placenta previa[32] suggest that implantation in the lower uterine segment does not affect the normal development of the utero-placental circulation and/or normal placental functions.

ACCRETA PLACENTATION

The phrase placenta accreta spectrum (PAS) was first used by Luke and colleagues[33] in 1966 to describe the different grades of abnormally adherent and invasive placentas. These include placenta adherenta or creta when the placenta is adherent but not invasive (**Fig. 1**A), placenta increta when the villi invade into the myometrium (**Fig. 1**B), and placenta percreta where the villi invade the full thickness of the myometrium into the serosal surface of the uterus and beyond (**Fig. 1**C). The first large series of abnormally adherent placenta accreta was published by Irving and Hertig in 1937.[34] They described their cases clinically as "the abnormal adherence of the afterbirth in whole or in parts to the underlying uterine wall with absence of spontaneous

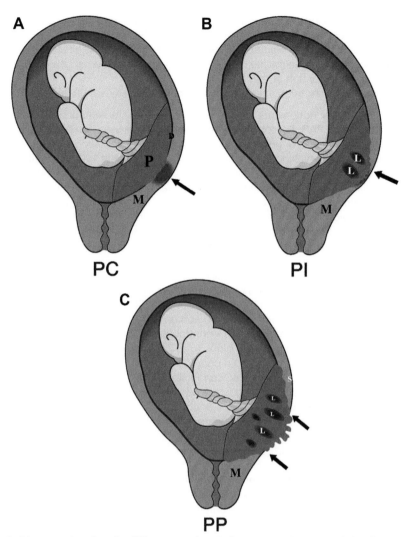

Fig. 1. Diagrams showing the different grades of placenta previa accrete. (*A*) Adherenta or creta (PC) where placental (P) villi adhere directly to the decidua (D, *dark red layer*) to the myometrium (M) without interposing decidua above a prior CD scar area (*arrow*). (*B*) Increta (PI), where the villi invade the myometrium in and around the scar area (*arrow*); (*C*) and per-creta (PP) where the villi invade the entire myometrium and cross the uterine serosa (S, *black layer*). Note the presence of lacunae (L) in both placenta increta and percreta. (*Courtesy of* E. Jauniaux, MD, PhD, FRCOG, London, UK.)

separation 60 min after birth," and histologically as "the complete or partial absence of the decidua basalis between the villi and the myometrium." Although, cases of inva-sive PAS were described earlier in the 20th century, many 21st century authors have used Irving and Hertig's definition to describe both abnormally adherent and invasive types of placentation, including a morbidly adherent placenta, a definition that was used in the 19th century to describe placental retention.[21,35,36] Modern au-thors have also used additional clinical descriptions for PAS, including:

Difficult manual or piecemeal removal of the placenta;

Retained placental fragments requiring curettage after vaginal birth;

Absence of spontaneous placental separation 30 minutes after vaginal birth, despite active management including bimanual massage of the uterus, use of oxytocin, and controlled traction of the umbilical cord; and

Heavy bleeding from the placental bed after placental removal during CD[37–40]

These clinical descriptions are similar to those of placental retention, and as most modern authors of PAS do not report on clinical criteria used for the diagnosis of the condition at birth and/or on detailed histopathologic confirmation of the diagnosis, not surprisingly the prevalence of PAS varies between 1 case in 100 births and 1 case in 10,000 births.[41] Furthermore, methodological inconsistencies between modern studies and the lack of differential diagnosis between adherent and invasive accreta placentation limit the analysis of diagnostic criteria, outcome data, and the impact of different management strategies. In an attempt to palliate for these methodological issues, which have hampered PAS epidemiology data analysis for several decades, the FIGO has recently proposed a classification and basic dataset for reporting new data.[42]

Like placenta previa, the main risk factors associated with the development of PAS are prior CD and IVF procedures (**Table 2**), and the risks of developing PAS in subsequent pregnancies increases with the number of prior CDs. Not surprisingly, the incidence of PAS increases exponentially in women with prior CD presenting with a placenta previa.[44] The UK national case-control study[45] found that the incidence of PAS rises from 1.7 cases per 10,000 births to 577 cases per 10,000 births in women presenting with a placenta previa and a prior CD (aOR 65.02; 95% CI: 16.58, 254.96). The Nordic countries population-based cohort study found that the single most important risk factor was placenta previa, which was reported in 49% of the cases (OR: 292.02, 95% CI; 196, 400) and the risk doubles in women with prior CD (OR 614; 95% CI: 372, 844).[46] Overall 4.1% of women with 1 prior CD, diagnosed prenatally with placenta previa, will have a PAS, and the incidence increases to 13.3% in women with at least 2 previous CDs.[43] IVF increases the risk for PAS between fourfold to 13-fold compared with spontaneous pregnancy.[45–47] Unlike placenta previa, the risk of PAS is not directly affected by maternal smoking, but it is also increased after minor uterine surgical procedures such as operative hysteroscopy, suction curettage, surgical termination, myomectomy, and endometrial ablation.[45,48] It is also associated with uterine pathologies such as bicornuate uterus, adenomyosis, and myotonic dystrophy.[49]

During the last century, 2 opposing views of how PAS occurs have prevailed. The first and oldest concept is that there is a primary defect of the trophoblast that is abnormally invasive right from the start at the time of implantation.[49] This concept goes back to the time when CD was rarely performed and was associated with high maternal morbidity and mortality. Most women delivered at home, and the main risk factors associated with accreta placentation were prior endometritis and/or placental manual delivery. Only 1 of the 18 cases personally treated by Irving and Hertig in 1937 occurred after a CD, and all their cases were reported as abnormally adherent with no macroscopic or histologic evidence of myometrial villous tissue invasion.[34] The second and more recent concept is that the trophoblast is normal but becomes excessively invasive secondary to implantation into an anatomically abnormal uterine bed such as from damage by a surgical scar.[20,50] This concept is supported by modern epidemiologic data showing that more than 90% of women diagnosed with invasive PAS have a history of CD, and present with placenta previa.[35,45,46,51]

Table 2
Clinical variables associated with placenta accreta spectrum in large epidemiologic studies and systematic reviews

Variables	Author, Year/Type of Study	Risk Calculation
Prior CD	Wu et al,[43] 2005/case-control study of 64,359 births	OR after 1 CD: 2.16 (95% CI 9.0–4.86) OR after 2 or more CDs: 8.6 (95% CI 3.53–21.07)
	Silver et al,[44] 2006/cohort study of 378,063 births and 83,754 CDs	OR after 2 CDs: 17.4 (95% CI 9.0–31.4) OR after ≥ 3 CDs: 55.9 (95% CI 25.0–110.3)
	Klar et al,[11] 2014SR&MA of prior CDs	Summary RR: 1.38 (95% CI:1.35–1.42) Summary OR: 2.19 (95% CI:1.09–4.43)
	Keag et al,[12] 2018/SR&MA of 705,108 prior CDs	OR: 2.95 (95% CI 1.32–6.60)
	Fitzpatrick et al,[45] 2012/case-control study of 134 cases of PAS	aOR: 14.41 (95% CI 5.63–36.85)
	Thurn et al,[46] 2016/cohort-study of 605,362 births	Overall OR: 8.8 (95% CI 6.1–12.6) OR after 1 CD: 6.6 (95% CI 4.4–9.8) OR after 2 CDs: 17.4 (95% CI 9.0–31.4) OR after ≥3 CDs: 55.9 (95% CI 25.0–110.3)
IVF	Fitzpatrick et al,[45] 2012/case-control study of 134 cases of PAS	aOR: 32.13 (95% CI 2.03–509.23)
	Thurn et al,[46] 2016/cohort-study of 605,362 births	OR: 3.1 (95% CI 1.6–5.8)
	Roque et al,[47] 2018/SR&MA of fresh embryo transfer	aOR: 3.51 (95% CI 2.04–6.05)
Other surgery	Fitzpatrick et al,[45] 2012/case-control study of 134 cases of PAS	aOR: 3.40 (95% CI 1.30–8.91)
	Baldwin et al,[48] 2018/cohort-study of 380,775 births.	RR for 1 procedure: 1.5 (99% CI 1.1–1.9) RR for 2: 2.7 (99% CI 1.7–4.4) RR for ≥3: 5.1 (95% CI 2.7–9.6)

Abbreviations: aOR, adjusted odds ratio; CD, cesarean delivery; MA, meta-analysis; OR, odds ratio; RR, relative risk; SR, systematic review.

In large and deep myometrial defects caused by multiple CDs, there is often an absence of re-epithelialization in the scar area.[52] A thin endometrial thickness is associated with low pregnancy rates after IVF irrespective of the causing factor,[53] suggesting that a large scar area does not constitute an ideal environment for implantation. There is a direct association between blastocyst implantation in a caesarean scar and the development of placenta previa accreta.[54–56] Because of the high risk of complications, few caesarean scar pregnancies are managed conservatively, and thus outcome data are limited to 69 cases in the international literature, with only 40 progressing to the third trimester.[56] High variability in study design and poor correlation with histopathologic findings at birth, including overdiagnosis of placenta percreta due to scar dehiscence, further limit the analysis of these data. These findings suggest that a blastocyst may get trapped within a uterine scar and may implant on its border where there is sufficient decidua to allow further development and placentation. Within this context, there are similarities between ectopic pregnancies where the blastocyst implants within the epithelium of the Fallopian tube and intrauterine scar placentation.

This points to the secondary defect in PAS being the absence of the normal decidual signals that regulate placentation and affect extravillous trophoblast (EVT) invasion and differentiation.[57] Histopathological studies have shown that EVT cells invade tubal vessels,[58] but subsequent development of the placenta in the tube differs from that in the uterus in so far as invasion of the tubal tissues is unrestrained, with penetration of the trophoblast into the serosa. A recent immuno-histochemical study has shown that EVT cells in tubal pregnancies show more pro-liferative and invasive characteristics[59] compared with their intrauterine counterparts. Similarly, in PAS, the EVT cells are increased in size and number, and the depth of their myometrial invasion is greater.[60] NK cells are absent in the nonpregnant and pregnant Fallopian tube, whereas in cases of ectopic pregnancy there are higher numbers of CD8[+] lymphocytes, CD68[+] macrophages, and CD11c[+] dendritic cells compared with nonpregnancy.[61] Leukocyte recruitment to the endometrium during the secretory phase is affected by the presence of scar tis-sue.[52] In both tubal ectopic and intrauterine accreta placentation, multinucleated giant cells are lower in number or totally absent,[60] indicating that the EVTs have not undergone their normal terminal differentiation.[62] These data suggest that accreta placentation is not caused by an inherently more aggressive trophoblast, but that migration is uncontrolled because of the absence of the physiologic mech-anisms arising from the maternal decidual cells (including immune cells) that nor-mally limit invasion. Hence, the result is abnormally deep placentation beyond the junction of the decidua and chorioallantoic placenta. A key question to address, therefore, is how does decidua induce EVT to form giant cells and limit the depth of invasion?

Invasion of larger vessels in the outer myometrium as far as the uterine serosa in PAS is most certainly also determined by abnormal access, rather than trophoblastic mal-function and points to the inherent ability of trophoblast to invade arteries, which is also characteristic of choriocarcinoma. The EVT invasion of the tissue around and within the wall of the radial, and even the arcuate, arteries leads to their excessive dilatation and to the entry of high-velocity blood flows inside the intervillous space.[62] Subplacental hypervascularity and the presence of intraplacental lacunae are the most prominent fea-tures of invasive PAS prenatally on ultrasound.[20,35,62] The entry of abnormally high-velocity blood flow into the placenta at the end of the first trimester when the intervillous circulation is established permanently distorts the normal anatomy of the definitive placenta, in particular the architecture of the lobules and destruction of interlobular sep-tae (**Fig. 2**). The villous tissue shows no morphologic changes in PAS compared with nonaccreta placentas, even in the invasive areas.[49,50] Various phenotypic changes in syncytiotrophoblast in PAS villous tissue have been reported, but wide variations in study design, accreta definition, number of cases studied, type of tissue investigated, and the extent of quantification of morphologic changes limit their interpretation.[50] These changes are most likely secondary to focal oxidative stress and/or mechanical shear stress within the intervillous space and the placental tissue above the invasive areas. Several authors have found that spiral artery remodeling is focally reduced.[60,63,64] The deficiency is seen more in PAS cases without local decidua, and remodeling is sometimes completely absent in the accreta area. The pathologic and phenotypic changes are hard to define, as the normal vascular architecture of the placental bed may be distorted in the scar area. Furthermore, these changes in remodeling of the utero-placental circulation in placenta accreta are not associated with any impact on placental or fetal growth, nor on the incidence of pre-eclampsia.[32]

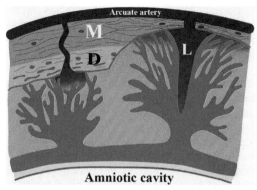

Fig. 2. Diagram showing a normal placental cotyledon (*left*) with decidua (D) and normal myometrium (M) and an increta cotyledon (*right*). The increta cotyledon anatomy is distorted with villi reaching the deep myometrial circulation and the formation of a lacuna (L). (*Courtesy of* E. Jauniaux, MD, PhD, FRCOG, London, UK.)

ABNORMAL INSERTION OF THE UMBILICAL CORD

The umbilical cord can be inserted centrally, eccentrically, or marginally on the placental disk, and VCI refers to an umbilical cord that is inserted into the membranes.[65,66] Vasa previa (VP) occurs when fetal vessels run through the membranes, over the cervix, and under the fetal presenting part (**Fig. 3**). VCI is found in approximately 1% of births, and 3% to 4% of women with a VCI also have a vasa previa.[67,68] Conversely, 90% of women with vasa previa have VCI.[65–68] VP is relatively uncommon in the general population and has been reported to occur in 1 case per 1200 births to 1 case in 5000 births.[67] Anomalies of the cord insertion are probably under-reported, as unlike the occurrence of a single umbilical artery cord that is systematically recorded by midwives at birth, they are only recorded when associated with perinatal complications.

In twin pregnancies, the incidence of VCI of one of the umbilical cords is 8 times more common than in singletons. Monochorionicity doubles the risk for VCI

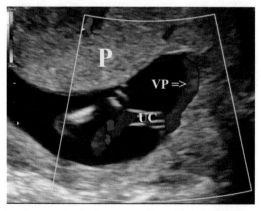

Fig. 3. Transabdominal longitudinal ultrasound view at 13 weeks of a velamentous umbilical cord (UC) inserted outside the placenta (P) with a vasa previa (VP) connecting the cord to the placenta. (*Courtesy of* E. Jauniaux, MD, PhD, FRCOG, London, UK.)

compared with dichorionicity.[69] IVF singleton pregnancies have a higher incidence of marginal cord insertion, VCI, and VP compared with spontaneously conceived singletons.[70] There is no difference in incidence between spontaneous and IVF twins.[71] Marginal and VCI without VP have been associated with small-for-gestational age in both singleton and twin pregnancies.[72–75] A noncentral cord insertion is associated with a sparser chorionic vascular distribution, which could lead to markedly reduced transport efficiency through hemodynamic effects on the feto-placental circulation.[76] The pathophysiology of abnormal cord insertion is uncertain, but the higher incidence in IVF pregnancies suggests that it could be the consequence of malrotation of the blastocyst at the time of implantation[77–87]. The molecular mechanisms that control blastocyst orientation are not fully understood, but it may be relevant that as the blastocyst enlarged expression of FGFR1 becomes restricted to the trophectoderm overlying the inner cell mass.[77] This finding indicates there may be subpopulations of trophectoderm that may have different adhesive properties. Whether this differentiation is affected by ART, or whether there are changes in endometrial receptivity caused by the hormonal regimens employed, is not known at present.

ABNORMAL PLACENTAL SHAPES AND PLACENTA EXTRACHORIOALIS

The mature placenta is often described as discoid; however, there has been considerable debate as to whether most are actually circular or ellipsoid.[65,66] The placenta can also be bilobate or multilobate (**Fig. 4**) or can present with an accessory lobe, defined as succenturiate if attached to the main placenta or spuria if not. There is a strong correlation between the shape of the placenta at the end of the first trimester and that at term,[78] suggesting that events during the first trimester are critical. Profound remodeling of the early placenta occurs with onset of the maternal circulation, and excessive or asymmetrical regression can lead to abnormal placental shapes and cord insertions.[79] Abnormal shapes may therefore be caused by aberrant onset of the maternal circulation, which in turn may reflect local variations in the extent of extravillous trophoblast invasion across the placental bed.

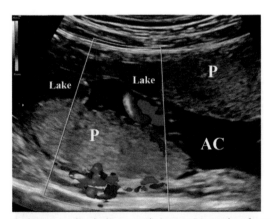

Fig. 4. Trans-abdominal, longitudinal ultrasound view at 20 weeks of gestation of a fundal bilobate placenta (P) with the umbilical cord inserted at the edge of the anterior lobe. Note the presence of lakes. AC, amniotic cavity. (*Courtesy of* E. Jauniaux, MD, PhD, FRCOG, London, UK.)

Placenta extrachorialis is characterized by the transition from the villous chorion to the membranes being not at the edge of the placenta but at some distance within the fetal surface.[65] If the transitional zone is made of a flat ring of membrane, the placenta is classified as circummarginate, whereas if it is plicated with a raised, rolled edge, it is classed as circumvallate. Placenta extrachorialis may occur if implantation and placentation are too superficial.[65]

Bilobate placenta and extrachorialis have been associated a higher incidence of anomalies of the cord insertion.[80,81] Bilobate placenta with VCI and succenturiate lobes are more commonly found in IVF pregnancies.[82,83] Succenturiate lobes of the placenta are more common in twin pregnancies compared with singletons, whereas placenta extrachorialis has the same incidence in both singletons and twins.[83] In singleton pregnancies, but not in twins, abnormally shaped placentas have been associated with a higher incidence of placental abruption, vasa previa, and retained placenta.[83] Increased variability in shape has been linked to reduced placental efficiency as estimated by the ratio of fetal to placental weight,[79] but there are no epidemiologic data supporting this hypothesis. Circumvallate placenta has been associated with a higher incidence of preterm delivery,[84] probably because of a lack of physiologic elasticity of the rolled edge of membranes during formation of the lower uterine segment in the third trimester of pregnancy.

SUMMARY AND FUTURE RESEARCH

The events taking place at the time of human implantation are not fully understood, but clearly have a profound impact on the correct formation of the placenta and on pregnancy outcome. An understanding of the factors determining where implantation occurs and how orientation of the blastocyst is regulated in normal pregnancies is critical in order to assess how these processes are perturbed in pathologic cases. Equally little is known about the molecular mechanisms restraining trophoblast invasion, but findings in ectopic pregnancies and PAS both indicate that the decidual and maternal immune cells play a key role. The lack of preclinical animal models limits systematic investigation, but the recent derivation of human endometrial and trophoblast organoids[85,86] and the ability to culture human blastocysts beyond the implantation stage[87] offer new opportunities to explore these otherwise inaccessible events.

Placenta previa and PAS should be diagnosed prior to delivery through antenatal screening in countries with well-resourced health care systems and access to specialist centers. However, they still pose considerable risks to maternal and fetal/neonatal health globally, and their incidence is rising in line with the rate of CD. Variations in placental shape and cord insertion present less of a challenge clinically, but indicate that implantation and placentation have been suboptimal. When excessive, such variations should alert health care professionals to the possibility of impaired fetal growth, vasa previa, and to the risk of recurrence in subsequent pregnancies.

ACKNOWLEDGMENTS

The authors are grateful to Mrs Angela Scott, Senior Graphic Designer, UCL Digital Media, for her support in making the diagrams included in this article.

DISCLOSURE

The authors have no conflict of interest to declare and nothing to disclose.

REFERENCES

1. Marr JP. Historical background of the treatment of placenta praevia. Bull Hist Med 1941;9:258–93.
2. Bell C. Placenta praevia. Trans Edinb Obstet Soc 1878;5:73–91.
3. Kerr JMM, Mackay WG. The diagnosis of placenta praevia with special reference to the employment of X-rays for this purpose. Trans Edinb Obstet Soc 1933;53:21–32.
4. McNair AJ. Placenta praevia, with vasa praevia: caesarean section. Proc R Soc Med 1921;14:195–6.
5. Forster DS. A case of placenta accreta. Can Med Assoc J 1927;17:204–7.
6. Hunt AB, Mussey RD, Faber JE. Circumvallate placenta. New Orleans Med Surg J 1947;100:203–7.
7. Jauniaux E, Alfirevic Z, Bhide AG, et al, Royal College of Obstetricians and Gynaecologists. Placenta praevia and placenta accreta: diagnosis and management: green-top guideline no. 27a. BJOG 2019;126:e1–48.
8. Ananth CV, Smulian JC, Vintzileos AM. The association of placenta previa with history of cesarean delivery and abortion: a meta-analysis. Am J Obstet Gynecol 1997;177:1071–8.
9. Getahun D, Oyelese Y, Salihu HM, et al. Previous cesarean delivery and risks of placenta previa and placental abruption. Obstet Gynecol 2006;107:771–8.
10. Marshall NE, Fu R, Guise JM. Impact of multiple cesarean deliveries on maternal morbidity: a systematic review. Am J Obstet Gynecol 2011;205:262.e1-8.
11. Klar M, Michels KB. Cesarean section and placental disorders in subsequent pregnancies - a meta-analysis. J Perinat Med 2014;42:571–83.
12. Keag OE, Norman JE, Stock SJ. Long-term risks and benefits associated with cesarean delivery for mother, baby, and subsequent pregnancies: systematic review and meta-analysis. PLoS Med 2018;15:e1002494.
13. Grady R, Alavi N, Vale R, et al. Elective single embryo transfer and perinatal outcomes: a systematic review and meta-analysis. Fertil Steril 2012;97:324–31.
14. Ginström Ernstad E, Bergh C, Khatibi A, et al. Neonatal and maternal outcome after blastocyst transfer: a population-based registry study. Am J Obstet Gynecol 2016;214:378.e1-10.
15. Qin J, Liu X, Sheng X, et al. Assisted reproductive technology and the risk of pregnancy-related complications and adverse pregnancy outcomes in singleton pregnancies: a meta-analysis of cohort studies. Fertil Steril 2016;105:73–85.e1-6.
16. Karami M, Jenabi E, Fereidooni B. The association of placenta previa and assisted reproductive techniques: a meta-analysis. J Matern Fetal Neonatal Med 2018;31:1940–7.
17. Aliyu MH, Lynch O, Wilson RE, et al. Association between tobacco use in pregnancy and placenta-associated syndromes: a population-based study. Arch Gynecol Obstet 2011;283:729–34.
18. Rombauts L, Motteram C, Berkowitz E, et al. Risk of placenta praevia is linked to endometrial thickness in a retrospective cohort study of 4537 singleton assisted reproduction technology births. Hum Reprod 2014;29:2787–93.
19. Shobeiri F, Jenabi E. Smoking and placenta previa: a meta-analysis. J Matern Fetal Neonatal Med 2017;30:2985–90.
20. Jauniaux E, Bhide A, Burton GJ. Pathophysiology of accreta. In: Silver R, editor. Placenta accreta syndrome. Portland (OR): CRC Press; 2017. p. 13–28.

21. Jauniaux E, Ayres-de-Campos D, FIGO Placenta Accreta Diagnosis and Management Expert Consensus Panel. FIGO consensus guidelines on placenta accreta spectrum disorders: introduction. Int J Gynaecol Obstet 2018;140:261–4.

22. Ananth CV, Demissie K, Smulian JC, et al. Placenta praevia in singleton and twin births in the United States, 1989 through 1998: a comparison of risk factor profiles and associated conditions. Am J Obstet Gynecol 2003;188:275–81.

23. Weis MA, Harper LM, Roehl KA, et al. Natural history of placenta previa in twins. Obstet Gynecol 2012;120:753–8.

24. Sahin Ersoy G, Zhou Y, Inan H, et al. Cigarette smoking affects uterine receptivity markers. Reprod Sci 2017;24:989–95.

25. Zhou Y, Gan Y, Taylor HS. Cigarette smoke inhibits recruitment of bone-marrow-derived stem cells to the uterus. Reprod Toxicol 2011;31:123–7.

26. Rzymski P, Rzymski P, Tomczyk K, et al. Metal status in human endometrium: relation to cigarette smoking and histological lesions. Environ Res 2014;132:328–33.

27. Jenabi E, Fereidooni B. The uterine leiomyoma and placenta previa: a meta-analysis. J Matern Fetal Neonatal Med 2017;21:1–5.

28. Weiner E, Miremberg H, Grinstein E, et al. The effect of placenta previa on fetal growth and pregnancy outcome, in correlation with placental pathology. J Perinatol 2016;36:1073–8.

29. Weiner E, Miremberg H, Grinstein E, et al. Placental histopathology lesions and pregnancy outcome in pregnancies complicated with symptomatic vs. non symptomatic placenta previa. Early Hum Dev 2016;101:85–9.

30. Ananth CV, Demissie K, Smulian JC, et al. Relationship among placenta previa, fetal growth restriction, and preterm delivery: a population-based study. Obstet Gynecol 2001;98:299–306.

31. Harper LM, Odibo AO, Macones GA, et al. Effect of placenta previa on fetal growth. Am J Obstet Gynecol 2010;203:330.e1-5.

32. Jauniaux E, Dimitrova I, Kenyon N, et al. Impact of placenta previa with placenta accreta spectrum disorder on fetal growth. Ultrasound Obstet Gynecol 2019;54:643–9.

33. Luke RK, Sharpe JW, Greene RR. Placenta accreta: the adherent or invasive placenta. Am J Obstet Gynecol 1966;95:660–8.

34. Irving C, Hertig AT. A study of placenta accreta. Surg Gynecol Obstet 1937;64:178–200.

35. Jauniaux E, Bhide A. Prenatal ultrasound diagnosis and outcome of placenta previa accreta after caesarean delivery: a systematic review and meta-analysis. Am J Obstet Gynecol 2017;217:27–36.

36. Collins SL, Chantraine F, Morgan TK, et al. Abnormally adherent and invasive placenta: a spectrum disorder in need of a name. Ultrasound Obstet Gynecol 2018;51:165–6.

37. Gielchinsky Y, Rojansky N, Fasouliotis SJ, et al. Placenta accreta–summary of 10 years: a survey of 310 cases. Placenta 2002;23:210–4.

38. Sheiner E, Levy A, Katz M, et al. Identifying risk factors for peripartum cesarean hysterectomy. A population-based study. J Reprod Med 2003;48:622–6.

39. Woodring TC, Klauser CK, Bofill JA, et al. Prediction of placenta accreta by ultrasonography and color Doppler imaging. J Matern Fetal Neonatal Med 2011;24:118–21.

40. Klar M, Laub M, Schulte-Moenting J, et al. Clinical risk factors for complete and partial placental retention: a case-control study. J Perinat Med 2014;41:529–34.

41. Jauniaux E, Bunce C, Grønbeck L, et al. Prevalence and main outcomes of placenta accreta spectrum: a systematic review and metaanalysis. Am J Obstet Gynecol 2019;221:208–18.

42. Jauniaux E, Ayres-de-Campos D, Langhoff-Roos J, et al, FIGO Placenta Accreta Diagnosis and Management Expert Consensus Panel. FIGO classification for the clinical diagnosis of placenta accreta spectrum disorders. Int J Gynaecol Obstet 2019;146:20–4.

43. Wu S, Kocherginsky M, Hibbard JU. Abnormal placentation: twenty-year analysis. Am J Obstet Gynecol 2005;192:1458–61.

44. Silver RM, Landon MB, Rouse DJ, et al, National Institute of Child Health and Human Development Maternal-Fetal Medicine Units Network. Maternal morbidity associated with multiple repeat cesarean deliveries. Obstet Gynecol 2006;107: 1226–32.

45. Fitzpatrick KE, Sellers S, Spark P, et al. Incidence and risk factors for placenta accreta/increta/percreta in the UK: a national case-control study. PLoS One 2012;7:e52893.

46. Thurn L, Lindqvist PG, Jakobsson M, et al. Abnormally invasive placenta-prevalence, risk factors and antenatal suspicion: results from a large population-based pregnancy cohort study in the Nordic countries. BJOG 2016; 123:1348–55.

47. Roque M, Valle M, Sampaio M, et al. Obstetric outcomes after fresh versus frozen-thawed embryo transfers: a systematic review and meta-analysis. JBRA Assist Reprod 2018;22:253–60.

48. Baldwin HJ, Patterson JA, Nippita TA, et al. Antecedents of abnormally invasive placenta in primiparous women: risk associated with gynecologic procedures. Obstet Gynecol 2018;131:227–33.

49. Jauniaux E, Jurkovic D. Placenta accreta: pathogenesis of a 20th century iatrogenic uterine disease. Placenta 2012;33:244–51.

50. Jauniaux E, Burton GJ. Pathophysiology of placenta accreta spectrum disorders: a review of current findings. Clin Obstet Gynecol 2018;61:743–54.

51. Jauniaux E, Chantraine F, Silver RM, et al, FIGO Placenta Accreta Diagnosis and Management Expert Consensus Panel. FIGO consensus guidelines on placenta accreta spectrum disorders: epidemiology. Int J Gynaecol Obstet 2018;140: 265–73.

52. Ben-Nagi J, Walker A, Jurkovic D, et al. Effect of cesarean delivery on the endometrium. Int J Gynaecol Obstet 2009;106:30–4.

53. Mahajan N, Sharma S. The endometrium in assisted reproductive technology: how thin is thin? J Hum Reprod Sci 2016;9:3–8.

54. Zosmer N, Fuller J, Shaikh H, et al. Natural history of early first-trimester pregnancies implanted in Cesarean scars. Ultrasound Obstet Gynecol 2015;46:367–75.

55. Cali G, Forlani F, Timor-Tritsch IE, et al. Natural history of Cesarean scar pregnancy on prenatal ultrasound: the crossover sign. Ultrasound Obstet Gynecol 2017;50:100–4.

56. Calì G, Timor-Tritsch IE, Palacios-Jaraquemada J, et al. Outcome of cesarean scar pregnancy managed expectantly: systematic review and meta-analysis. Ultrasound Obstet Gynecol 2018;51:169–75.

57. Pollheimer J, Vondra S, Baltayeva J, et al. Regulation of Placental extravillous trophoblasts by the maternal uterine environment. Front Immunol 2018;13:2597.

58. Randall S, Buckley CH, Fox H. Placentation in the fallopian tube. Int J Gynecol Pathol 1987;6:132–9.

59. Gao T, Liang Y, Tang H, et al. The increased level of Tspan5 in villi suggests more proliferation and invasiveness of trophoblasts in tubal pregnancy. Eur J Obstet Gynecol Reprod Biol 2018;228:38–42.
60. Khong TY, Robertson WB. Placenta creta and placenta praevia creta. Placenta 1987;8:399–409.
61. Shaw JL, Fitch P, Cartwright J, et al. Lymphoid and myeloid cell populations in the non-pregnant human Fallopian tube and in ectopic pregnancy. J Reprod Immunol 2011;89:84–91.
62. Jauniaux E, Collins SL, Burton GJ. Placenta accreta spectrum: Pathophysiology and evidence-based anatomy for prenatal ultrasound imaging. Am J Obstet Gynecol 2018;218:75–87.
63. Tantbirojn P, Crum CP, Parast MM. Pathophysiology of placenta creta: the role of decidua and extravillous trophoblast. Placenta 2008;29:639–45.
64. Hannon T, Innes BA, Lash GE, et al. Effects of local decidua on trophoblast invasion and spiral artery remodeling in focal placenta creta - an immunohistochemical study. Placenta 2012;33:998–1004.
65. Fox H, Sebire NJ. Pathology of the placenta. 3rd edition. Philadelphia: : Saunders-Elsevier; 2007.
66. Benirschke K, Burton GJ, Baergen RN. Pathology of the human placenta. 6th edition. Berlin: : Springer-Verlag; 2012.
67. Jauniaux E, Alfirevic Z, Bhide AG, et al, Royal College of Obstetricians and Gynaecologists. Vasa praevia: diagnosis and management: green-top guideline no. 27b. BJOG 2019;126:e49–61.
68. Melcer Y, Maymon R, Jauniaux E. Vasa previa: prenatal diagnosis and management. Curr Opin Obstet Gynecol 2018;30:385–91.
69. Jauniaux E, Melcer Y, Maymon R. Prenatal diagnosis and management of vasa previa in twin pregnancies: a case series and systematic review. Am J Obstet Gynecol 2017;216:568–75.
70. Ruiter L, Kok N, Limpens J, et al. Incidence of and risk indicators for vasa praevia: a systematic review. BJOG 2016;123:1278–87.
71. Gavriil P, Jauniaux E, Leroy F. Pathologic examination of placentas from singleton and twin pregnancies obtained after in vitro fertilization and embryo transfer. Pediatr Pathol 1993;13:453–62.
72. Sinkin JA, Craig WY, Jones M, et al. Perinatal outcomes associated with isolated velamentous cord insertion in singleton and twin pregnancies. J Ultrasound Med 2018;37:471–8.
73. Allaf MB, Andrikopoulou M, Crnosija N, et al. Second trimester marginal cord insertion is associated with adverse perinatal outcomes. J Matern Fetal Neonatal Med 2018;26:1–6.
74. Kalafat E, Thilaganathan B, Papageorghiou A, et al. Significance of placental cord insertion site in twin pregnancy. Ultrasound Obstet Gynecol 2018;52:378–84.
75. Ismail KI, Hannigan A, O'Donoghue K, et al. Abnormal placental cord insertion and adverse pregnancy outcomes: a systematic review and meta-analysis. Syst Rev 2017;6:242.
76. Yampolsky M, Salafia CM, Shlakhter O, et al. Centrality of the umbilical cord insertion in a human placenta influences the placental efficiency. Placenta 2009;30:1058–64.
77. Niakan KK, Eggan K. Analysis of human embryos from zygote to blastocyst reveals distinct gene expression patterns relative to the mouse. Dev Biol 2013;375:54–64.

78. Salafia CM, Yampolsky M, Shlakhter A, et al. Variety in placental shape: when does it originate? Placenta 2012;33:164–70.
79. Burton GJ, Jauniaux E, Charnock-Jones DS. The influence of the intrauterine environment on human placental development. Int J Dev Biol 2010;54:303–12.
80. Nordenvall M, Sandstedt B, Ulmsten U. Relationship between placental shape, cord insertion, lobes and gestational outcome. Acta Obstet Gynecol Scand 1988;67:611–6.
81. Baulies S, Maiz N, Muñoz A, et al. Prenatal ultrasound diagnosis of vasa praevia and analysis of risk factors. Prenat Diagn 2007;27:595–9.
82. Suzuki S, Igarashi M. Clinical significance of pregnancies with succenturiate lobes of placenta. Arch Gynecol Obstet 2008;277:299–301.
83. Suzuki S, Igarashi M, Inde Y, et al. Abnormally shaped placentae in twin pregnancy. Arch Gynecol Obstet 2010;281:65–9.
84. Taniguchi H, Aoki S, Sakamaki K, et al. Circumvallate placenta: associated clinical manifestations and complications-a retrospective study. Obstet Gynecol Int 2014;2014:986230.
85. Turco MY, Gardner L, Hughes J, et al. Long-term, hormone-responsive organoid cultures of human endometrium in a chemically defined medium. Nat Cell Biol 2017;195:568–77.
86. Turco MY, Gardner L, Kay RG, et al. Trophoblast organoids as a model for maternal-fetal interactions during human placentation. Nature 2018;564:263–7.
87. Haider S, Meinhardt G, Saleh L, et al. Self-renewing trophoblast organoids recapitulate the developmental program of the early human placenta. Stem Cell Reports 2018;11:537–51.

Key Infections in the Placenta

Maria Laura Costa, MD, PhD[a],*, Guilherme de Moraes Nobrega[a],
Arthur Antolini-Tavares, MD[b]

KEYWORDS

- Placenta • Congenital infection • TORCH

KEY POINTS

- Congenital infections are an important cause of morbidity and mortality worldwide. Understanding pathogen characteristics, routes of transmission, and placental infection can guide effective interventions to control the burden of disease, especially in under-resourced settings.
- The recent Zika virus epidemic represents a warning toward the possibility of new emerging viruses. Scientists and policy makers should both be prepared to face new challenges.
- Infection of placental trophoblast cells can induce proinflammatory responses, cell death, and impaired remodeling of decidual spiral arteries, compromising the adequacy of uteroplacental blood flow.

INTRODUCTION

Knowledge of the role of the placenta in infections during pregnancy and mechanisms of vertical transmission have evolved greatly in the past decades. For many years, the classic paradigm of reproductive immunology, considering the antigenically foreign fetus in contact with the pregnant mother, was based on the theories of "anatomical separation of fetus from mother; antigenic immaturity of the fetus and immunologic inertness of the mother."[1] These concepts were confronted by mechanisms of transplacental infection. Despite many signaling pathways being suggested to explain how immune modulation and response to infections interact,[2] much is yet unknown and new questions arise as novel epidemics bring attention to unpredicted outcomes.[2,3]

The consequences of placental infections have been known for centuries, including abortions, preterm births, dysfunction, and abnormal development of the newborn. The first associations of such outcomes with infections by a range of pathogens,

[a] Department of Obstetrics and Gynecology, School of Medicine, University of Campinas, Rua Alexander Fleming 101, Campinas, São Paulo 13084-881, Brazil; [b] Department of Pathological Anatomy, School of Medicine, University of Campinas, Rua Alexander Fleming 101, Campinas, São Paulo 13084-881, Brazil
* Corresponding author.
E-mail address: mlaura@unicamp.br

Obstet Gynecol Clin N Am 47 (2020) 133–146
https://doi.org/10.1016/j.ogc.2019.10.003
0889-8545/20/© 2019 Elsevier Inc. All rights reserved.

obgyn.theclinics.com

however, only came about in the late nineteenth and early twentieth centuries, with advances in the area of human medicine.[2] Since then, studies have been exposing the repercussions that infections can cause in pregnancy and within the placenta.[4–6] The placenta as a complex organ presents several responses to infection, depending on the nature of the pathogen involved.[7,8]

During pregnancy, the placenta acts as an immunologic and physical barrier to many molecules, particles, and even other organisms, such as fungi and bacteria. This characteristic is especially a result of the histologic organization of the organ, making a maternal-fetal barrier.[2,4,7] Several viral, bacterial, parasitic, and other infections, however, can affect this organ in a significant way, disturbing the natural homeostasis and causing a breakdown of the placental barrier.[4]

In order to understand the consequences, it is key to remember the placental structure. In summary, the placenta is a branching villous structure. Villi are composed of 2 layers of specialized trophoblast cells, the inner layer of mononuclear cytotrophoblasts that can replicate and fuse into the outer layer of multinucleated syncytiotrophoblasts, which cover the total surface of the villous placenta and is bathed in maternal blood. The site of placental implantation in the uterus undergoes significant modification and decidualization, forming a dense cellular matrix in which there is an invasion of extravillous trophoblasts that ultimately penetrate the walls of maternal arterioles, transforming spiral arteries to facilitate maternal blood flow to the intervillous space.[9]

Congenital infections are an important cause of mortality and morbidity worldwide, especially in low-income settings.[2] This review aims to discuss the main pathways of infections and associated adverse maternal and fetal outcomes, considering the TORCH pathogens, including Zika virus (ZIKV). TORCH stands for *Toxoplasma gondii* infection, other (*Treponema pallidum*, *Listeria monocytogenes*, and parvovirus B19, among others, including ZIKV), rubella, cytomegalovirus (CMV), and herpes simplex viruses type 1 and (HSV)-1 and type 2 (HSV-2).

TORCH—*TOXOPLASMA GONDII*

Toxoplasmosis is the most frequent protozoa infection worldwide and a public health issue, especially in under-resourced settings. The reported prevalence of infection in continental Europe, Central America, and South America ranges from 30% to 90%.[10]

T gondii is a coccidian protozoa whose definitive host are felines. Humans acquire the infection by consuming sporulated oocysts from water, soil, or food contaminated by feces of these animals.[11] Most infections are asymptomatic or mild (flu-like), with relevant consequences in vulnerable groups, such as pregnant women. Only 10% to 20% of infected pregnant women have symptoms. The parasites are recognized by trophoblast surface receptors and then invade these cells, where they can multiply and further release within the villous stroma causing placental and fetal infection. In vitro studies suggest that the extravillous trophoblasts are the most vulnerable to infection, followed by villous cytotrophoblasts and rarely syncytiotrophoblasts.[7]

In the first trimester, most likely due to infectious resistance of the syncytiotrophoblast, the risk of transplacental infection is approximately 1 in 6; however, when infection occurs, there can be devastating consequences. During the second and third trimesters, transmission is higher, between one-third and two-thirds, but less severe. Early infections cause abortions and highly destructive lesions that occur with intracranial calcifications, ventriculomegaly, microcephaly, hydrocephalus, chorioretinitis, hepatosplenomegaly, and cardiomegaly, commonly with cardiac failure and hydrops, with postnatal sequelae, such as blindness, cognitive deficit, and deafness.[12] Late infection is either discrete or inapparent at birth, although deficiencies may cause long-term consequences, such as ocular disease.[10]

Although there are 3 genotypes of *T gondii*, type II is the most common in Europe and the United States, and the major one responsible for congenital infection.[13] In these cases, tachyzoites and pseudocysts can be found, respectively, in areas of active inflammation and hypocellular tissues, such as the brain and umbilical cord, under conventional microscopy or with staining, such as periodic acid–Schiff.[7] The placenta shows lymphohistiocytic chronic villitis, with severe and diffuse inflammation and granulomas (**Fig. 1**). Such findings can occur with other parasitic (*T cruzi*), viral (varicella), and mycobacterial infections. The villi are immature, with increased Hofbauer cells in the villous stroma, chorion, and Wharton jelly.[7]

The main diagnostic method in pregnant women is serologic assay: immunoglobulin (Ig)M and IgG titers within 2 weeks of infection and determination of their respective avidity. The recommendation is to test women at high risk for toxoplasmosis, such as those in endemic areas and, if acute infection is suspected, therapy with spiramycin should be started for fetal prophylaxis to prevent cross-placental infection. The combined therapy with pyrimethamine, sulfadiazine, and folinic acid should be considered as treatment of women with highly suspected or confirmed fetal infection, such as those with positive amniotic fluid polymerase chain reaction (PCR).[14]

TORCH—OTHER—SYPHILIS

Syphilis is caused by *Treponema pallidum*, a mobile spiral spirochete, that promotes low immunogenic recognition, through an outer membrane of proteins that lacks lipopolysaccharide and has few exposed lipoproteins. This spirochete, however, promotes adherence to host cells and facilitates perivascular infiltration; tissue destruction results mainly from the host's immune response to infection.[7] Humans are the only natural hosts, with infection established by congenital transmission or through sexual contact.

Treponema pallidum is the third most common sexually transmitted bacterial disease in the United States, with infections by *Chlamydia trachomatis* and *Neisseria gonorrhoeae* numbers 1 and 2, respectively.[15] There are 5.6 million new cases of syphilis every year worldwide[16] and this prevalence yields 2 million new cases of congenital syphilis annually. This high incidence is disconcerting because effective treatment can eliminate 98% of congenital infections if instituted 30 days before delivery. Syphilis has become a re-emerging congenital infection not only in the United States,[17] but

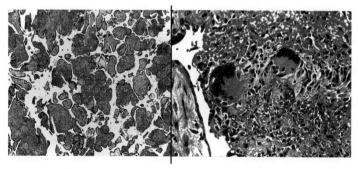

Fig. 1. Toxoplasmosis. Intensely destructive chronic granulomatous villitis on a 16-week stillbirth ([*left*] 4× objective), with numerous immune multinucleated giant cells ([*right*] 40× magnification). (*Courtesy of* A. Antolini-Tavares, São Paulo, Brazil.)

universally in high-income, middle-income, and low-income countries.[18] Thus, syphilis infection occurs throughout the world, with burden of disease and highest prevalence in eastern and southern Africa.

Transmission risk during pregnancy is directly associated with the stage of syphilis.[16] The secondary stage of the disease in the untreated mother is the most prone to cause vertical infection with nearly 100% of colonized patients yielding infection. This high penetrance of infection is due to the greater number of spirochetes in the bloodstream of women with secondary syphilis, among the 4 stages of syphilis that include primary, secondary, latent, and tertiary disease. Syphilis during pregnancy can cause prematurity, low birth weight, stillbirth, early neonatal death, or congenital infection in infants.[16] There is as high as a 40% risk of stillbirth if the infection occurs early in gestation.[7]

Pathologic findings of the placenta may be subtle and nonspecific. For example, gross evaluation presents placental thickening and pallor, which are secondary to a fetal anemia which can evolve to hydrops.[19] The histologic triad of a syphilitic infection of the chorionic villi includes

- Enlarged, edematous, and hypercellular villi and an immature villous core histomorphology containing prominent stromal and Hofbauer cells
- Capillary fetal vessels showing marked endovascular and perivascular connective tissue secondary to vasculitis), with an onion-skin appearance after fixation and viewing in light microscopy, acute and/or chronic villitis associated, or both[12,20]

In term pregnancies, findings frequently include chronic lymphohistiocytic villitis, with foci of necrosis, similar to *Treponema* lesions of other organs in infected patients. Necrotizing funisitis, acute chorioamnionitis, and plasma cell deciduitis result from the tendency of spirochetes to attach to components of basement membranes and extracellular matrix when amniotic fluid infection is present.[7] Thus, the presence of excess numbers of immature villi, numerous Hofbauer cells, and chronic villitis with local acute vasculitis indicates the need for investigation of a newborn for congenital syphilis. Established methods for spirochete identification in villi include silver staining, such as the Warthin-Starry and Steiner methods, PCR, or immunohistochemistry for treponemal antigens. Silver staining methods for spirochetes are positive in only half of cases when there is the classical triad,[21] described previously, underscoring vigilant use of other methods in pursuing suspicious findings.

For the immediate diagnosis of a candidate patient, dark-field microscopy or direct immunofluorescence is used if mucosal ulcers are observed in the primary or secondary phase of syphilis. Moreover, serology is very sensitive in the secondary and late (tertiary) phases of syphilis. Penicillin is the drug of choice and should be used in penicillin allergic patients after desensitization; however, some investigators recommend doxycycline if a patient is allergic to penicillin and desensitization is not an option. Safe sex practices should be encouraged, and sexual partners of infected patients should be treated. No vaccine is available.[22]

TORCH—OTHER—*LISTERIA MONOCYTOGENES*

L monocytogenes is a rod-shaped, gram-positive bacterium, of the order Bacillales, and *Filo firmicutes* is a human pathogen. This facultative, anaerobic, intracellular bacterium normally results from a severe blood-borne infection in humans to cause the disease listeriosis.[23] The microorganism is found in soil and decaying plant matter, and humans become infected when these agents contaminate ingested food, such as poorly cooked meats, seafood, soft cheeses, milk and other dairy products, and raw vegetables.[24]

Once the pathogen is acquired, infection is commonly established in the intestinal tract, causing mild symptoms in adults. Progression to the clinical features of intestinal listeriosis is marked by fever, diarrhea, and flulike symptoms. *Listeria*, however, also can be invasive, in which the bacterium spreads through the hematogenous route reaching other sites in the organism.[25] The disease is especially debilitating in the elderly, in immunocompromised patients, and, especially, in pregnant women.[24]

In pregnant women, symptoms include headache, confusion, and even convulsions, in addition to fever and muscle pain. The pathogen can reach the placenta by the hematogenous route, attaching to the villous syncytiotrophoblast to penetrate the villous surface, leading to placental microabcesses and, ultimately, fetal infection.[26] The placental infection occurs mainly by cell-to-cell transmission, occurring among placental cellular populations susceptible to Listeria infection, including syncytiotrophoblasts, cytotrophoblasts, and decidual cells.[2,23] Untreated, Listeriosis during pregnancy can cause fetal death, preterm delivery, and neonatal infection, sepsis, and meningitis, mainly because of fetoplacental formation of widespread acute villitis with abscesses. Treatment is based on the use of high-dose wide-spectrum antibiotics, such as ampicillin, penicillin, and amoxicillin, in suspected or confirmed cases. Prevention is focused on avoiding the consumption of any potentially contaminated food, along with sanitary surveillance.[24,25,27]

TORCH—OTHER—MALARIA

Malaria is second only to tuberculosis as the most common cause of death due to infectious disease worldwide. Therefore, malaria is a major public health problem, with great impact in under-resourced settings. This is especially true in sub-Saharan Africa, where local characteristics are ideal for the efficacious spread of severe malaria infection. In light of the mobility of all populations around the world, travel from endemic regions to developed countries is inevitable and raises the need to understand the pathophysiology and treatment of this disease process.

There are 4 human malaria parasites: *Plasmodium vivax, Plasmodium ovale, Plasmodium malariae,* and *Plasmodium falciparum. Plasmodium falciparum* is the most hazardous protozoan parasite responsible for the disease, and this parasite effectively spreads by the malarian vector, the mosquito *Anopheles gambiae.*[28] The effectiveness of this combination causes malaria infection in pregnancy to reach a prevalence of more than 25%. Identified risk factors in high-transmission areas include primigravidae, younger age, and multiple pregnancy.[29]

Estimates of the contribution of malaria to mortality are limited; however, a few studies suggest that malaria infection might be associated with up to 25% of all maternal deaths in endemic areas, especially those exposing women to coinfection by human immunodeficiency virus/acquired immunodeficiency virus. Importantly, severe malarial disease in pregnancy associates with a mortality approaching 50%.[30] Moreover, malaria infection during pregnancy can lead to increased rates of abortion, fetal growth restriction, stillbirth, prematurity, low birth weight, neonatal death, and an increased risk of infant malaria.[31] Complications in the mothers are related to severe anemia and multiorgan dysfunction.

Placental infection by malaria is recognized by the sequestration of malarial parasites in erythrocytes in the intervillous space. Placental blood infection often is higher than that in peripheral blood, and the placental infection can persist in the absence of peripheral blood parasitemia and after antimalarial treatment.[28] Pathologic disruptions of the placenta are caused by immune reaction toward erythrocyte infection, with infiltration of monocyte cells and increased release of tumor necrosis factor α and interferon γ, and signaling through Toll-like receptor 4. This leads to suboptimal placental perfusion, reduced trophoblast invasion, and alteration in angiogenic factors. The risk of placental infection increases with first-trimester parasitemia.[28,32,33] The histopathology of villi includes excessive perivillous fibrinoid deposits, proliferation of cytotrophoblast cells, and thickening of the trophoblastic basement membrane.[34]

There currently are no approaches to prevent malaria in pregnant women in endemic or epidemic areas. The main strategies recommended are to treat bed nets with insecticide and to intermittently treat presumptive infections with antimalarial medications, for example, provide 2 or more doses of chemoprophylaxis after 20 weeks' gestation to reduce subclinical malarial load. Unfortunately, such strategies yield poor adherence among women.[30] Infection with *Plasmodium vivax* can also have an adverse impact on pregnancy outcomes,[35] but the role of chemoprophylaxis, intermittent treatment, or both in management needs to be further studied.[36]

TORCH—OTHER—PARVOVIRUS B19

Found throughout the world, parvovirus B19 is transmitted by droplets as the smallest single-stranded DNA virus known and is the source of a childhood infectious erythema, dubbed fifth disease. Fortunately, two-thirds of the adult population are immune by age 40. Infection by parvovirus depends on the presence of mitotically active cells that replicate, such as the erythroid lineage of cells. The virus is cytolytic and promotes inflammatory responses with flu-like symptoms and a maculopapular rash. Included in the differential diagnosis in adults is rubella with arthralgia and late-stage arthritis with circulating immune complexes.[37–41]

There is no means of control or treatment, but the infection can be detected by either PCR or enzyme-linked immunosorbent assay (ELISA). Parvovirus B19 can cross the placental barrier to cause fetal anemia and fetal hydrops, with transmission rates of 25% to 50% and fetal death in 5% to 10%, if infection occurs before 20 weeks of gestation. The critical period for infection is from 13 weeks to 16 weeks, when there is an intense hepatic extramedullary hematopoiesis in the fetus. One in 9 of the fetuses so affected develop hydrops due to the destruction of red blood cells and increased central venous pressure,[12] and 10% progress to stillbirth without hydrops. In cases of unexplained stillbirth, immunohistochemistry to localize viral capsids can identify the virus. In other cases, the phenotype of the fetus is similar to fetal erythroblastosis, or immune hydrops, but with circulating, nucleated erythrocytes containing viral inclusions called giant normoblasts (**Fig. 2**). The pathology of the placenta shows villous edema, erythroblastosis, and Hofbauer cell hyperplasia, but lymphocytic infiltration is uncommon and villitis is undetectable.[12]

Diagnosis of maternal infection is usually performed by parvovirus B19–specific IgM and IgG antibodies, or both, and fetal infection is confirmed by PCR assay of parvovirus in the amniotic fluid or fetal blood. When a recent parvovirus B19 infection is diagnosed during pregnancy, the woman should be referred to a maternal-fetal medicine specialist and counseled about risks of fetal transmission, fetal loss, and hydrops. Serial ultrasounds are recommended to detect the development of evolving hydrops from a severe fetal anemia.[42]

TORCH—OTHER—ZIKA VIRUS

ZIKV is an arbovirus of the genus *Flavivirus*, of the family Flaviridae. Like all flaviviruses, ZIKV carries a positive-sense single-stranded RNA genome[43] and has a lipid envelope with surface viral glycoproteins, with antigenic similarity to other members of this viral

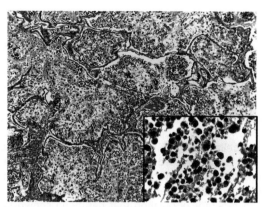

Fig. 2. Parvovirus. Primigravida with skin rash at 20 weeks delivered a 26-week hydropic stillbirth. The placenta was thick and heavy. At optical microscopy, immature foci were seen (10× objective), besides nucleated red blood cells with giant viral nuclear inclusions ([*inset*] 10× objective). (*Courtesy of* A. Antolini-Tavares, São Paulo, Brazil.)

family, such as dengue virus, yellow fever virus, West Nile virus, and Japanese encephalitis virus.[44] ZIKV remains in the wild among nonhuman primates and hematophagous mosquitoes, such as *Aedes africanus* and *Aedes serratus*.[43] In urban areas, ZIKV is transmitted to humans mainly by the bite of *Aedes aegypti*, and direct transmission through sexual intercourse, blood transfusion, and direct contact also are reported.[3]

ZIKV was first isolated from Rhesus sentinel monkeys in 1947 and from mosquitoes of the genus *Aedes* in 1948, both from the Zika Forest, Uganda. In 1952, it was described as a human-onset pathogen, with the first outbreak characterized in Nigeria in 1954.[45] Since then, ZIKV has spread to several regions of the globe, such as Asia, Oceania, and the Americas.[3] Until the beginning of the twenty-first century, ZIKV was described as a pathogen that caused sporadic cases of mostly mild diseases in Africa and Southeast Asia.[3,46] This scenario changed in 2007, with the introduction of a new variant of Asian lineage, on Yap Island in Micronesia.[47] Since then, the virus spread to French Polynesia in 2013, causing more than 32,000 cases, and to other Pacific islands, reaching Brazil in 2014.[43] From the northeast of Brazil, ZIKV spread to the rest of the country and to other American countries, culminating in the detection of ZIKV in more than 70 countries around the world in 2016 and causing a great epidemic in Brazil that affected pregnant women to a great degree.[3]

Up to 80% of patients infected with ZIKV are asymptomatic,[47] the main clinical features associated with ZIKV infection being the development of a febrile exanthem, characterized by low fever, maculopapular rash, nonpurulent conjunctivitis, arthralgias of the small joints of the hands and feet, myalgia, and prostration.[48] The incubation period of the clinical manifestations may vary from 4 days to 10 days, and the duration of the disease from 5 days to 7 days, with viremia detectable until 5 days after the onset of symptoms.

A wide range of complications may be associated with maternal ZIKV infection, including fetal and neonatal neurologic and ocular abnormalities, fetal growth restriction, stillbirth, and perinatal death. Among the neurologic abnormal findings in the fetus, there are cases of microcephaly with pronounced brain damage, mainly characterized by reduction of cortical development and atrophy, arthrogryposis, and hypoplasia of the cerebellum and cerebellar vermis.[49] The most severe cases of fetal neurologic changes usually are associated with ZIKV infection in the first trimester, but there are reported cases of microcephaly associated with infection in the second and third trimesters.[3] Complications associated with ZIKV also include Guillain-Barré syndrome, which results in a marked subacute, flaccid paralysis in adults.[50] In pregnancies, infection by ZIKV can lead to congenital morpho-functional dysfunctions and neurologic syndromes in newborns, named congenital Zika syndrome.[3]

Placental infection occurs in cells that are most susceptible to the virus, which includes Hofbauer cells, villous cytotrophoblasts, basal decidual cells, endothelial cells, and amnion-chorionic cells[8,51] (**Fig. 3**). ZIKV infection occurs to a lesser degree in syncytiotrophoblast cells. Once infected with ZIKV, viral RNA can be detected in the placenta months after the first symptoms.[52] In the placenta and other organs, the viral particle of ZIKV is recognized and internalized by contact with TIM and TAM receptors in their membrane, a receptor population that has been shown to have differential expression in the placenta.[53]

Placental tissue damage caused by this pathogen is reflected by a deciduitis, chronic villitis, increased perivillous fibrin, villous edema, and increased prominence of cytotrophoblast cells (**Fig. 4**). There currently is no available treatment, and recommendations are aimed at attenuating maternal symptoms, surveillance of fetal condition, and counseling on risks for adverse outcomes. Vaccines are in development but a few have reached phase 1 in clinical trials.[54]

TORCH—RUBELLA VIRUS

Rubella virus (RV) is a vaccine-preventable cause of congenital infection. RV is an RNA virus from the Togoviridae family (species *rubivirus*) that replicates only in humans. The viral structure is known to be spherical with spikes formed by its envelope proteins called E1 and E2.[8] Transmission occurs by aerosols disseminated from person to person, and the virus spreads from the respiratory tract, with infection of lymphocytes and alveolar macrophages, to lymph nodes, skin, joints, and other organs. The infection is commonly manifested as a mild, measles-like exanthem. Joint pain and lymphadenopathy reflect a response toward immune defense and are a consequence of circulating RV-specific immune complexes of antibodies directed against the E1 and E2 antigens.[8]

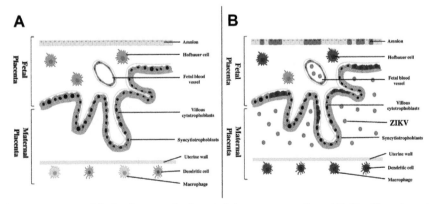

Fig. 3. ZIKV. Simplified schemes of placental transverse section. (*A*) Healthy placental cellular environment. (*B*) ZIKV infection routes in placenta by cell type susceptibility, showing infected cells in red. (Created with BioRender.com.)

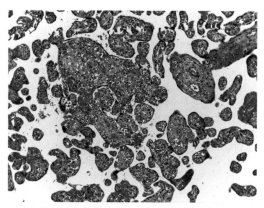

Fig. 4. ZIKV. Focal chronic lymphohistiocytic villitis with focal trophoblast destruction and fibrin deposition (10× objective). (*Courtesy of* M.L. Costa, MD, PhD, São Paulo, Brazil.)

Infection immediately before conception or within the first 10 weeks of pregnancy causes multiple fetal defects in up to 90% of cases, which can result in stillbirth. Fetal infection is rare if maternal rubella occurs after the sixteenth week of gestation, although hearing deficits may occur with infection as late as 20 weeks of gestation. Congenital rubella syndrome is characterized by defects in eyes (such as cataracts, chorioretinitis, glaucoma, microphthalmia, and pigmentary retinopathy), hearing (sensorineural deafness), heart (such as patent ductus arteriosus or ventricular septal defects and peripheral pulmonary artery stenosis), and brain (microcephaly). Newborns who survive may suffer developmental disabilities.[55,56]

The diagnostic test for recent postnatal infection is the detection of RV-specific IgM by ELISA. During the acute phase, a 4-fold rise in RV-specific IgG is also diagnostic for rubella infection.[57] Viral detection can be performed on oral fluids, throat swabs, nasopharyngeal secretions, or urine.

Placental pathology features villous necrosis, vascular inflammation, and enlarged Hofbauer cells, with intense acute and chronic villitis. RV inclusions can be identified within decidual cells, extravillous trophoblasts, endothelial cells, and amnion.[7] Infected endothelial cells can facilitate viral dissemination and have a further impact on the transport functions of the placenta, leading to fetal growth restriction.[8]

Vaccination is clearly the intervention to avoid the burden of rubella infection. In 2011, the World Health Organization provided guidance to strengthen routine immunization for rubella worldwide, including an initial vaccination campaign for offspring aged 9 months to 14 years. Global partners have set targets to eliminate rubella and congenital rubella syndrome in at least 5 of the 6 World Health Organization regions by 2020.[58] Unfortunately, this worthy goal seems unrealistic. Globally, travelers have enabled rubella to enter countries that had previously eliminated the virus, leading to new outbreaks and endemic transmission.[59,60]

TORCH—CYTOMEGALOVIRUS

CMV is a double-stranded DNA virus within the family of the herpes virus, which commonly causes asymptomatic infection but with devastating consequences in vulnerable groups, such as pregnant women. The seroprevalence of CMV is 60% for the American population[61] and increases with age. CMV is the most common cause of congenital infection, reaching 2.2%, among all infants born worldwide.[62,63]

CMV infection in the first or second trimester results in substantial damage to brain development and deafness.[64]

CMV transmission can occur through exposure to blood and most body secretions, where infection of epithelial cells, T cells and macrophages, decidua, extravillous trophoblasts, and villous cytotrophoblasts occurs. Viral cytopathic effects yield cytomegalic inclusions, dubbed owl's eye (**Fig. 5**), in capillary endothelium and stromal cells of the placenta, yielding bulky villi with delayed maturation. Virus detection has been demonstrated in up to 15% of fetal and placental tissues.[65] The histopathologic findings may diminish as infection progresses and the inclusions are not always easily identified. End-stage changes in the placental injury include chronification, vascular obliteration with stromal sclerosis, thrombosis, hemosiderosis, multifocal calcifications, and chronic lymphoplasmacytic villitis. Immunohistochemistry may assist in the assignment of etiology for such histologic changes but immunohistochemistry is less sensitive than molecular techniques to evaluate for infection nevertheless.[7]

Seroconversion is commonly used as the marker of primary CMV infection, although other assays using cultured fibroblasts, antigenic assays, PCR, or cytology may be useful. Congenital CMV infection is best identified by isolating the CMV virus from the neonate's urine in the first week of life.[66] There currently is no available vaccine for CMV: treatment of serious acute infection is initially with ganciclovir.[66]

TORCH—HERPES SIMPLEX VIRUS

HSV-1 and HSV-2 represent a large family of DNA viruses, transmitted through epithelial mucosal cells and skin breaks to persist latent in nerve tissues. HSV-1 and HSV-2 are worldwide and highly prevalent, especially in Africa, Southeast Asia, and Western Pacific.[55] Genital HSV-2 is the most frequent sexually transmitted infection in US women of reproductive age.[67] HSV-1 is commonly found in orofacial lesions, and oral sex has the potential for transmission to cause genital infection. Therefore, HSV-1 and HSV-2 can both lead to genital lesions and viral shedding.[55] This fact is of great relevance during pregnancy, because most neonatal herpes infections result from exposure to HSV shed during childbirth.[68]

Although HSV neonatal infection is rare, such infections create significant morbidity, mortality, risk of neurologic impairment, and risk of disseminated disease or disease of the skin, eyes, and mucosa.[68] A protective mechanism during pregnancy exists in the

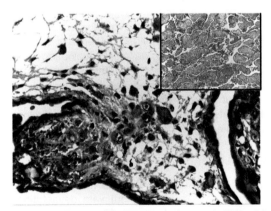

Fig. 5. CMV. Classical CMV owl's eye inclusions in a placental villus with a diffuse vascular destruction chronic villitis (16-week stillbirth). Main picture on a 40× objective; inset is on a 4× one. (*Courtesy of* A. Antolini-Tavares, São Paulo, Brazil.)

form of maternal IgG antibodies, which can cross the placenta to provide immunity to herpes in the neonate. This phenomenon also explains why the risk of neonatal herpes is greater when primary maternal infection happens close to term, when the virus can shed from the genital tract to infect the newborn but maternal IgG antibodies are not yet produced.[55]

Placental histopathologic findings with herpes infection can be nonspecific and mild, because the presence of viral inclusions is rare. Syncytiotrophoblast is resistant to HSV colonization because this trophoblast phenotype does not express the HSV entry mediators HveA, HveB and HveC. In contrast, extravillous cytotrophoblast expresses all 3 mediators and, therefore, can be infected by HSV.[69]

Antiviral therapy is recommended for documented acute, primary herpes infections any time in pregnancy and during the last 4 weeks of pregnancy in patients with known histories of infection to reduce viral shedding and HSV recurrence at delivery.[70] Cesarean section is indicated for recurrent lesions when delivery is indicated. Among cases of asymptomatic HSV in labor, invasive procedures are commonly discouraged yet active management should be considered if rupture of membranes occur before the onset of labor.[55]

DISCLOSURE

This work was supported by Grant CNPq # 409605/2016 - Conselho Nacional de Desenvolvimento Científico e Tecnológico (CNPq).

REFERENCES

1. Billington WD. The immunological problem of pregnancy: 50 years with the hope of progress. A tribute to Peter Medawar. J Reprod Immunol 2003;60(1):1–11.
2. Arora N, Sadovsky Y, Dermody TS, et al. Microbial vertical transmission during human pregnancy. Cell Host Microbe 2017;21(5):561–7.
3. Proenca-Modena JL, Milanez GP, Costa ML, et al. Zika virus: lessons learned in Brazil. Microbes Infect 2018;20(11–12):661–9.
4. Vinturache AE, Gyamfi-Bannerman C, Hwang J, et al. Maternal microbiome - A pathway to preterm birth. Semin Fetal Neonatal Med 2016;21(2):94–9.
5. Burton GJ, Jauniaux E. Pathophysiology of placental-derived fetal growth restriction. Am J Obstet Gynecol 2018;218(2):S745–61.
6. Phipps EA, Thadhani R, Benzing T, et al. Pre-eclampsia: pathogenesis, novel diagnostics and therapies. Nat Rev Nephrol 2019;15(5):275–89.
7. Heerema-McKenney A. Defense and infection of the human placenta. Apmis 2018;126(7):570–88.
8. Pereira L. Congenital viral infection: traversing the uterine-placental interface. Annu Rev Virol 2018;5(1):273–99.
9. Nelson DM. How the placenta affects your life, from womb to tomb. Am J Obstet Gynecol 2015;213(4):S12–3.
10. Aguirre AA, Longcore T, Barbieri M, et al. The one health approach to toxoplasmosis: epidemiology, control, and prevention strategies. Ecohealth 2019. https://doi.org/10.1007/s10393-019-01405-7.
11. Kim K, Weiss LM. Toxoplasma gondii: the model apicomplexan. Int J Parasitol 2004;34(3):423–32.
12. Faye-Petersen OM, Heller DS, Joshi VV. Handbook of placental pathology. 2nd edition. Oxfordshire (UK): Taylor & Francis; 2006.
13. Lindsay DS, Dubey JP. Toxoplasma gondii: the changing paradigm of congenital toxoplasmosis. Parasitology 2011;138(14):1829–31.

14. Paquet C, Yudin MH. Toxoplasmosis in pregnancy: prevention, screening, and treatment. J Obstet Gynaecol Can 2018;40(8):e687–93.

15. Nelson R. Congenital syphilis and other STIs rise in the USA. Lancet Infect Dis 2018;18(11):1186–7.

16. Peeling RW, Mabey D, Kamb ML, et al. Syphilis. Nat Rev Dis Primers 2017;3: 17073.

17. Virginia B, John S, Elizabeth T, et al. Increase in incidence of congenital syphilis — United States, 2012–2014. MMWR Morb Mortal Wkly Rep 2015;64(44):1233–40.

18. Spiteri G, Unemo M, Mårdh O, et al. The resurgence of syphilis in high-income countries in the 2000s: a focus on Europe. Epidemiol Infect 2019;147:e143.

19. Macé G, Castaigne V, Trabbia A, et al. Fetal anemia as a signal of congenital syphilis. J Matern Fetal Neonatal Med 2014;27(13):1375–7.

20. Kitt E, May RM, Steenhoff AP. Rash and hepatosplenomegaly in a newborn. JMM Case Rep 2017;4(6):10–1.

21. Genest DR, Choi-Hong SR, Tate JE, et al. Diagnosis of congenital syphilis from placental examination: comparison of histopathology, steiner stain, and polymerase chain reaction for Treponema pallidum DNA. Hum Pathol 1996;27(4):366–72.

22. Taylor M, Gliddon H, Nurse-Findlay S, et al. Revisiting strategies to eliminate mother-to-child transmission of syphilis. Lancet Glob Health 2018;6(1):e26–8.

23. Vázquez-Boland JA, Krypotou E, Scortti M. Listeria placental infection. MBio 2017;8(3):1–6.

24. Imanishi M, Routh JA, Klaber M, et al. Estimating the attack rate of pregnancy-associated listeriosis during a large outbreak. Infect Dis Obstet Gynecol 2015; 2015:1–5.

25. Centers for Disease Control and Prevention (CDC). Vital signs: listeria death, illnesses, and outbreaks - United States 2009-2011. Morb Mortal Wkly Rep 2013; 62(22):448–52. Available at: http://www.cdc.gov/mmwr/preview/mmwrhtml/mm6222a4.htm?s_cid=mm6222a4_w.

26. Lamond N, Freitag N. Vertical transmission of listeria monocytogenes: probing the balance between protection from pathogens and fetal tolerance. Pathogens 2018;7(2):52.

27. Lamont RF, Sobel J, Mazaki-Tovi S, et al. Listeriosis in human pregnancy: a systematic review. J Perinat Med 2011;39(3):227–36.

28. Uneke CJ. Impact of placental Plasmodium falciparum malaria on pregnancy and perinatal outcome in sub-Saharan Africa: I: introduction to placental malaria. Yale J Biol Med 2007;80(2):39–50.

29. Desai M, TerKuile F, Nosten F, et al. Epidemiology and the burden of malaria in pregnancy. Lancet Infect Dis 2007;7(February):93–104.

30. Schantz-Dunn J, Nour NM. Malaria and pregnancy: a global health perspective. Rev Obstet Gynecol 2009;2(3):186–92.

31. De Beaudrap P, Turyakira E, Nabasumba C, et al. Timing of malaria in pregnancy and impact on infant growth and morbidity: a cohort study in Uganda. Malar J 2016;15:92.

32. Fried M, Duffy PE. Malaria during pregnancy. Cold Spring Harb Perspect Med 2017;7(6).

33. Pandya Y, Penha-Gonçalves C. Maternal-fetal conflict during infection: lessons from a mouse model of placental malaria. Front Microbiol 2019;10:1126.

34. Matteelli A, Caligaris S, Castelli F, et al. The placenta and malaria. Ann Trop Med Parasitol 1997;91(7):803–10.

35. Bardají A, Martínez-Espinosa FE, Arévalo-Herrera M, et al. Burden and impact of Plasmodium vivax in pregnancy: a multi-centre prospective observational study. Plos Negl Trop Dis 2017;11(6):e0005606.

36. World Health Organization. WHO Expert Committee on Malaria. World Health Organ Tech Rep Ser 2000;892:i–v, 1–74. Available at: http://europepmc.org/abstract/MED/10892307.

37. Xiong Y, Tan J, Liu Y, et al. The risk of maternal parvovirus B19 infection during pregnancy on fetal loss and fetal hydrops: a systematic review and meta-analysis. J Clin Virol 2019;114:12–20.

38. Kontomanolis EN, Fasoulakis Z. Hydrops fetalis and the parvovirus B-19. Curr Pediatr Rev 2018;14(4):239–52.

39. Pistorius LR, Smal J, de Haan TR, et al. Disturbance of cerebral neuronal migration following congenital parvovirus B19 infection. Fetal Diagn Ther 2008;24(4):491–4.

40. Klugman D, Berger JT, Sable CA, et al. Pediatric patients hospitalized with myocarditis: a multi-institutional analysis. Pediatr Cardiol 2010;31(2):222–8.

41. Courtier J, Schauer GM, Parer JT, et al. Polymicrogyria in a fetus with human parvovirus B19 infection: a case with radiologic-pathologic correlation. Ultrasound Obstet Gynecol 2012;40(5):604–6.

42. Crane J, Mundle W, Boucoiran I, et al. Parvovirus B19 infection in pregnancy. J Obstet Gynaecol Can 2014;36(12):1107–16.

43. Musso D, Gubler DJ. Zika virus. Clin Microbiol Rev 2016;29(3):487–524.

44. Turrini F, Ghezzi S, Pagani I, et al. Zika virus: are-emerging pathogen with rapidly evolving public health implications. New Microbiol 2016;39(2):86–90.

45. Macnamara FN. Zika virus: a report on three cases of human infection during an epidemic of jaundice in nigeria. Trans R Soc Trop Med Hyg 1954;48(2).

46. Faye O, Freire CCM, Iamarino A, et al. Molecular evolution of Zika virus during its emergence in the 20th century. PLoS Negl Trop Dis 2014;8(1):36.

47. Duffy MR, Chen TH, Hancock WT, et al. Zika virus outbreak on yap island, federated states of Micronesia. N Engl J Med 2009;360(24):2536–43.

48. Cao-Lormeau VM, Blake A, Mons S, et al. Guillain-Barré syndrome outbreak associated with Zika virus infection in french polynesia: a case-control study. Lancet 2016;387(10027):1531–9.

49. Chimelli L, Melo ASO, Avvad-Portari E, et al. The spectrum of neuropathological changes associated with congenital Zika virus infection. Acta Neuropathol 2017;133(6):983–99.

50. Tiwari SK, Dang J, Qin Y, et al. Zika virus infection reprograms global transcription of host cells to allow sustained infection. Emerg Microbes Infect 2017;6(4):e24.

51. Simoni MK, Jurado KA, Abrahams VM, et al. Zika virus infection of Hofbauer cells. Am J Reprod Immunol 2017;77(2).

52. Driggers RW, Ho CY, Korhonen EM, et al. Zika virus infection with prolonged maternal viremia and fetal brain abnormalities. Obstet Anesth Dig 2017;37(1):51.

53. Tabata T, Petitt M, Puerta-Guardo H, et al. Zika virus targets different primary human placental cells, suggesting two routes for vertical transmission. Cell Host Microbe 2016;20(2):155–66.

54. Poland GA, Kennedy RB, Ovsyannikova IG, et al. Development of vaccines against Zika virus. Lancet Infect Dis 2018;18(7):e211–9.

55. Silasi M, Cardenas I, Kwon J-Y, et al. Viral infections during pregnancy. Am J Reprod Immunol 2015;73(3):199–213.

56. Yazigi A, De Pecoulas AE, Vauloup-Fellous C, et al. Fetal and neonatal abnormalities due to congenital rubella syndrome: a review of literature. J Matern Fetal Neonatal Med 2017;30(3):274–8.
57. Versalovic J, Carroll KC, Funke G, et al, editors. Manual of clinical microbiology. 10th edition. Washington, DC: American Society of Microbiology; 2011. Available at: http://www.asmscience.org/content/book/10.1128/9781555816728.
58. Grant GB, Reef SE, Patel M, et al. Progress in Rubella and congenital rubella syndrome control and elimination - worldwide, 2000-2016. MMWR Morb Mortal Wkly Rep 2017;66(45):1256–60.
59. Martínez-Quintana E, Castillo-Solórzano C, Torner N, et al. Congenital rubella syndrome: a matter of concern. Rev Panam Salud Publica 2015;37(3):179–86.
60. Zimmerman LA, Muscat M, Singh S, et al. Progress toward measles elimination - European Region, 2009-2018. MMWR Morb Mortal Wkly Rep 2019;68(17): 396–401.
61. Zhang LJ, Hanff P, Rutherford C, et al. Detection of human cytomegalovirus DNA, RNA, and antibody in normal donor blood. J Infect Dis 1995;171(4):1002–6.
62. Marin LJ, Santos de Carvalho Cardoso E, Bispo Sousa SM, et al. Prevalence and clinical aspects of CMV congenital Infection in a low-income population. Virol J 2016;13(1):148.
63. Barron SD, Pass RF. Infectious causes of hydrops fetalis. Semin Perinatol 1995; 19(6):493–501. https://doi.org/10.1016/S0146-0005(05)80056-4.
64. Weichert A, Vogt M, Dudenhausen JW, et al. Evidence in a human fetus of micrognathia and cleft lip as potential effects of early cytomegalovirus infection. Fetal Diagn Ther 2010;28(4):225–8.
65. Iwasenko JM, Howard J, Arbuckle S, et al. Human cytomegalovirus infection is detected frequently in stillbirths and is associated with fetal thrombotic vasculopathy. J Infect Dis 2011;203(11):1526–33.
66. Rawlinson WD, Hamilton ST, van Zuylen WJ. Update on treatment of cytomegalovirus infection in pregnancy and of the newborn with congenital cytomegalovirus. Curr Opin Infect Dis 2016;29(6):615–24.
67. Looker KJ, Magaret AS, May MT, et al. Global and regional estimates of prevalent and incident herpes simplex virus type 1 infections in 2012. PLoS One 2015; 10(10):e0140765.
68. Looker KJ, Magaret AS, May MT, et al. First estimates of the global and regional incidence of neonatal herpes infection. Lancet Glob Health 2017;5(3):e300–9.
69. Koi H, Zhang J, Makrigiannakis A, et al. Syncytiotrophoblast is a barrier to maternal-fetal transmission of herpes simplex virus1. Biol Reprod 2004;67(5): 1572–9.
70. Sheffield JS, Hollier LM, Hill JB, et al. Acyclovir prophylaxis to prevent herpes simplex virus recurrence at delivery: a systematic review. Obstet Gynecol 2003;102(6):1396–403.

Fetal Membranes, Not a Mere Appendage of the Placenta, but a Critical Part of the Fetal-Maternal Interface Controlling Parturition

Ramkumar Menon, PhD, MS[a], John J. Moore, MD[b],*

KEYWORDS

- Amniochorion • Oxidative stress • Preterm birth • pPROM • Senescence • Aging
- GM-CSF

KEY POINTS

- Fetal membranes (FMs) protect the fetus and maintain pregnancy.
- FM senescence (mechanism of aging) and senescence-associated inflammation are associated with labor at term.
- Premature FM senescence in response to pregnancy-associated risk factors, such as infection, is associated with preterm premature rupture of the fetal membranes (pPROM).
- Inflammation-induced FM weakening requires the generation of the critical intermediate, granulocyte-macrophage colony-stimulating factor.
- Prevention of pPROM may be possible in the future with success in ongoing research into biomarkers for susceptibility to pPROM and therapeutic agents to prevent it.

Obstetricians, neonatologists, and reproductive scientists have collectively performed much research in pregnancy and parturition. These authors contend, however, that a major knowledge gap remains, specifically in the area of fetal membranes (FMs). Furthermore, the authors suggest that this gap is partly responsible for high rates of adverse pregnancy outcomes, specifically, spontaneous preterm births (PTBs), birth before 37 weeks' gestation. Approximately 10% of all pregnancies end as preterm births. Universal approaches to diagnose and manage preterm labor have not significantly reduced the risk or the impact. In addition to the immediate mortality and

[a] Department of Obstetrics and Gynecology, Perinatal Research Division, The University of Texas Medical Branch, MRB 11.138, 301 University Boulevard, Galveston, TX 77555, USA; [b] Case Western Reserve University School of Medicine, 2500 MetroHealth Drive, Cleveland, OH 44109, USA
* Corresponding author. Department of Pediatrics and Reproductive Biology, Division of Neonatology, MetroHealth Medical Center, 2500 MetroHealth Drive, Cleveland, OH 44109.
E-mail address: jjm6@case.edu

Obstet Gynecol Clin N Am 47 (2020) 147–162
https://doi.org/10.1016/j.ogc.2019.10.004
0889-8545/20/© 2019 Elsevier Inc. All rights reserved.

morbidity, preterm birth contributes to lifelong health issues of premature babies.[1] Advanced diagnostic and management strategies of identifying high-risk women, better access to medical care, and revolutionary advancements in research fields are in place, but PTB rates still remain relatively high.[1]

Why can the incidence of PTB not be reduced? Fetal-maternal uterine tissues have been structurally and functionally (mechanisms and pathways) well studied in an attempt to understand the mechanisms that maintain pregnancy and pathways leading to parturition.[2–4] This knowledge is critical to reducing the risk of complications during pregnancy. Interventions and management strategies, however, have been generally targeted to the maternal reproductive tissues (cervix, endometrial decidua, and myometrium).[2,5–7] This approach has not been successful in reducing PTBs.

This article asks, is it possible that the targeted tissues are not the primary initiators of parturition and the process of preterm parturition is already too far advanced such that targeting secondarily involved maternal reproductive tissues is not effective? The authors suggest that a knowledge gaps exists in understanding of the involvement of a specific reproductive tissue in PTBs.

In this review, the authors highlight the existence of what is considered a black hole in knowledge. A tissue is described that is frequently ignored and often inaccurately referred to as just part of the placenta, that is, FMs (placental membranes/amniochorionic membrane). Although FMs have received some attention recently due to increasing interest in using the membrane as a model to understand immune, endocrine, mechanical, and cellular aspects of pregnancy and parturition,[8,9] nonetheless, FMs are minimally studied and often referred to as "dead tissue" in the perinatal medicine and reproductive biology fields.[10] Hence, their potential role as tissue that maintains pregnancy and is critically involved in parturition is ignored.

FETAL MEMBRANES, AN OFTEN IGNORED CRITICAL UTERINE TISSUE

The FMs are not placenta and do not follow the placental developmental trajectory. They have their own developmental origin during embryogenesis and growth during in-utero life. FMs might be described as an organism in-between the fetus and the mother, performing unique functions different from the placenta. FMs provide structural framework to the uterine cavity and provide immune, antimicrobial, endocrine, and mechanical protection to the growing fetus.[8,9] FMs exhibit longevity that matches the in-utero fetal maturation and then undergo senescence (mechanism of aging). As they age, FMs perform yet another critical function where they produce a unique inflammatory biochemical profile that functions as a fetal signal for readiness for parturition. This signal propagates from the fetus to the mother either by diffusion or via extracellular vesicles (exosomes).[11–15] Thus, FMs initially protect pregnancy and then ultimately promote parturition while sacrificing their own existence. It is, therefore, logical to think that dysfunctional FMs can be detrimental to pregnancy. Certain adverse events during pregnancy are linked to functional and mechanical failures of the FMs. Fetal inflammatory signals associated with aging also can be augmented by inflammatory conditions at the fetal-maternal interface related to infection, decidual bleeding, or premature cervical ripening.[3,15] This review expands on the function of the FMs and how their aging can promote parturition at term. Additionally, how their possible premature aging and the impact of biochemical and inflammation-induced inflammatory processes can cause structural, mechanical, and functional disruption, contributing to preterm birth and other adverse pregnancy outcomes, are discussed.

SO, WHAT ARE FETAL MEMBRANES?

The FMs are tissues that provide mechanical support, compartmentalization, and immunologic protection (from the mother) for the growing fetus until their disruption and rupture at parturition (**Fig. 1**).[16,17] The major cellular components of the FMs are a solid layer of amnion epithelial cells (AECs) facing the fetus and a dense layer of chorion cytotrophoblasts at the maternal-fetal interface. These 2 cellular sheets are sandwiched together and organized by a collagen-rich extracellular matrix (ECM) that contains, and is constructed by, fibroblast cells.[18,19] Collagen is a major component of the FM ECM. The collagen structure is organized in 2 important ways. First, there is a layer of collagen in the amnion just below the AEC layer. Second, there are bands of collagen, described as rivets in their original description,[20] which bind the amnion cells, passing through the collagen layer, to fibroblasts closer to the maternal facing side of the amnion. These collagen rivets hold all the components of the amnion together. Balanced collagenolytic remodeling modulates membrane

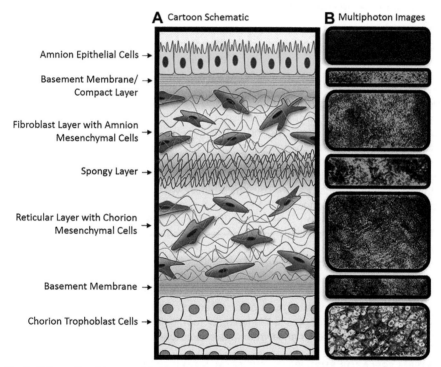

Fig. 1. Schematic of human fetal (amniochorionic) membrane. (*A*) Human fetal membrane comprises a single layer of cuboidal epithelial cells that is near the fetus and constantly bathed in amniotic fluid. Amnion epithelium is connected to the ECM by type IV collagen-rich basement membrane. FM amnion and chorion components are demarcated by the spongy layer. Dispersed in the ECM are amnion mesenchymal and chorion mesenchymal cells. Another layer of basement membrane connects chorion ECM to chorion trophoblast cells. (*B*) Multiphoton images of human fetal membranes. Shown here are nonlinear optical microscopy images of unstained human fetal membrane layers. Live imaging of unstained fetal membrane tissue using multiphoton autofluorescence and second harmonic generation microscopy reveal cellularity and collagen contents (*green*) of human FMs. The colors in the figure are pseudocolor representation of cells and matrices.

homeostasis during pregnancy.[3,10] Reactive oxygen species from intrauterine redox reactions maintain their structural and functional integrity.[21] Simply put, the chorion cytotrophoblast layer provides protection for the fetus against the mother's immune system. The amnion layer provides compartmentalization allowing an amniotic fluid layer to separate the fetus from both the placenta and the FMs. This allows the fetus to escape the uterus at parturition. The collagen-rich ECM holds the FM structure together during pregnancy but, importantly, degrades to allow parturition.

Other than the immune protection, these FM functions are not those of the placenta, whose major function is transport of nutrients and wastes. The FMs thus are not part of the placenta, either structurally or functionally. Although attached to the placenta, the amnion has a completely separate embryologic origin and the chorion deviates from the placenta in structure and function by the first month of pregnancy. Membranes develop in parallel with the fetus, becoming fully formed with the fusion of the amnion and chorion by the fifteenth week of gestation.[22]

PHYSIOLOGIC AGING OF FETAL MEMBRANES DURING GESTATION AND ITS RELATIONSHIP TO NORMAL PARTURITION

FM cells proliferate and transition to maintain cellular integrity during gestation. FMs grow with the fetus through active cell proliferation and maintain their structural and functional integrity through remodeling. Remodeling of FMs takes place at recently discovered sites, called *biologic microfractures*.[17,23] Microfractures are wounds that develop due to FM cell shedding, gap formation, and collagen matrix degradation. Microfractures heal by cellular transitions and by nascent collagen matrix production.[24] This is likely part of the mechanism by which FMs heal after fetoscopic surgeries in a majority of cases. During active growth and multiplication, membrane cells undergo replicative senescence, a mechanism associated with aging. This is a telomere-dependent process as telomere lengths are progressively decreased (biological markers of cellular aging) in FM cells. Senescence of FMs is well correlated with fetal growth and maturation. This has been shown in both animal models and human pregnancy.[25–29] Senescent FMs show a unique inflammatory profile (senescence-associated secretory phenotype [SASP]) as well as senescence-induced cellular injury that generates damage-associated molecular pattern markers (DAMPs).[30,31] Both SASP and DAMPs are prolabor inflammatory mediators that are propagated from senescent FMs to maternal uterine tissues via extracellular vesicles that cause parturition-related changes.[32–34] Thus, FMs not only protect the fetus during pregnancy but also ensure fetal delivery by informing the mother about fetal maturation through biochemical signals sent via endocrine and or paracrine pathways. Normally FM aging contributes to the timing of term delivery and concomitant rupture of the FMs. Major problems arise when this occurs prematurely.

PRETERM PRELABOR RUPTURE OF THE FETAL MEMBRANES, AN UNDERSTUDIED PHENOTYPE OF SPONTANEOUS PRETERM BIRTHS

Approximately 60% of all preterm deliveries are spontaneous PTBs where the causality is unclear. Recent advancement in technology has provided multitudes of promising diagnostic markers to predict imminent preterm labor in asymptomatic women.[35–38] No similar markers are available, however, to predict preterm prelabor rupture of the FMs (pPROM). At term, FMs either rupture naturally (spontaneous rupture of membranes) or are artificially ruptured by delivering personnel (artificial rupture of membranes) to induce delivery. pPROM, however, prior to 37 weeks' gestation, precedes approximately 40% of all spontaneous PTBs.[39–41] In the United States, approximately 175,000 pPROM cases occur each year, making it the most common pregnancy complication, more than all reported cases of indicated PTBs (preeclampsia, intrauterine growth restriction, gestational diabetes mellitus, and so forth).[40] Irrespective of the gestational age at delivery, morbidity and mortality rates associated with pPROM are higher than other spontaneous PTBs.[42,43] Several tests, such as pooling, ferning, nitrazine, and AmniSure (QIAGEN), are available to confirm that pPROM has occurred. Despite the availability of a plethora of tests confirming its occurrence, there are no reliable markers or methods to predict pPROM before it occurs.[44–47] Several reports have identified significant predisposing associations that increase the risk of pPROM, including reproductive tract infections, behavioral factors, environmental toxins, genetic factors, and obstetric complications.[48–52] The authors suggest that because the underlying causes and pathways of pPROM are poorly understood, attempts to develop screening or interventions have been largely unsuccessful.[53] Because of the importance of the control and timing of the FM rupture, especially in pPROM, the remainder of this review discusses this function of the FMs.

THE CAUSALITY OF PRETERM PRELABOR RUPTURE OF THE FETAL MEMBRANES, AN UNTAPPED AREA OF RESEARCH WITH NO PROGRESS IN CLINICAL TRANSLATIONAL MEDICINE

pPROM is traditionally considered a disease caused by intraamniotic infection. Approximately 70% of pPROM cases have an infectious association due to positive amniotic fluid culture or positive polymerase chain reaction for microbial DNA from intraamniotic pathogens.[48,51,54,55] Weakening of the amniochorion ECM by collagen degradation is one of the key events predisposing to rupture. Both endogenous and exogenous factors activate collagen degradation. The intrinsic factors include pathologic aging, a local variation in membrane thickness, and a reduction in collagen content along with the host or fetal inflammatory response. The extrinsic factors include effects of infection and intrauterine bleeding, including those associated with preterm cervical remodeling.[56]

INTRINSIC FACTORS: PATHOLOGIC AGING OF FETAL MEMBRANES PROMOTES PRETERM PRELABOR RUPTURE OF THE FETAL MEMBRANES AND PRETERM BIRTHS

Premature activation of senescence and attrition of telomeres often are seen in pPROM FMs and not as often in preterm labor when FMs are intact (**Fig. 2**).[26,31] Infection, inflammation, and oxidative stress (OS) can accelerate premature aging of the FMs, where untimely inflammatory signaling can cause membrane rupture or preterm labor. Aging-related studies on FMs showed that membrane aging is much more pronounced and the number of microfractures is far greater in pPROM than in preterm labor. Similarities between term labor and pPROM suggest that pPROM is associated with premature aging pathology. Premature aging of FMs is not absent in preterm labor, but aging is not as noticeable. Membrane aging in pPROM could be due to maternal conditions that result in OS because OS is one of the major accelerators of the aging process. OS-inducing risk factors include, but are not limited to, poor nutrition, high body mass index (BMI), behavioral factors (cigarette smoking and drug and alcohol abuse), environmental pollutants, psychosocial stressors, toxic chemical exposures, prior history, twin gestation, ethnicity/race, and genetics.[48,57–59] All these risk factors can induce OS and accelerate SASP and DAMP-mediated FM weakening, predisposing them to rupture. The authors postulate that the presence of these risk factors predisposes them to premature weakening that, in turn, compromises antimicrobial defense. This paves the way for genital mycoplasmas and other

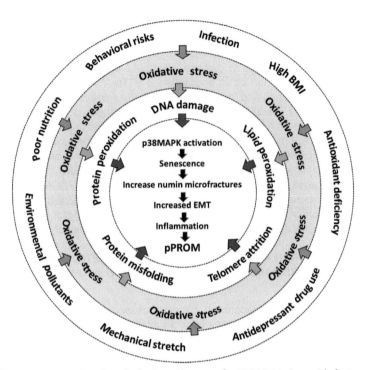

Fig. 2. Senescence-associated pathologic pathways of pPROM. Various risk factors during pregnancy (as shown in the outer layer) can induce OS in human fetal membranes (shaded layer). OS has an impact on cellular function by causing damages to various cellular elements and organelles, as shown in the third layer. OS-induced damages can lead to stress signaler pathway activation. In FMs, stress signaling is activated by p38MAPK. Various studies have shown that p38MAPK-mediated senescence is associated with increased biological microfracture formation, transition of AECs into amnion mesenchymal cells (EMT) and their accumulation in the ECM. Amnion mesenchymal cells are highly vulnerable to OS damages and increase localized inflammation. Senescence of cells also contribute to SASP, a form of inflammation marked by cytokines, chemokines, and MMPs capable of degrading ECM matrix and weakening the membrane (inner layer). Thus, pPROM results from cellular biological changes resulting from risk factor–induced, OS-mediated damages. These damages produce a terminal pathway causing inflammation that leads to ECM degradation and weakening of membrane predisposing them to rupture. EMT, epithelial mesenchymal transition.

cervical-vaginal colonizers to ascend to the membranes, cross over to the amniotic cavity and start colonization, infection, and inflammation. Although colonization of bacteria is a poor OS inducer, the host immune response can attract neutrophils and other immune cells that cause inflammation (histologic chorioamnionitis). Inflammation essentially is an inseparable component of OS and thus infection-associated inflammation can produce further damage to FMs.

Failure of antibiotics to reduce the risk of preterm birth after pPROM is partially explained by this theory:

1. Infection may not be the primary cause, but rather a consequence, of OS and OS-induced damage to FMs that compromise FM antimicrobial defense function.
2. Persistence of underlying risk or risk-induced damage to tissues is not corrected by antibiotics.

3. Persistent inflammation in tissues results in nonreversible senescence and increased SASP markers.

The authors, however, do not argue that infection is not associated with pPROM and antibiotics should be withheld. Based on the points listed previously, the authors suggest that infection may be a secondary causal factor in a major subset of pPROM where FM functions are compromised. Similarly, membrane-weakening agents, such as thrombin, arising from decidual hemorrhage, and granulocyte macrophage colony-stimulating factor (GM-CSF), arising from senescence-associated inflammation, are well described mediators of membrane weakening.[43,50] Antimicrobial interventions are doomed to failure if underlying primary causal factors are not investigated or are ignored.

EXTRINSIC FACTORS

The rupture of FMs at parturition usually occurs in the FM region overlying the cervix. Biomechanical studies have shown that the FMs overlying most of the uterine surface are strong enough to withstand the strongest possible uterine contractions without rupture.[60] More than 3 decades ago, however, the FM region overlying the cervix was noted to be different from the other areas and showed more evidence of collagen remodeling and cell death compared with the remaining regions of the FMs.[61–65] Subsequently, this region also was demonstrated to be significantly weaker than the remaining FM areas and in many cases with 10% of the rupture strength of the rest of the FMs.[66,67] As term approaches, the entire FM undergoes changes and becomes weaker but especially the pericervical region.[68] This overall weakening with increasing gestation, especially in the last month of pregnancy, may be related to aging and senescence, as described previously.

CERVICAL REMODELING AND FETAL MEMBRANE RUPTURE

Recent biomechanical modeling studies suggest that cervical remodeling may be largely responsible for the normal development of focal weakness of the pericervical region of the FMs. These studies suggest that the pericervical region undergoes enormous mechanical strain as the cervix shortens and remodels. This can and often does result in separation of the amnion and chorion and eventually detachment from the uterine surface of the chorion with attached decidua.[69,70] This tissue disruption results in both decidual bleeding and inflammation that can lead directly to FM weakening and additional cervical remodeling.[71]

EXTERNAL INFLAMMATORY CHALLENGES AND FETAL MEMBRANE RUPTURE

An in vitro model system studied over the past decade has shown that inflammatory challenges to the FMs from almost any source causes FM weakening (**Fig. 3**).[72] Inflammation/infection with the release of cytokines, such as tumor necrosis factor (TNF) and interleukin (IL)-1, or inflammation related to decidual bleeding, releasing thrombin and other factors, all weaken FMs. Interestingly, inflammation modifies FMs biochemically to resemble the naturally occurring pericervical weak region of the FMs.[73,74] Most important, GM-CSF has been found to be the critical intermediate for all inflammation-induced FM weakening processes.[75] GM-CSF is produced in a concentration-dependent manner by TNF, IL-1, or thrombin. The weakening effects of all these agents are blocked by GM-CSF neutralizing antibody. In addition, GM-CSF directly weakens FMs in a concentration-dependent manner.[75] GM-CSF acts on the choriodecidua to produce specific proteases and decrease specific protease inhibitors that are

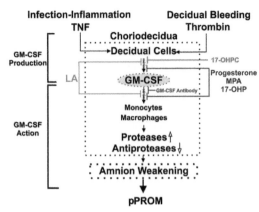

Fig. 3. FM weakening pathway based on work with the authors' model system. (1) TNF (modeling inflammation) and thrombin (modeling decidual bleeding/abruption) weaken FMs in vitro. (2) TNF and thrombin induce production of the critical intermediate GM-CSF by decidual cells. GM-CSF neutralizing antibody blocks both TNF and thrombin-induced weakening. (3) GM-CSF recruits and activates mononuclear cells and then activates macrophages, which produce proteases to cause FM weakening. (4) Progestogens (P4, MPA, and OHP) inhibit FM weakening both by inhibition of GM-CSF production and GM-CSF action. 17-OHPC, however, inhibits FM weakening only by inhibition of GM-CSF production (not GM-CSF action) and thus may be less efficacious in clinical use than other agents. (5) LA inhibits FM weakening by inhibiting both GM-CSF production by TNF/thrombin and also inhibiting GM-CSF downstream weakening activity. 17-OHPC, 17α-hydroxyprogesterone caproate; LA, lipoic acid; MPA, medroxyprogesterone acetate; OHP, 17α-hydroxyprogesterone; P4, progesterone.

thought to directly weaken the ECM of both the chorion and amnion. These inflammation-induced weakening processes can occur at any time during gestation, superimposed on the ongoing changes that FMs undergo with aging. In addition, cell senescence also produces GM-CSF and thus feeds into the inflammation-induced FM weakening pathway.

WHAT HAS BEEN LEFT OUT?

The authors' concern is that it is not known what has been left out. The authors think that the following questions have merit and require additional focused research:

1. Do FMs have the potential to inhibit uterine contractions? Work suggesting this was started by Collins 3 decades ago but not continued after her death.[76,77]
2. How do the FMs fight off small inflammatory challenges that might otherwise produce FM weakening, rupture, and labor onset?
3. How, and to what extent, do the FMs communicate with the fetus and mother? Recent FM studies have shown extracellular vesicles, specifically exosomes, as a possible mediator of fetal-maternal communication during pregnancy and parturition.[14,78–82] FM exosomes carry SASP and DAMPs in response to OS and can traverse through tissues, reaching maternal uterine tissues to cause functional changes.[12,79] Usefulness of exosomes in liquid biopsy for biomarkers and functional indicators also are being investigated.[83]

The authors are excited to state that preliminary and emerging research suggests that the FMs perform all the actions indicated above.

CAN PRETERM PRELABOR RUPTURE OF THE FETAL MEMBRANES BE PREDICTED PRIOR TO OCCURRENCE?

As discussed previously, current laboratory tests are performed to diagnose pPROM after the fact and not to predict women who are at high risk for pPROM prospectively. Clearly, prediction is extremely important.

Static risk factors, such as prior history, BMI, and nutritional, behavioral, and other socioeconomic, geographic, and genetic factors, are not changing during pregnancy. These factors can be used to create a high-risk profile for screening. These women can be followed-up using biomarkers indicative of developing risk of pPROM. The next question is, are there any biomarkers worthy of developing to predict underlying membrane weakening?

FMs are a source of various biochemical markers, many of which are constitutively produced whereas others are inducible.[84] Fetal immune response often mimics that seen in amniotic fluid,[85] but documentation reveals the production of a unique biomarker signature in preterm labor and pPROM.[86] This further exposes the FMs' unique contribution to the PTB pathway. A comprehensive search of literature published between 1967 and 2013 by the authors' group led to a list of biomarkers studied in human FMs.[84] The extensive research on FM biomarkers and the various classes of biomarkers highlights the significance of fetal response that are essential in maintenance of normal of pregnancy. Biomarker production highlights FMs' capability to respond to multiple stimuli and produce a plethora of biochemicals that can potentially determine host response in adverse pregnancy conditions.

Matrix metalloproteinases (MMPs), enzymes that degrade FM ECM, are elevated in the amniotic fluid in pPROM cases; however, amniocentesis for diagnostic purposes is not a practical strategy. Salivary MMP activities are elevated in pPROM cases and correlate well with membrane level MMP increase and activation. An increase in salivary protease has been shown to be independent of periodontal disease status in women with pPROM and could be developed as a biomarker.[87] As discussed previously, OS markers (F2-isoprostanes, pro-oxidants, and antioxidants) and OS-induced tissue damage markers (eg, 8-oxoguanine), GM-CSF, HMGB1, cell-free telomere fragments, and so forth can be developed as potential biomarkers of pPROM based on longitudinal sample studies. Many of them also are indicative of maternal risk exposures or developing pathologies.[57] As discussed previously, recent advances in extracellular vesicles (exosomes) as a biomarker has been promising. Senescent FM cells generate exosomes loaded with unique inflammatory cargoes, and fetal exosomes are detectable in the maternal circulation. Although FM specificity of these exosomes has yet to be proved, research is advancing in this area. Multiple recent publications have shown that exosomes predictive of PTBs can be detected in maternal blood as early as 12 weeks of pregnancy.[35] Similarly, microRNA and proteome-based markers also have been developed to predict PTBs in the first or early second trimester of pregnancy. Similarly, pPROM biomarkers could be developed and can be detected early prior to its occurrence. Understanding the fundamental mechanisms of pPROM pathology is the key in developing biomarkers and interventional targets.

IF A METHOD TO IDENTIFY LIKELY PRETERM PRELABOR RUPTURE OF THE FETAL MEMBRANES BECOMES AVAILABLE, CAN FETAL MEMBRANES BE TARGETED THERAPEUTICALLY?

With reasonable research progress, the authors speculate that patients with a significant likelihood (30%–50%) of delivering prematurely due to pPROM could be identified by a combination of clinical (previous pPROM and so forth) and biological markers. In parallel, the mechanisms leading to pPROM could be better defined. Then, if the resulting delivery is extremely preterm, pharmacologic intervention is reasonable. In terms of therapeutics, some progress has been made despite the lack of an animal model for pPROM. Using an in vitro human FM explant model, the authors have examined the ability of several agents to inhibit FM weakening induced by inflammation (modeled by TNF/IL-1β) or decidual bleeding (modeled by thrombin).[72] More recently, the authors have used the same model system to examine the inhibition of FM weakening by GM-CSF, which has been demonstrated to be a critical intermediate in the weakening pathway for both TNF and thrombin. As stated previously, GM-CSF is both necessary and sufficient for their FM weakening action.[75] Several analogs of progesterone have been trialed with some success in blocking inflammation-induced FM weakening.[87] Ironically, the least successful progesterone analog trialed was 17 hydroxyprogesterone caproate.[42] Two other anti-inflammatory agents have been trialed in this in vitro model, α-lipoic acid, which was effective, and vitamin C, which was not effective.[88] Several other anti-inflammatory dietary agents have been investigated by the Lappas group using generation of proteases as an endpoint.[89,90] N-acetylcysteine, another inflammatory agent has been used in a small clinical study.[91] To date, these agents either have not been trialed in clinical studies or have not been specifically targeted against pPROM.

ISSUES RELATED TO STUDY OF FETAL MEMBRANES

Studies to understand pPROM causality, mechanisms, biomarkers, and intervention strategies are underfunded in significant part because (1) there is not a pertinent animal model for pPROM and (2) FMs are difficult to obtain, in particular pPROM FMs, in a physiologic condition for study. PPROM FMs are unavailable until delivery, which often is well after the rupture has occurred (hours–weeks), at which point they have undergone postrupture degradation, infection, and trauma. These are useless for study. In addition, the pressure to avoid late preterm birth has resulted in available FMs, which are much more likely to be ragged and meconium-stained. These FMs also are useless for study. These facts have led to the persistence of a condition with no diagnostic markers to determine high-risk subjects for pPROM or appropriate intervention strategies to reduce the risk of pPROM.

There are new methodologies. In addition to the in vitro human FM model system, described previously,[72] recent advances in 3-dimensional culture and the emerging field of organ-on-chip technology provide hope for FM biologists. In these models, specifically organ-on-chips, various FM cell types can be maintained on nude (cell-free) ECM. This microfluidic system can be connected to amniotic fluid or maternal circulation with decidual cells to recreate in vitro scenarios. These models are useful in testing various matrix rigidities for cell and matrix growth, shear stress and stretch effects, elasticity of cells and matrix, proliferation, transition, and even differentiation (representing stem cell properties of membrane cells) and development of microfractures partly mimicking pPROM.[92] Such models, currently funded by the National Institutes of Health (NIH)/National Institute of Child Health and Human Development (NICHD), are under investigation for cellular communication and changes in response to infection, immune cell trafficking, and drug delivery responses. These are advantageous over currently used 2-dimensional culture systems that are limited to a single cell type, where interactive and proliferative features are hardly reproducible.

TIMES, HOWEVER, ARE CHANGING

This review is intended to create awareness about a tissue—the FMs—that plays a major role in pregnancy maintenance and promoting parturition at term. Although attached, FMs are not just part of the placenta. FM dysfunctions are associated with and may be a cause of adverse pregnancy outcomes. Healthy FMs are necessary for healthy fetal growth as well as the future health of the child. A small but determined cadre of investigators has uncovered the information discussed in this article. This puts FMs in a new light in relation to the major health issues of prematurity and infant mortality. A new organization, the Fetal Membrane Society (https://www.fetalmembraneclub.org/) recently was formed and will pursue this agenda.

ACKNOWLEDGMENTS

The authors would like to acknowledge Lauren Richardson, PhD (postdoctoral fellow, the Menon laboratory, and secretary general, Fetal Membrane Society), for her help with **Figs. 1** and **2**.

DISCLOSURE

R. Menon is supported by grants from (NIH/NICHD 1R03HD098469-01), NIH/1R21AI140249-01A1. J.J. Moore is supported by Burroughs Wellcome Fund Prematurity Research Grant #1015024.

REFERENCES

1. Beck S, Wojdyla D, Say L, et al. The worldwide incidence of preterm birth: a systematic review of maternal mortality and morbidity. Bull World Health Organ 2010; 88:31–8.
2. Romero R, Dey SK, Fisher SJ. Preterm labor: one syndrome, many causes. Science 2014;345:760–5.
3. Menon R, Bonney EA, Condon J, et al. Novel concepts on pregnancy clocks and alarms: redundancy and synergy in human parturition. Hum Reprod Update 2016;22:535–60.
4. Conde-Agudelo A, Papageorghiou AT, Kennedy SH, et al. Novel biomarkers for the prediction of the spontaneous preterm birth phenotype: a systematic review and meta-analysis. BJOG 2011;118:1042–54.
5. Keelan JA, Coleman M, Mitchell MD. The molecular mechanisms of term and preterm labor: recent progress and clinical implications. Clin Obstet Gynecol 1997; 40:460–78.
6. Elovitz MA. Anti-inflammatory interventions in pregnancy: now and the future. Semin Fetal Neonatal Med 2006;11:327–32.
7. Behrman RE, Butler AS for Institute of Medicine (US) Committee on Understanding Premature Birth and Assuring Healthy Outcomes. Preterm birth: causes, consequences, and prevention. Washington, DC: National Academies Press; 2007.
8. Martin LF, Richardson LS, da Silva MG, et al. Dexamethasone induces primary amnion epithelial cell senescence through telomere-P21 associated pathway. Biol Reprod 2019;100(6):1605–16.
9. Menon R, Richardson LS, Lappas M. Fetal membrane architecture, aging and inflammation in pregnancy and parturition. Placenta 2019;79:40–5.
10. Menon R. Human fetal membranes at term: dead tissue or signalers of parturition? Placenta 2016;44:1–5.

11. Jin J, Menon R. Placental exosomes: a proxy to understand pregnancy complications. Am J Reprod Immunol 2018;79:e12788.
12. Hadley EE, Sheller-Miller S, Saade G, et al. Amnion epithelial cell derived exosomes induce inflammatory changes in uterine cells. Am J Obstet Gynecol 2018;219(5):478.e1-21.
13. Salomon C, Nuzhat Z, Dixon CL, et al. Placental exosomes during gestation: liquid biopsies carrying signals for the regulation of human parturition. Curr Pharm Des 2018;24:974–82.
14. Sheller-Miller S, Trivedi J, Yellon SM, et al. Exosomes cause preterm birth in mice: evidence for paracrine signaling in pregnancy. Sci Rep 2019;9:608.
15. Menon R, Mesiano S, Taylor RN. Programmed fetal membrane senescence and exosome-mediated signaling: a mechanism associated with timing of human parturition. Front Endocrinol (Lausanne) 2017;8:196.
16. Bryant-Greenwood GD. The extracellular matrix of the human fetal membranes: structure and function. Placenta 1998;19:1–11.
17. Richardson L, Vargas G, Brown T, et al. Redefining 3Dimensional placental membrane microarchitecture using multiphoton microscopy and optical clearing. Placenta 2017;53:66–75.
18. Malak TM, Ockleford CD, Bell SC, et al. Confocal immunofluorescence localization of collagen types I, III, IV, V and VI and their ultrastructural organization in term human fetal membranes. Placenta 1993;14:385–406.
19. Mossman HW. Classics revisited: comparative morphogenesis of the fetal membranes and accessory uterine structures 1. Placenta 1991;12:1–5.
20. Ockleford CD, McCracken SA, Rimmington LA, et al. Type VII collagen associated with the basement membrane of amniotic epitelium forms giant anchoring rivets with penetrate a massive laminina reticularis. Placenta 2013;34:727–37.
21. Burton GJ. Oxygen, the Janus gas; its effects on human placental development and function. J Anat 2009;215:27–35.
22. Jones CJ, Fox H. Ultrastructure of the placenta in prolonged pregnancy. J Pathol 1978;126:173-9.
23. Richardson LS, Vargas G, Brown T, et al. Discovery and characterization of human amniochorionic membrane microfractures. Am J Pathol 2017;187(12): 2821–30.
24. Richardson L, Jeong S, Kim S, et al. Amnion membrane organ-on-chip: an innovative approach to study cellular interactions. FASEB J 2019;33(8):8945–60.
25. Menon R, Behnia F, Polettini J, et al. Placental membrane aging and HMGB1 signaling associated with human parturition. Aging (Albany NY) 2016;8(2): 216–30.
26. Menon R, Yu J, Basanta-Henry P, et al. Short fetal leukocyte telomere length and preterm prelabor rupture of the membranes. PLoS One 2012;7:e31136.
27. Bonney EA, Krebs K, Saade G, et al. Differential senescence in feto-maternal tissues during mouse pregnancy. Placenta 2016;43:26–34.
28. Polettini J, Dutta EH, Behnia F, et al. Aging of intrauterine tissues in spontaneous preterm birth and preterm premature rupture of the membranes: a systematic review of the literature. Placenta 2015;36(9):969–73.
29. Polettini J, Richardson LS, Menon R. Oxidative stress induces senescence and sterile inflammation in murine amniotic cavity. Placenta 2018;63:26–31.
30. Menon R, Boldogh I, Hawkins HK, et al. Histological evidence of oxidative stress and premature senescence in preterm premature rupture of the human fetal membranes recapitulated in vitro. Am J Pathol 2014;184:1740–51.

31. Dutta EH, Behnia F, Boldogh I, et al. Oxidative stress damage-associated molecular signaling pathways differentiate spontaneous preterm birth and preterm premature rupture of the membranes. Mol Hum Reprod 2016;22:143–57.

32. Behnia F, Taylor BD, Woodson M, et al. Chorioamniotic membrane senescence: a signal for parturition? Am J Obstet Gynecol 2015;213(3):359.e1-16.

33. Polettini J, Behnia F, Taylor BD, et al. Telomere fragment induced amnion cell senescence: a contributor to parturition? PLoS One 2015;10:e0137188.

34. Bredeson S, Papaconstantinou J, Deford JH, et al. HMGB1 promotes a p38MAPK associated non-infectious inflammatory response pathway in human fetal membranes. PLoS One 2014;9:e113799.

35. Cantonwine DE, Zhang Z, Rosenblatt K, et al. Evaluation of proteomic biomarkers associated with circulating microparticles as an effective means to stratify the risk of spontaneous preterm birth. Am J Obstet Gynecol 2016;214:631.e1-11.

36. Kearney P, Boniface JJ, Price ND, et al. The building blocks of successful translation of proteomics to the clinic. Curr Opin Biotechnol 2018;51:123–9.

37. Ngo TTM, Moufarrej MN, Rasmussen MH, et al. Noninvasive blood tests for fetal development predict gestational age and preterm delivery. Science 2018;360:1133–6.

38. D'Silva AM, Hyett JA, Coorssen JR. Proteomic analysis of first trimester maternal serum to identify candidate biomarkers potentially predictive of spontaneous preterm birth. J Proteomics 2018;178:31–42.

39. Mercer BM. Preterm premature rupture of the membranes: diagnosis and management. Clin Perinatol 2004;31:765–82, vi.

40. Ananth CV, Vintzileos AM. Epidemiology of preterm birth and its clinical subtypes. J Matern Fetal Neonatal Med 2006;19:773–82.

41. Mercer BM, Rabello YA, Thurnau GR, et al. The NICHD-MFMU antibiotic treatment of preterm PROM study: impact of initial amniotic fluid volume on pregnancy outcome. Am J Obstet Gynecol 2006;194:438–45.

42. Kumar D, Moore RM, Mercer BM, et al. In an in-vitro model using human fetal membranes, 17-alpha hydroxyprogesterone caproate is not an optimal progestogen for inhibition of fetal membrane weakening. Am J Obstet Gynecol 2017;217:695.e1-14.

43. Puthiyachirakkal M, Lemerand K, Kumar D, et al. Thrombin weakens the amnion extracellular matrix (ECM) directly rather than through protease activated receptors. Placenta 2013;34:924–31.

44. Kacerovsky M, Musilova I, Hornychova H, et al. Bedside assessment of amniotic fluid interleukin-6 in preterm prelabor rupture of membranes. Am J Obstet Gynecol 2014;211:385.e1-9.

45. Cooper AL, Vermillion ST, Soper DE. Qualitative human chorionicgonadotropin testing of cervicovaginal washings for the detection of preterm premature rupture of membranes. Am J Obstet Gynecol 2004;191:593–6 [discussion: 596–7].

46. Trochez-Martinez RD, Smith P, Lamont RF. Use of C-reactive protein as a predictor of chorioamnionitis in preterm prelabour rupture of membranes: a systematic review. BJOG 2007;114:796–801.

47. Kalafat E, Yuce T, Tanju O, et al. Preterm premature rupture of membrane assessment via transperineal ultrasonography: a diagnostic accuracy study. J Matern Fetal Neonatal Med 2016;29:3690–4.

48. Goldenberg RL, Culhane JF, Iams JD, et al. Epidemiology and causes of preterm birth. Lancet 2008;371:75–84.

49. Mercer BM, Crouse DT, Goldenberg RL, et al, Eunice Kennedy Shriver National Institute of Child Health and Human Development Maternal-Fetal Medicine Units

Network. The antibiotic treatment of PPROM study: systemic maternal and fetal markers and perinatal outcomes. Am J Obstet Gynecol 2012;206:145.e1-9.

50. Romero R, Friel LA, Velez Edwards DR, et al. A genetic association study of maternal and fetal candidate genes that predispose to preterm prelabor rupture of membranes (PROM). Am J Obstet Gynecol 2010;203:361.e1-30.

51. Kacerovsky M, Vrbacky F, Kutova R, et al. Cervical microbiota in women with preterm prelabor rupture of membranes. PLoS One 2015;10:e0126884.

52. Faucett AM, Metz TD, DeWitt PE, et al. Effect of obesity on neonatal outcomes in pregnancies with preterm premature rupture of membranes. Am J Obstet Gynecol 2016;214:287.e1-5.

53. Menon R, Richardson LS. Preterm prelabor rupture of the membranes: a disease of the fetal membranes. Semin Perinatol 2017;41:409–19.

54. Cousens S, Blencowe H, Gravett M, et al. Antibiotics for pre-term pre-labour rupture of membranes: prevention of neonatal deaths due to complications of pre-term birth and infection. Int J Epidemiol 2010;39(Suppl 1):i134–43.

55. Kacerovsky M, Pliskova L, Bolehovska R, et al. The microbial load with genital mycoplasmas correlates with the degree of histologic chorioamnionitis in preterm PROM. Am J Obstet Gynecol 2011;205:213–7.

56. Murtha AP, Menon R. Regulation of fetal membrane inflammation: a critical step in reducing adverse pregnancy outcome. Am J Obstet Gynecol 2015;213:447–8.

57. Menon R. Oxidative stress damage as a detrimental factor in preterm birth pathology 14. Front Immunol 2014;5:567.

58. Behnia F, Peltier MR, Saade GR, et al. Environmental pollutant polybrominated diphenyl ether, a flame retardant, induces primary amnion cell senescence. Am J Reprod Immunol 2015;74(5):398–406.

59. Behnia F, Sheller S, Menon R. Mechanistic differences leading to infectious and sterile inflammation. Am J Reprod Immunol 2016;75(5):505–18.

60. Joyce EM, Diaz P, Tamarkin S, et al. In -vivo stretch of term human fetal membranes. Placenta 2016;38:57–66.

61. Gomez-Lopez N, Hernandez-Santiago S, Lobb AP, et al. Normal and premature rupture of fetal membranes at term delivery differ in regional chemotactic activity and related chemokine/cytokine production. Reprod Sci 2013;20:276–84.

62. Malak TM, Bell SC. Structural characteristics of term human fetal membranes: a novel zone of extreme morphological alteration within the rupture site. Br J Obstet Gynaecol 1994;101:375–86.

63. Reti NG, Lappas M, Riley C, et al. Why do membranes rupture at term? Evidence of increased cellular apoptosis in the supracervical fetal membranes. Am J Obstet Gynecol 2007;196:484.e1-10.

64. Lappas M, Odumetse TL, Riley C, et al. Pre-labour fetal membranes overlying the cervix display alterations in inflammation and NF-kappaB signalling pathways. Placenta 2008;29:995–1002.

65. McLaren J, Taylor DJ, Bell SC. Increased concentration of pro-matrix metalloproteinase 9 in term fetal membranes overlying the cervix before labor: implications for membrane remodeling and rupture. Am J Obstet Gynecol 2000;182:409–16.

66. El Khwad M, Stetzer B, Moore RM, et al. Term human fetal membranes have a weak zone overlying the lower uterine pole and cervix before onset of labor. Biol Reprod 2005;72:720–6.

67. El Khwad M, Pandey V, Stetzer B, et al. Fetal membranes from term vaginal deliveries have a zone of weakness exhibiting characteristics of apoptosis and remodeling. J Soc Gynecol Investig 2006;13:191–5.

68. Rangaswamy N, Abdelrahim A, Moore RM, et al. Biomechanical characteristics of human fetal membranes; preterm fetal membranes are stronger than term fetal membranes. Gynecol Obstet Fertil 2011;39:373–7.

69. Arikat S, Novince RW, Mercer BM, et al. Separation of amnion from choriodecidua is an integral event to the rupture of normal fetal membranes and constitutes a significant component of the work required. Am J Obstet Gynecol 2006;194: 211–7.

70. Strohl A, Kumar D, Novince R, et al. Decreased adherence and spontaneous separation of fetal membrane layers–amnion and choriodecidua—a possible part of the normal weakening process. Placenta 2010;31(1):18–24.

71. Fernandez M, House M, Jambawalikar S, et al. Investigating the mechanical function of the cervix during pregnancy using finite element models derived from high-resolution 3D MRI. Comput Methods Biomech Biomed Engin 2016;19: 404–17.

72. Kumar D, Moore RM, Mercer BM, et al. The physiology of fetal membrane weakening and rupture: Insights gained from the determination of physical properties revisited. Placenta 2016;42:59–73.

73. Kumar D, Schatz F, Moore RM, et al. The effects of thrombin and cytokines upon the biomechanics and remodeling of isolated amnion membrane, in vitro. Placenta 2011;32:206–13.

74. Kumar D, Fung W, Moore RM, et al. Proinflammatory cytokines found in amniotic fluid induce collagen remodeling, apoptosis, and biophysical weakening of cultured human fetal membranes. Biol Reprod 2006;74:29–34.

75. Kumar D, Moore RM, Nash A, et al. Decidual GM-CSF is a critical common intermediate necessary for thrombin and TNF induced in-vitro fetal membrane weakening. Placenta 2014;35:1049–56.

76. Collins PL, Idriss E, Moore JJ. Fetal membranes inhibit prostaglandin but not oxytocin-induced uterine contractions. Am J Obstet Gynecol 1995;172(4 Pt 1): 1216–23.

77. Collins PL, Moore JJ, Idriss E, et al. Human fetal membranes inhibit calcium L-channel activated uterine contractions. Am J Obstet Gynecol 1996;175:1173–9.

78. Sheller-Miller S, Urrabaz-Garza R, Saade G, et al. Damage-Associated molecular pattern markers HMGB1 and cell-Free fetal telomere fragments in oxidative-Stressed amnion epithelial cell-Derived exosomes. J Reprod Immunol 2017; 123:3–11.

79. Sheller-Miller S, Lei J, Saade G, et al. Feto-maternal trafficking of exosomes in murine pregnancy models. Front Pharmacol 2016;7:432.

80. Jin J, Richardson L, Sheller-Miller S, et al. Oxidative stress induces p38MAPK-dependent senescence in the feto-maternal interface cells. Placenta 2018;67: 15–23.

81. Sheller-Miller S, Choi K, Choi C, et al. Cre-reporter mouse model to determine exosome communication and function during pregnancy. Am J Obstet Gynecol 2019;221(5):502e1–e12.

82. Menon R, Debnath C, Lai A, et al. Circulating exosomal miRNA profile during term and preterm birth pregnancies - a longitudinal study. Endocrinology 2018;160(2): 249–75.

83. Kumar D, Springel E, Moore RM, et al. Progesterone inhibits in vitro fetal membrane weakening. Am J Obstet Gynecol 2015;213:520.e1-9.

84. Menon R, Noda Nicolau N, Bredeson S, et al. Fetal membranes: potential source of preterm birth biomarkers. In: Preedy VR, PV, editors. General methods in

biomarker research and their applications. Springer Science Publisher; 2015. p. 483–529.

85. Fortunato SJ, Menon RP, Swan KF, et al. Inflammatory cytokine (interleukins 1, 6 and 8 and tumor necrosis factor-alpha) release from cultured human fetal membranes in response to endotoxic lipopolysaccharide mirrors amniotic fluid concentrations. Am J Obstet Gynecol 1996;174:1855–61.

86. Brou L, Almli LM, Pearce BD, et al. Dysregulated biomarkers induce distinct pathways in preterm birth. BJOG 2012;119:458–73.

87. Menon R, McIntyre JO, Matrisian LM, et al. Salivary proteinase activity: a potential biomarker for preterm premature rupture of the membranes. Am J Obstet Gynecol 2006;194:1609–15 [discussion: 1615].

88. Kumar D, Moore RM, Sharma A, et al. In an in-vitro model using human fetal membranes, α-lipoic acid inhibits inflammation induced fetal membrane weakening. Placenta 2018;68:9–14.

89. Wijesuriya YK, Lappas M. Potent anti-inflammatory effects of honokiol in human fetal membranes and myometrium. Phytomedicine 2018;49:11–22.

90. Morwood CL, Lappas M. The citrus flavone nobiletin reduces pro-inflammatory and pro-labour mediators in fetal membranes and myometrium: implications for preterm birth. PLoS One 2014;9(9):e108390.

91. Shahin AY, Hassanin IM, Ismail AM, et al. Effect of oral N-acetyl cysteine on recurrent preterm labor following treatment for bacterial vaginosis. Int J Gynaecol Obstet 2009;104(1):44–8.

92. Richardson L, Menon R. Proliferative, migratory, and transition properties reveal metastate of human amnion cells. Am J Pathol 2018;188:2004–15.

Evidence for Corpus Luteal and Endometrial Origins of Adverse Pregnancy Outcomes in Women Conceiving with or Without Assisted Reproduction

Kirk P. Conrad, MD[a,b,*]

KEYWORDS

- Decidua • Trophoblast • Preeclampsia • Endometrium spectrum disorders
- In vitro fertilization • Autologous frozen embryo transfer • Relaxin

KEY POINTS

- Preeclampsia may arise in some women from insufficient or defective decidualization before and during early pregnancy that, in turn, disrupts decidual immune cell populations and activity, thereby compromising placental formation and/or function.
- The transcriptomics of choriodecidua (chorionic villous samples) and cultured endometrial stromal cells decidualized in vitro derived from midsecretory biopsies of women who experienced severe preeclampsia overlapped significantly with the transcriptomics of midsecretory biopsies from women with recurrent implantation failure, recurrent miscarriage, and endometriosis.
- Women who conceived using artificial (programmed) in vitro fertilization (IVF) protocols had widespread dysregulation of cardiovascular function in the first trimester and were at increased risk for several adverse pregnancy outcomes, including hypertensive disorders of pregnancy and preeclampsia. These IVF protocols preclude the development of a corpus luteum, which is a key regulator of endometrial function.

Continued

INTRODUCTION

Adverse pregnancy outcomes may have antecedents in the preconception and periconception periods and the first trimester of pregnancy. This idea was

---

[a] Department of Physiology and Functional Genomics, D.H. Barron Reproductive and Perinatal Biology Research Program, University of Florida College of Medicine, 1600 Southwest Archer RD, PO Box 100274, M552, Gainesville, FL 32610-0274, USA; [b] Department of Obstetrics and Gynecology, University of Florida College of Medicine, 1600 Southwest Archer RD, PO Box 100294, N3-9, Gainesville, FL 32610-0274, USA
* Department of Physiology and Functional Genomics, University of Florida College of Medicine, 1600 Southwest Archer RD, PO Box 100274, M552, Gainesville, FL 32610-0274.
E-mail address: kpconrad@ufl.edu

Obstet Gynecol Clin N Am 47 (2020) 163–181
https://doi.org/10.1016/j.ogc.2019.10.011
0889-8545/20/© 2019 Elsevier Inc. All rights reserved.

Continued

- The lack of circulating corpus luteal product(s) (eg, relaxin, a potent vasodilator and stimulus of decidualization) could have an adverse impact on the maternal cardiovascular system directly and/or compromise decidualization, thereby increasing the risk of hypertensive disorders of pregnancy and preeclampsia.

supported by studies implicating dysregulation of endometrial maturation (decidualization) during the secretory phase and early pregnancy in the genesis of preeclampsia (PE).[1-4] The concept of endometrium spectrum disorders then emerged,[3] which was underpinned by the integration of multiple endometrial transcriptomic databases available in the public domain.[5] These bioinformatics analyses provided evidence for dysregulation of molecular pathways in common among the classic endometrial disorders—recurrent implantation failure (RIF), recurrent miscarriage (RM), endometriosis (OSIS)—and one of the great obstetric or placental syndromes, PE.[5,6] Conceivably, other adverse pregnancy outcomes that may arise from placental pathology, including normotensive intrauterine growth restriction and preterm birth, also fall within the continuum of endometrial spectrum disorders affecting implantation, placentation, or both, depending on the specific molecular pathways disrupted and the severity of disruption.[3] Although the genesis of the great obstetric syndromes, including PE, is likely multifactorial, in some women these disease entities may have antecedents in endometrial dysregulation during early pregnancy or even before pregnancy.

In vitro fertilization (IVF) is another setting in which preconception and periconception as well as early pregnancy factors may have an impact on obstetric outcome. In pregnancies conceived by IVF using artificial (programmed) cycles (ACs) involving hypothalamic-pituitary suppression and development of the endometrium with estradiol and progesterone, a corpus luteum (CL) does not develop.[7] These IVF protocols were observed to perturb endometrial gene expression in the midsecretory phase[8,9] and to be associated with greater risk of postterm delivery, large-for-gestational-age infants, and macrosomia as well as placental accreta.[10,11] In addition, ACs were linked to maternal hemodynamic dysregulation in the first trimester and hypertensive disorders of pregnancy and PE.[12,13] Because the CL is a key regulator of endometrial function, including decidualization in the secretory phase and early pregnancy, one potential explanation for increased incidence of these adverse obstetric outcomes is that, despite luteal support with exogenous estradiol and progesterone, the absence of other crucial circulating CL factors(s) negatively affects endometrial maturation in IVF ACs.[7,10,12] Another potential, albeit not mutually exclusive, explanation is that the dosage and timing of estradiol and progesterone administration for luteal support are suboptimal.[8,9]

In this review, the molecular evidence of impaired decidualization in PE and the emerging concept of endometrial spectrum disorders, in which dysregulated decidualization of PE, RIF, RM, and OSIS demonstrated significant overlap of molecular pathology, are presented. In addition, the discovery of dysregulated maternal hemodynamics during the first trimester of IVF ACs, as well as the association with increased risk for hypertensive disorders of pregnancy and PE, are also presented in the context of the CL or, more precisely, the lack thereof, in cases of ACs.

ENDOMETRIUM SPECTRUM DISORDERS: A NEW AND EMERGING CONCEPT
Molecular Evidence of Impaired Endometrial Maturation in Preeclampsia

One widely held theory is that PE originates within the placental bed during early gestation in many women. Normally, the fetal extravillous trophoblast emanating from the anchoring villous tips invade the gestational endometrium (decidua) and inner third of the myometrium, remodeling the uterine spiral arteries from low-caliber, high-resistance blood vessels to high-caliber, low-resistance blood vessels. These physiologic changes of the spiral arteries facilitate increased maternal blood flow into the intervillous space. In contrast, PE often is associated with impaired trophoblast invasion and spiral artery remodeling, thereby restricting blood flow into the intervillous space, leading to placental ischemia. These placentation deficiencies may not be unique to PE, as they have also been described, albeit not universally so, in late sporadic miscarriage, normotensive fetal growth restriction, placental abruption, and preterm labor.[6]

The classical view of the biological consequences of spiral artery remodeling, or lack thereof, as discussed previously, recently has been called into question. Revised computational modeling suggested that spiral artery remodeling is unlikely to contribute substantially to reducing uterine vascular resistance and increasing blood flow in normal pregnancy (NP); rather, the (proximal) radial artery is a more significant resistance site.[14] Computational modeling further revealed that spiral artery remodeling in NP reduces the velocity of increased blood flow into the intervillous space, thereby protecting delicate villi from mechanical damage and increasing the transit time of blood flow through the intervillous space, allowing for adequate exchange of oxygen and nutrients across the syncytiotrophoblast layer.[15] According to this model, failure of spiral artery remodeling in PE would lead to the opposite chain of events, that is, mechanical damage of villi by high-velocity blood flow and rapid transit time of blood flow through the intervillous space precluding adequate oxygen and nutrient exchange across the syncytiotrophoblast layer.[15] Nevertheless, regardless of which model is apropos, each predicts that failure to remodel spiral arteries would impair placental function. In both scenarios, ischemia-reperfusion injury also would occur as a consequence of spontaneous and hormone-induced constriction or relaxation of spiral arteries that were not remodeled and retained vascular smooth muscle.

Because uterine invasion and spiral artery remodeling by trophoblast can be deficient in PE, this fetal cell has been intensively investigated. Moreover, the paternal genetic contribution to disease etiology could be manifest, at least in part, through impairment of trophoblast invasion. The seminal work of Fisher[16] revealed the extensive molecular and functional aberrations of the extravillous trophoblast in early-onset, severe PE as investigated at the end of pregnancy in situ and after trophoblast isolation in vitro. A potential caveat to this methodological approach, however, is that molecular pathology at the end of pregnancy may be more related to the phenotypic expression of the disease, which typically emerges at that time or may even be a consequence of the disease (eg, sFLT1 conceivably could be injurious to endometrium in addition to endothelium). Therefore, the molecular pathology of tissues procured at delivery is likely to be unrelated to the molecular etiology that caused the disease months before, when the physiologic processes of uterine trophoblast invasion and spiral arterial remodeling transpired. That is, the large temporal gap between the acquisition of placental tissues for molecular studies at delivery and the critical period of trophoblast invasion and spiral artery remodeling occurring in early pregnancy may preclude any insights into the molecular genesis of PE. One potential solution to this conundrum is prospective acquisition of early placental tissues (surplus chorionic villous samples [CVSs]) months before onset of clinical manifestations.

Although the advent of noninvasive prenatal screening has markedly reduced the number of CVS procedures performed worldwide, collaboration among large medical centers with the greatest volume of CVS cases annually could lead to acquisition of sufficient sample numbers for molecular and functional investigation of PE etiology targeting the trophoblast.

Another potentially relevant tissue that has received little attention in the context of adverse pregnancy outcomes is the maternal decidua (soil), which extravillous trophoblasts (seed) invade (discussed previously). Conceivably, insufficient or defective endometrial maturation (decidualization) that begins in the secretory phase and continues after implantation may impede trophoblast invasion and spiral artery remodeling, thereby contributing to the genesis of PE.[1,17] This alternative but not mutually exclusive hypothesis is perhaps intuitive or self-evident, in light of the close apposition of endometrial stromal, glandular epithelial, and maternal immune cells with trophoblast and spiral arteries in the placental bed. Furthermore, the maternal inheritance pattern of PE could be manifest, at least in part, through dysregulation of decidualization. Normally, massive molecular and functional changes occur in endometrial stromal and epithelial cells, spiral arteries, and immune cells during decidualization in the secretory phase and early pregnancy. Implantation and placentation depend on the optimal and timely progression of decidualization. Decidualization of the glandular epithelium is prerequisite to histiotrophic nutrition during early gestation prior to onset of maternal blood flow; uterine natural killer (NK) cells become the major immune cell type in the placental bed and assume an immunomodulatory rather than cytotoxic phenotype, and they initiate spiral artery remodeling and stimulate trophoblast invasion; uterine macrophages accumulate and they adopt an M2 or alternatively active rather than proinflammatory phenotype; and T-regulatory cells contribute to immune tolerance at the maternal-fetal interface in the face of the fetoplacental semiallograft.[3,18] In essence, decidualization is preparation of the soil for the seed, that is, embryo implantation and subsequent placentation. Impairment of this process as one possible etiology of PE seems a reasonable hypothesis to explore.

In order to investigate relevant reproductive tissue temporally related to decidualization, trophoblast invasion, and spiral artery remodeling, the author and coworkers prospectively obtained surplus CVSs at approximately 11.5 gestational weeks in women who developed PE with severe features (sPE) or who experienced NP outcome 5 months to 6 months later.[1] These tissue samples were snap frozen in liquid nitrogen and ultimately analyzed by DNA microarray. Contrary to the hypothesis, a molecular signature consistent with ischemia or ischemia-reperfusion was not detected; rather, many genes identified as biomarkers of decidualization were down-regulated in the CVSs from women who developed sPE relative to NP outcome, including insulin-like growth factor binding protein-1 (IGFBP-1), glycodelin [progesterone-associated endometrial protein], prolactin, and interleukin-15. These initial observations prompted a wider text mining approach, which revealed many other dysregulated decidual genes that, in turn, provided the justification for a formal bioinformatics reanalysis of the raw data from the CVS microarray data.[2]

The bioinformatics reanalysis of the CVS microarray data revealed 396 differentially expressed genes (DEGs) between CVSs from sPE and NP-CVSs, of which 154, or 40%, overlapped with DEGs, changing during endometrial maturation either in the secretory phase or in early pregnancy ($P = 4.7 \times 10^{-14}$), the latter DEGs obtained by reanalyzing publicly available microarray data sets of normal decidualization. Moreover, approximately 73% of these 154 DEGs changed in the opposite direction compared with normal endometrial maturation ($P = .01$), and 75% overlapped significantly with DEGs between proliferative versus late secretory endometrium or DEGs between decidualized versus nondecidualized endometrium obtained from tubal ectopic pregnancies ($P = 4.4 \times 10^{-9}$). Neither of these endometrial tissues contains extravillous trophoblast, thus suggesting a primary role for dysregulated decidualization. In addition, 16 DEGs normally up-regulated in uterine compared with peripheral NK cells were down-regulated in sPE compared with NP-CVSs ($P<.0001$). DEGs normally up-regulated in uterine relative to peripheral macrophages were down-regulated in sPE versus NP-CVSs ($P = 9.5 \times 10^{-13}$) and vice versa ($P = 1.1 \times 10^{-6}$).[3] Taken together, these observations suggested deficient or defective endometrial maturation, including uterine NK cells and macrophages, may precede the development of sPE. The concept that dysregulated decidualization may be involved in the genesis of PE is supported by 6 studies published throughout the past 10 years or so, which demonstrated a reduction of circulating concentrations of IGFBP-1 during early pregnancy in women who later developed PE (reviewed by Conrad and colleagues[3]).

Another notable finding from the CVS microarray study was that the average mRNA expression of a cohort of 20 decidual genes uniquely up-regulated in normal late secretory compared with proliferative endometrium were down-regulated in sPE versus NP-CVSs by approximately 2-fold ($P<.0001$)[2]. This observation suggested that the dysregulation of endometrial maturation in the women who developed PE with severe features may have started before pregnancy during the secretory phase. The idea that endometrial pathology may reside in the secretory endometrium was strongly reinforced by Garrido-Gomez and coworkers,[4] who reported marked impairment of in vitro decidualization of endometrial stromal cells isolated and then cultured from midsecretory endometrial biopsies of women who experienced sPE during the previous 1 year to 5 years. In fact, there was significant overlap of DEGs that arose from sPE-CVSs versus NP-CVSs, as reported by Rabaglino and Conrad,[5] with the DEGs observed by Garrido-Gomez and coworkers,[4] in cultured endometrial stromal cells decidualized in vitro that were derived from women who experienced prior sPE versus NP.

A priori, decidual tissue at delivery is likely to be markedly dissimilar from decidual tissue in the secretory phase or early pregnancy (discussed previously). This important point was highlighted by additional bioinformatics analysis of differential gene expression in these temporally disconnected decidual tissues from women who experienced sPE versus NP, insofar as there was little or no overlap.[5] Thus, designing strategies to address the molecular genesis of PE, which resides in the secretory endometrium and/ or placental bed of early pregnancy, based on the molecular pathology of delivered tissue may be misleading and unlikely to lead to preventative or early corrective measures.

In summary, emerging evidence supports the concept that PE may arise at least in some women from dysregulated decidualization, including aberrant endometrial immune cell number and/or function in the secretory phase and during early pregnancy[1,2,4] **(Fig. 1)**. In delivered placentas, decidual function also is perturbed, which may contribute to or arise from deleterious circulating placental factors like sFLT1 (see Deepak and colleagues[19]; and reviewed by Conrad and colleagues[3]). But, as discussed previously, the transcriptomics of delivered decidua are distinct from those of early pregnancy or the secretory phase in women who developed PE and, as such, may not be relevant to disease etiology.[3,5] Perhaps not totally unexpected in light of this potential link between aberrant decidualization and PE, an elegant recently published study by Dunk and colleagues provided evidence that intrauterine growth restriction, another disease entity classified under the great obstetric or placental syndromes, also may have origins in impaired decidualization.[20]

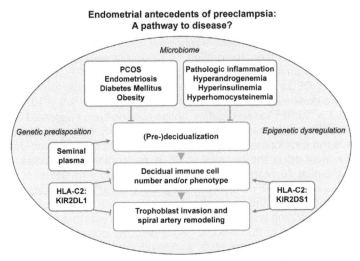

Fig. 1. Aberrant decidualization in the late secretory phase and during early pregnancy may play a role in the development of PE for some women. See Refs.[3,5] for details. (*From* Conrad KP, Rabaglino MB, Post Uiterweer ED. Emerging role for dysregulated decidualization in the genesis of PE. Placenta 2017;60:125; with permission.)

Evidence for Common Molecular Pathways of Dysregulated Endometrial Maturation in Preeclampsia, Recurrent Implantation Failure, Recurrent Miscarriage, and Endometriosis

Because dysregulated decidualization was associated with PE, the author asked the question whether there might be molecular overlap with other endometrial disorders.[5] To this end, 8 microarray databases in the public domain from normal and pathologic endometrium or decidua were analyzed. A significant proportion of the DEGs up-regulated or down-regulated in CVSs from women who experienced PE with severe features compared with NP, or in cultured endometrial stromal cells decidualized in vitro derived from midsecretory biopsies of women who experienced severe PE relative to NP (discussed previously), demonstrated overlap with, and the same directional change as, DEGs in RIF, RM, and OSIS compared with their respective control tissues.[5]

In order to further explore this idea, a functional analysis and pathway-driven approach was taken.[5] The cytokine-cytokine receptor interaction pathway (264 genes) was one of the most prominent and significant molecular pathways in common among normal and pathologic endometrium. Principal component analysis was used to compare gene expression in this pathway among the different normal and pathologic endometrial tissues represented by 8 microarray databases (**Fig. 2**). CVSs and in vitro decidualized endometrial stromal cells derived from midsecretory phase biopsies of women who suffered sPE segregated with the 3 endometrial disorders. In contrast, decidua procured at delivery from women affected by sPE clustered with normal endometrium, indicating that the expression pattern of the genes of these tissues at least in the cytokine-cytokine receptor pathway more resembled the normal than pathologic endometrium. Of course, other molecular pathways in the decidua obtained at delivery from women who suffered sPE may be abnormal. Overall, however, the DEGs affected in delivered tissues were not overlapping with those found in the CVS or in vitro decidualized endometrial stromal cells from midsecretory phase

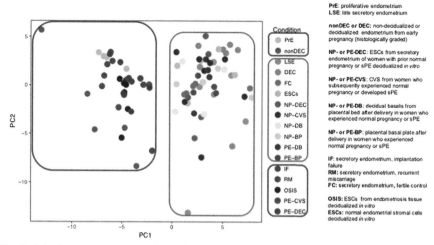

Fig. 2. Principal component analysis of genes belonging to the cytokine-cytokine receptor interaction pathway. Principal component plots show that normal endometrial samples obtained from healthy women (shades of green, n = 36), decidual tissues obtained postdelivery from women with PE (shades of pink, n = 8), and NP (shades of yellow, n = 8) formed a distinct cluster. Endometrial samples from women with pathologic endometrium (shades of red, n = 25) and samples from nondecidualized endometrium (nonDEC) or proliferative endometrium (PrE) (shades of blue, n = 9) formed another distinct cluster. The analysis was applied to 264 genes belonging to the cytokine-cytokine receptor interaction pathway. LSE, late-secretory endometrium; DEC, approximately 9-week gestational endometrium with confluent decidualization; FC, midsecretory endometrium from fertile controls; ESCs, endometrial stromal cells isolated from midsecretory biopsies of healthy women, cultured, and decidualized in vitro; PE-CVS and NP-CVS, CVSs obtained from women at approximately 11.5 gestational weeks who developed sPE or experienced NP; PE-DEC and NP-DEC, midsecretory endometrial biopsies obtained from women between 1 year and 5 years after a pregnancy either complicated by PE with severe features or an uncomplicated pregnancy; endometrial stromal cells were subsequently isolated, cultured, and decidualized in vitro; PE-DB and NP-DB, decidual tissue obtained by placental bed biopsy after cesarean section; PE-BP and NP-BP, decidual tissue harvested from the basal plate of delivered placentas; IF, secretory endometrium from women with RIF; RM, secretory endometrium from women with RM; and OSIS, endometrial stromal cells isolated from ovarian endometriomas, cultured and decidualized in vitro. (*From* Rabaglino MB, Conrad KP. Evidence for shared molecular pathways of dysregulated decidualization in PE and endometrial disorders revealed by microarray data integration. FASEB J 2019;33(11):11682-95; with permission.)

biopsies of women who suffered sPE. In the same vein, proliferative endometrium and nondecidualized early pregnancy endometrium, as histologically assessed, clustered with pathologic endometrium in the context of the cytokine-cytokine receptor interaction pathway.

Taken together, integration of multiple microarray data sets derived from normal and pathologic endometrium suggested that, at least in some women, PE may be part of a continuum of endometrial disorders involving varying degrees of molecular dysregulation affecting implantation, placentation, or both. Other disease entities classified as placental syndromes also may fall along this continuum (**Fig. 3**). That PE has, in common with the classic endometrial disorders, many DEGs and gene pathways strengthens the concept that the genesis of the disease may reside in the decidua at least for some women. Viewing PE in this light also may partly explain why women

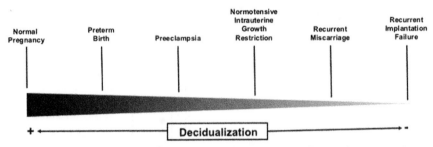

Endometrial Antecedents of Adverse Pregnancy Outcomes:
A Pathway to Disease?

Normal Pregnancy — Preterm Birth — Preeclampsia — Normotensive Intrauterine Growth Restriction — Recurrent Miscarriage — Recurrent Implantation Failure

+ ←——————— **Decidualization** ——————→ –

Fig. 3. Endometrium spectrum disorders. A significant number of DEGs that were either up-regulated or down-regulated in CVSs from women who experienced sPE compared with NP demonstrated overlap with, and the same directional change as, DEGs in RIF, RM, and OSIS relative to their respective control tissues. Similarly, a significant number of DEGs that were either up-regulated or down-regulated in cultured endometrial stromal cells decidualized in vitro derived from midsecretory biopsies of women who experienced severe PE compared with NP demonstrated overlap with, and the same directional change, as DEGs in RIF, RM, and OSIS compared with their respective control tissues. These findings gave rise to the notion of endometrium spectrum disorders, in which disease phenotype may be determined in part by which endometrial molecular pathways are disrupted and the severity of the disruption.

with OSIS who become pregnant experience increased PE risk as reported by some, but not all, investigators. Similarly, RM also was associated with increased PE risk (see Rabaglino and Conrad[5] for citations).

IN VITRO FERTILIZATION: ADVERSE PREGNANCY OUTCOMES
Hypertensive Disorders of Pregnancy and Preeclampsia

An association between IVF and hypertensive disorders of pregnancy or PE has been thoroughly documented (**Tables 1–3**). Several groups of researchers reported increased frequency of hypertensive disorders of pregnancy or PE in frozen embryo transfer (FET) versus fresh embryo transfer (ET). The FET protocol(s) were not delineated, however, and whether donor gametes were included or not was specified in only 1 of the studies.[21–23] In the investigation by Opdahl and colleagues,[23] relative risks (RRs) for hypertensive disorders of pregnancy were 7.0% and 4.7%, respectively, for FET and spontaneous pregnancy (adjusted odds ratio [AOR] 1.41; 95% CI, 1.27–1.56 [adjusted for maternal age, parity, birth year, infant sex, and country]). The same investigators also noted higher risk in siblings conceived by FET versus fresh ET (AOR 2.39; 95% CI, 1.48–3.86). More recently, the risk of PE also was found increased for autologous FET in ACs versus fresh ET.[24–26] In 1 of these studies, patients with polycystic ovary syndrome (PCOS) were randomized to FET-AC or fresh ET cycles.[24] Finally, in another investigation, autologous FET-NC and FET-stimulated cycles were used, and the investigators observed no significant differences in the rate of hypertensive disorders among women conceiving by FET-NC, FET-stimulated cycle, fresh ET, or spontaneous conception.[27] Taken together, these studies suggested that FET, in particular FET-AC, protocols may be associated with increased

Table 1
Singleton live births from frozen embryo transfer versus fresh embryo transfer

Study	Notes	In Vitro Fertilization Protocols	Hypertensive Disorders of Pregnancy	Preeclampsia
Wennerholm et al,[27] 1997, Sweden, Single IVF center, 1990–1995	Donor oocytes excluded; slow-freeze cryopreservation; results for singletons and twins combined	FET-NC (82%) or FET-stimulated cycle (18%); fresh ET; spontaneous conception cohorts, n = 209 each	aFET-NC/stimulated cycle 7.2%; afresh FET 7.7%; aspontaneous conception 6.2%; P = NS	
Wikland et al,[21] 2010, Fertility Center Scandinavia, 2006–2008	Exclusion of donor gametes or embryos not specified; both FET-NC and FET-AC used	Vitrified BC, n = 106, vs fresh BC, n = 207; Vitrified BC vs slow-freeze, early-cleavage stage, n = 206	11.8% vs 5.4%; P = .088; 11.8% vs 5.5%; P = .092	
Sazonova et al,[44] 2012, Sweden, All IVF clinics, 2002–2006	Donor oocytes excluded; cyropreservation method(s) and FET protocol(s) not specified; single and double ET	FET, n = 2348, vs fresh ET, n = 8944; FET vs spontaneous pregnancy, n = 571,914		5.6% vs 4.5%; AOR 1.32; 95% CI, 1.07–1.63; 5.6% vs 2.8%; AOR 1.25; 95% CI, 1.03–1.51
Ishihara et al,[22] 2014, Japanese ART registry database, 2008–2010	Donor gametes and embryos disallowed in Japan; cyropreservation method(s) and FET protocol(s) not specified	FET, n = 31,249, vs fresh ET, n = 16,909	2.8% vs 1.8%; AOR 1.58; 95% CI, 1.35–1.86; P<.001	
Opdahl et al,[23] 2015, Nordic population-based cohorts, 1988–2007	Exclusion of donor gametes or embryos, cyropreservation method(s), and FET protocol(s) not specified	FET, n = 6444; fresh ET, n = 39,878; Mothers with sibling pairs discordant for hypertensive disorders and ART method, n = 100	bFET RR 7.0%; AOR 1.41; 95% CI, 1.27–1.56; bFresh ET RR 5.7%; AOR 1.12; 95% CI, 1.06–1.18; cFET vs fresh ET: AOR 2.39; 95% CI, 1.48–3.86	

(continued on next page)

Table 1
(continued)

Study	Notes	In Vitro Fertilization Protocols	Hypertensive Disorders of Pregnancy	Preeclampsia
Chen et al,[24] 2016, China Multicenter RCT, 2013–2015	Donor oocytes excluded; donor sperm included; vitrification cryopreservation	Patients with PCOS randomized to receive FET-AC, n = 368, vs fresh ET, n = 320		FET-AC 4.4% vs fresh ET 1.4%; RR = 3.12; 95% CI, 1.26–7.73; P = .009 No severe or preterm PE
Barsky et al,[25] 2016 US single IVF center, 2009–2014	Donor oocytes excluded; vitrification cryopreservation	FET-AC, n=109, vs fresh ET, n=289		7.6% vs 2.6%; P = .023; AOR 3.1; 95% CI, 1.2–8.4 sPE 4.59% vs 1.73% No preterm PE
Sites et al,[26] 2017, US National Assisted Reproductive Technology Surveillance System, 2005–2010	Autologous oocytes; slow-freeze cyropreservation	FET-AC, n=1052, vs fresh ET, n=7453		7.51% vs 4.29%; P<.0001; AOR 2.17; 95% CI, 1.67–2.82; P<.0001 PE with preterm delivery 2.76% vs 1.48%; P = .002; AOR 2.19; 95% CI, 1.43–3.35; P = .0003. sPE 2.95% vs 1.41%; P = .0002
von Versen-Höynck et al,[12] 2019 Single IVF center, 2011–2017	Donor oocytes excluded; cryopreservation method(s) not specified	FET-AC, n = 94, vs FET-NC, n = 127		PE 12.8% vs 3.9%; P = .02; AOR 3.33; 95% CI, 1.20–11.94; P = .03 sPE 9.6% vs 0.8%; P<.001; AOR 15.05; 95% CI, 2.59–286.27; P = .01 No preterm PE

Study	Notes	Comparison	Outcome	
Saito et al,[28] 2019 Japanese ART registry database, 2004	Donor gametes and embryos disallowed in Japan; method(s) of cryopreservation not specified	FET-AC, n = 24,225, vs FET-NC, n = 10,755 (each >96% singleton)	4.0% vs 3.0%; P<.001; AOR 1.43; 95% CI, 1.14–1.80	
Ginstrom Ernstad et al,[10] 2019, Sweden IVF registries, 2005–2015	Exclusion of donor eggs or embryos not specified; slow freeze and vitrification cryopreservation (OR adjusted for method of cryopreservation)	FET-AC, n = 1446, vs FET-NC, n = 6297	10.5% vs 6.1%; aOR 1.78; 95% CI, 1.43–2.21	8.2% vs 4.4%
		FET-AC vs FET-stimulated cycle, n = 1983	10.5% vs 6.6%; aOR 1.61; 95% CI, 1.22–2.10	8.2% vs 4.3%
		FET-stimulated cycle vs FET-NC	aOR 1.05; 95% CI, 0.84–1.31	
		Fresh ET, n = 24,365	5.2%	3.7%
		Spontaneous conception, n = 1,127,566	3.9%	2.8%

IVF + intracytoplasmic sperm injection combined except where noted.
Abbreviations: ART, assisted reproductive technology; BC, blastocyst; ICSI, intracytoplasmic sperm injection; NS, nonsignificant.
a Singletons + twins combined.
b Reference: 268,599 single spontaneously conceived pregnancies (1.00); RR 4.7%.
c Reference: fresh cycles (1.00).

Table 2
Incidence of hypertensive disorders of pregnancy (%) according to in vitro fertilization protocol

Publication	In Vitro Fertilization Protocols or Spontaneous Conception			
	Frozen Embryo Transfer–Artificial Cycle	Frozen Embryo Transfer–Natural Cycle	Fresh Embryo Transfer	Spontaneous Conception
Wennerholm et al,[27] 1997		7.2[a]	7.7	6.2
Wikland et al,[21] 2010[b]	11.8[b]		5.5	
Ishihara et al,[22] 2014[c]	2.8[c]		1.8	
Opdahl et al,[23] 2015[c]	7.0[c]		5.7	4.7
Saito et al,[28] 2019	4.0	3.0		
Ginstrom Ernstad et al,[10] 2019	10.5	6.1	5.2	3.9
Mean ± SEM (%)	7.2 ± 1.8%	5.4 ± 1.3%	5.2 ± 1.0%	4.9 ± 0.7%

Omitting FET-AC for Wikland and colleagues, 2010; Ishihara and colleagues, 2015; and Opdahl and colleagues, 2014, due to uncertain status of FET protocol, yielded a similar mean: 7.3%.
[a] 82% FET-NC.
[b] Combination of FET-AC and FET-NC.
[c] Presuming mostly FET-AC, although protocols not specified.

rates of hypertensive disorders of pregnancy and PE, as compiled from **Table 1** and summarized in **Tables 2** and **3**, respectively.

In a recently published prospective study, von Versen-Hoynck and colleagues recruited women during early pregnancy with singleton intrauterine pregnancies who conceived using autologous oocytes and delivered live born infants (n = 878).[12] No participants had an infertility diagnosis of premature ovarian failure or were recipients of donor oocytes or embryos. After adjustment for several PE risk

Table 3
Incidence of preeclampsia (%) according to in vitro fertilization protocol

Publication	In Vitro Fertilization Protocols or Spontaneous Conception			
	Frozen Embryo Transfer–Artificial Cycles	Frozen Embryo Transfer–Natural Cycles	Fresh Embryo Transfer	Spontaneous Conception
Sazonova et al,[44] 2012	5.6[a]		4.5	2.8
Chen et al,[24] 2016	4.4		1.4	
Barsky et al,[25] 2016	7.6		2.6	
Sites et al,[26] 2017	7.5		4.3	
von Versen-Höynck et al,[12] 2019	12.8	3.9	4.7	4.9
Ernstad et al,[10] 2019	8.2	4.4	3.7	2.8
Mean ± SEM (%)	7.7 ± 1.2	4.2	3.5 ± 0.5	3.5 ± 0.7

Omitting Sazonova 2012 yielded a similar mean ± SEM: 8.1 ± 1.4.
[a] FET protocols not specified.

factors (ie, maternal age, nulliparity, history of hypertension, body mass index [BMI], PCOS, and pregestational and gestational diabetes), women conceiving by FET in ACs, in which a CL did not develop, had increased risk for PE (AOR 2.73; 95% CI, 1.14–6.49) and sPE (AOR 6.45; 95% CI, 1.94–25.09) compared with subfertile women with 1 CL. In a subanalysis of FET in ACs compared with FET in modified natural cycles (NCs) with 1 CL, the AORs were 3.55 (95% CI, 1.20–11.94) for developing PE and 15.05 (95% CI, 2.59–286.27) for sPE. Importantly, women conceiving by fresh ET in ovarian stimulation cycles who had multiple CL did not show increased PE risk. This study was the first to evaluate PE risk in IVF from the standpoint of CL status. The findings implicated absence of the CL as a possible contributor to the development of PE (see **Tables 1** and **3**).

In a parallel study, the author serially evaluated cardiovascular function in women before, during, and after pregnancies, who conceived after controlled ovarian stimulation (COS) (>1 CL), autologous FET, or fresh donor oocyte–derived embryos transferred in ACs (0 CL) or spontaneous conceptions (1 CL).[12,13] Significant attenuation of the gestational changes in numerous cardiovascular parameters during the first trimester were observed in women who conceived by IVF without a CL, which mostly recovered during the second trimester. These findings were consistent with the hypothesis that circulating CL factor(s) mediate cardiovascular adaptations to pregnancy during the first trimester in spontaneous pregnancy, and placental factors supersede after the corpus luteal–placental shift.[7] The cardiovascular adaptations to pregnancy in the IVF participants with multiple CL were comparable to those observed in spontaneous pregnancies. Although an association was established between absent CL, dysregulated cardiovascular adaptations in the first trimester, and increased PE risk, whether these factors were causally linked remains to be proved.

A recent comprehensive publication from Sweden based on a retrospective registry study of singleton pregnancies after autologous FET reported a frequency of 8.2% for PE in ACs (0 CL; n = 1446) compared with 4.4% in NCs (1 CL; n = 6297)—AOR 1.78 (95% CI, 1.–2.21 [adjusted for maternal age, BMI, parity, year of birth of infant, maternal smoking, chronic hypertension, child's sex, level of maternal education, and years of involuntary childlessness]).[10] The women conceiving by fresh ET with multiple CL (n = 24,365) showed a lower rate of PE closer to that of spontaneous conceptions (n = 1,127,566)—3.7% and 2.8%, respectively. Similar trends were observed for hypertensive disorders of pregnancy.[10] Additional published studies demonstrated that women conceiving by autologous FET in ACs had increased risk for hypertensive disease of pregnancy or PE compared with autologous FET in NCs or fresh ET in ovarian stimulation cycles. A potential etiologic role for absent CL in the elevated risk of hypertensive disorders of pregnancy or PE in ACs, however, was not hypothesized in these reports (see Refs.[24–26,28]; see **Tables 1–3**).

In summary, although not yet confirmed by a rigorous clinical randomized controlled trial (RCT) comparing autologous FET-AC and FET-NC or modified NC, the emerging data suggest that use of IVF protocols, which lead to suppression of CL formation, may increase PE risk. These data are concerning due to the immediate-term and long-term detrimental consequences of PE for both mother and child. Thus, in addition to prepregnancy maternal characteristics in many IVF patients, such as older maternal age and subfertility, absence of the CL as an etiologic factor in the impaired maternal cardiovascular adaptations during early pregnancy and increased PE risk also should be considered [12,13]. The absence of critical circulating CL factor(s) is perhaps the most likely explanation for the dysregulation of maternal cardiovascular function observed during early pregnancy in women conceiving by IVF without a CL, in part because either full recovery or partial recovery subsequently transpired after the corpus luteal–placental shift coincident with secretion of placental factors.[12,13] But, whether the absence of CL factor(s) and of their vasodilatory and prodecidualizing attributes, or the possibility of suboptimal luteal support with estrogen and progesterone for endometrial preparation in ACs (dose and/or timing [discussed previously]),[5,8] or both underlie increased PE risk is less clear. Ultimately, if replacement of the missing CL factor(s) (eg, relaxin) restores maternal cardiovascular function in early pregnancy and reduces PE risk, then this approach might be an alternative preventative strategy to autologous FET in an NC for some women and perhaps the only approach available for women who have ovarian failure requiring donor oocytes or embryos to conceive. Mild ovarian stimulation, which would permit CL development in an FET cycle, might be used in women who do not ovulate on a regular basis.

The absence of a CL and circulating CL product(s) likely contributes to the increased risk of PE in autologous FET-AC versus FET-NC. Whether or not cryopreservation, in addition to absence of a CL, may confer added risk of PE in FET-AC compared with fresh ET, however, is difficult to test. Close examination of the study by Sites and colleagues[26] in the context of CL status may shed some light on this question. Autologous fresh ET (>1 CL) and autologous FET in an AC (0 CL) yielded rates of PE of 4.29% and 7.51%, respectively (see **Tables 1** and **3**). The difference could have been a consequence of embryo state (fresh vs frozen) and/or CL number (>1 CL vs 0 CL). Donor fresh ET and FET in ACs yielded rates of PE of 12.13% and 10.78%, respectively[26] (use of ACs for donor FETs was standard of care according to Sites CK, personal communication, 2019). These PE rates were not significantly different, which suggested that the freeze/thaw manipulation of embryos did not confer increased risk for PE (although a ceiling effect cannot be excluded). Comparing autologous (4.29%) and donor (12.13%) fresh ET revealed that the difference, 7.17%, was PE risk attributable to donor (vs autologous) and CL (>1 CL vs 0 CL) effects. Comparing autologous (7.51%) and donor frozen (10.78%) ET, both using ACs (0 CL), revealed that the difference, 4.62%, was the contribution to PE attributable to donor (vs autologous) effect, alone. Thus, the difference between the PE rates attributable to donor and CL effects (7.17%) and donor (4.62%) effect, 2.55%, must be due to the CL effect alone. Although any conclusion based on these rough estimates must be regarded cautiously, the AC (0 CL), in addition to a donor embryo source, appeared to account for the considerably higher rates of PE in women who were recipient of donor oocyte–derived embryos.

WHY IS IN VITRO FERTILIZATION ASSOCIATED WITH INCREASED RISK OF ADVERSE PREGNANCY OUTCOMES?
Artificial (Programmed) Cycles

The emerging evidence suggests that perhaps not all IVF protocols are created equal with respect to increased risk for hypertensive disorders of pregnancy and PE. Although IVF protocols were frequently not presented in sufficient detail in many of the publications, after close inspection of those in which they were delineated, the balance of evidence implicated the AC protocol. That is, elevated risk for hypertensive disorders of pregnancy and PE primarily resulted from FET-AC, not FET-NC or FET-stimulated or fresh ET cycles (see **Table 1**). Perhaps not coincidentally, the maternal hemodynamic adaptations to pregnancy were perturbed in AC but not COS cycle protocols.[12,13] Close inspection of the grand averages of the rates for hypertensive disorders of pregnancy and PE, listed in **Table 1**, further highlights that increased risk is associated with the AC (see **Tables 2** and **3**).

In most of the studies that reported increased risk for PE in autologous FET-AC protocols, the gestational age of PE onset and the severity of disease were not specified (see **Table 1**). A few, however, did provide these details. Chen and coworkers[24] observed increased risk for term, but not preterm, PE and sPE; increased frequency of term, but not preterm PE and sPE were noted by both von Versen-Höynck and colleagues[12] and Barsky and colleagues[25]; and Sites and coworkers[26] reported increased incidence of both preterm PE and term PE and sPE in autologous FET-AC. Although the number of studies are too few to draw any definite conclusions, with the exception of Sites and coworkers, term PE both with and without severe features was associated with autologous FET-AC protocols. A recent theory for the pathogenesis of term PE proposes that it arises from villous overcrowding, which leads to compression of intervillous spaces that, in turn, impedes blood flow, causing placental ischemia. That is, villous growth outstrips uterine capacity[29] (discussed previously).

Women with low circulating relaxin concentration in early pregnancy were observed to be at increased risk of developing late-onset PE ($\geq$34 weeks).[30] Possibly, the vasodilatory attributes of relaxin are important in some women to mitigate the physiologic rise in circulating vasoconstrictors, such as sFLT1, thereby restraining the normal restoration of the maternal circulation to the nonpregnant state of relative vasoconstriction toward the end of pregnancy.[13,31,32] Circulating sFLT1 and the sFLT1/placental growth factor ratios were significantly higher at the end of pregnancy in women conceiving by IVF, especially for AC (0 CL) protocols,[33] perhaps reflecting villous overcrowding and placental ischemia. Whereas circulating relaxin is absent in ACs, concentrations are either comparable to spontaneous pregnancy or markedly higher in COS cycles, the latter possibly explaining the equivalent rates of PE in COS and spontaneous pregnancies, as discussed previously (see **Tables 1** and **3**).

The finding by Sites and colleagues[26] of increased preterm, in addition to term, PE after autologous FET-AC protocol should not be ignored (discussed previously). This investigation may have identified increased risk for both term PE and preterm PE due to larger cohort sizes and hence, increased study power. On the surface, however, it is difficult to reconcile preterm PE and term PE based on a common decidual etiology. Preterm PE is widely believed to be associated with impaired trophoblast invasion and spiral artery remodeling, whereas recent theory suggests that term PE does not involve deficient placentation but rather villous overcrowding (discussed previously). Conceivably, villous overcrowding might be exacerbated by post-term delivery and larger placentas associated with large-for-gestational-age or macrosomic infants—adverse pregnancy outcomes also associated with IVF ACs (see Refs.[10,34]). Post-term delivery itself has been associated with increased PE and eclampsia risk,[35] presumably as a consequence of the mechanisms, outlined previously, being exacerbated by prolonged time for placental growth.[29] Enhanced frequency of large for gestational age and macrosomia in autologous FET during ACs also are consistent with the increased risk of term PE, insofar as it is not infrequently accompanied by a large-for-gestational-age fetus[36,37] and large placenta.[38] Whether term PE may be associated with excessive trophoblast invasion, albeit to lesser degree than accreta spectrum disorders that also occur more frequently in IVF ACs (eg, see article by Kaser and colleagues[11]), is not known.

On the one hand, excessive trophoblast invasion is observed in tubal pregnancy and accreta spectrum disorders, in which decidua is deficient and/or dysregulated.[39–41] On the other hand, dysregulated decidualization is associated with preterm sPE, in which trophoblast invasion is deficient[2–4] (discussed previously). These apparently disparate actions of the decidua on trophoblast invasion are difficult to reconcile mechanistically, that is, how can decidual pathology lead to both excessive and deficient trophoblast invasion? One potential explanation is that activation of different molecular pathways accounts for these divergent actions of the decidua on trophoblast behavior that may be regulated, at least in part, by factors derived from the CL, or lack thereof. A priori, it seems logical to presume that decidual pathology would not be restricted to one phenotypic expression of excessive trophoblast invasion as in some cases of placental accreta disorders, but rather different molecular pathology could also arise, which leads to impaired trophoblast invasion frequently observed in preterm PE.

FUTURE INVESTIGATIONS

In light of the association between dysregulated decidualization and PE, the underlying molecular mechanism(s) of the pathologic decidua now need to be identified in order to design prophylactic or corrective interventions. Eventually, efforts to improve decidualization before and during early pregnancy might be indicated in those women at increased risk for the disease (eg, by administration of hormones known to promote decidualization). Finally, circulating or urinary biomarkers or a panel of biomarkers reflecting endometrial dysfunction might be helpful in identifying women at increased risk (eg, low circulating IGFBP-1 or glycodelin before and/or during early pregnancy).[3]

Given the perturbed maternal physiology and increased risk of several adverse pregnancy outcomes in IVF cycles involving autologous FET in ACs, what can be done to intervene? Careful inspection of the data revealed that the increased risk for hypertensive disorders of pregnancy and PE was not observed in FET using NCs, stimulated cycles, or in COS cycles. Based on this revelation, it is reasonable to propose that a large, multisite RCT be conducted comparing pregnancy outcomes between autologous FET-AC and FET-NC, FET-modified NC, or FET-stimulated cycles.[12] In a subgroup of patients, maternal physiology could be intensively investigated in order to determine whether it would be normal after FET-NC, FET-modified NC, or FET-stimulated cycles in contrast to FET-AC, as predicted.[7,12,13,42] If an RCT confirms the hypothesis that maternal physiology and pregnancy outcome will be improved, then FET-NC, FET-modified NC, or FET-stimulated cycles might be preferred protocols in many women. A common denominator is the absence of a CL in IVF ACs, whereas at least 1 CL develops in FET-NC, FET-modified NC, and FET-stimulated cycles.[7,12,13] All CL product(s) are missing in FET-AC (except for E2 and P4 administered for luteal support), and, therefore, the absence of any 1 or several of them could underlie the dysregulated maternal cardiovascular adaptations to pregnancy and increased risk for adverse pregnancy outcomes. Both the cardiovascular system and endometrium are known targets of at least 1 CL factor that is not replaced in AC protocols, relaxin (discussed previously).[42,43] Therefore, including the missing CL factor(s) like relaxin with E2 and P4 for luteal support in ACs might be investigated in order to determine whether the addition of CL factor(s) like relaxin to the IVF medical regimen would correct the dysregulated maternal cardiovascular physiology and reduce the risk for adverse pregnancy outcomes. For women with ovarian failure for which IVF NCs are unattainable, replacing the missing CL factor(s) may be the only option.

ACKNOWLEDGMENTS

This work was supported by P01 HD065647-01A1 from the National Institute of Child Health and Human Development, and the J. Robert and Mary Cade Professorship of Physiology.

DISCLOSURE

Dr K.P. Conrad discloses use patents for relaxin.

REFERENCES

1. Founds SA, Conley YP, Lyons-Weiler JF, et al. Altered global gene expression in first trimester placentas of women destined to develop preeclampsia. Placenta 2009;30(1):15–24.
2. Rabaglino MB, Post Uiterweer ED, Jeyabalan A, et al. Bioinformatics approach reveals evidence for impaired endometrial maturation before and during early pregnancy in women who developed preeclampsia. Hypertension 2015;65(2): 421–9.
3. Conrad KP, Rabaglino MB, Post Uiterweer ED. Emerging role for dysregulated decidualization in the genesis of preeclampsia. Placenta 2017;60:119–29.
4. Garrido-Gomez T, Dominguez F, Quinonero A, et al. Defective decidualization during and after severe preeclampsia reveals a possible maternal contribution to the etiology. Proc Natl Acad Sci U S A 2017;114:E8468–77.
5. Rabaglino MB, Conrad KP. Evidence for shared molecular pathways of dysregulated decidualization in preeclampsia and endometrial disorders revealed by microarray data integration. FASEB J 2019;33(11):11682–95.
6. Brosens I, Pijnenborg R, Vercruysse L, et al. The "Great Obstetrical Syndromes" are associated with disorders of deep placentation. Am J Obstet Gynecol 2011; 204(3):193–201.
7. Conrad KP, Baker VL. Corpus luteal contribution to maternal pregnancy physiology and outcomes in assisted reproductive technologies. Am J Physiol Regul Integr Comp Physiol 2013;304(2):R69–72.
8. Altmae S, Tamm-Rosenstein K, Esteban FJ, et al. Endometrial transcriptome analysis indicates superiority of natural over artificial cycles in recurrent implantation failure patients undergoing frozen embryo transfer. Reprod Biomed Online 2016; 32(6):597–613.
9. Young SL, Savaris RF, Lessey BA, et al. Effect of randomized serum progesterone concentration on secretory endometrial histologic development and gene expression. Hum Reprod 2017;32(9):1903–14.
10. Ginstrom Ernstad E, Wennerholm UB, Khatibi A, et al. Neonatal and maternal outcome after frozen embryo transfer: Increased risks in programmed cycles. Am J Obstet Gynecol 2019;221(2):126.e1-8.
11. Kaser DJ, Melamed A, Bormann CL, et al. Cryopreserved embryo transfer is an independent risk factor for placenta accreta. Fertil Steril 2015;103(5):1176–84.e2.
12. von Versen-Höynck F, Schaub AM, Chi YY, et al. Increased preeclampsia risk and reduced aortic compliance with in vitro fertilization cycles in the absence of a corpus luteum. Hypertension 2019;73(3):640–9.
13. Conrad KP, Petersen JW, Chi YY, et al. Maternal cardiovascular dysregulation during early pregnancy after in vitro fertilization cycles in the absence of a corpus luteum. Hypertension 2019;74(3):705–15.
14. Clark AR, James JL, Stevenson GN, et al. Understanding abnormal uterine artery Doppler waveforms: a novel computational model to explore potential causes within the utero-placental vasculature. Placenta 2018;66:74–81.
15. Burton GJ, Woods AW, Jauniaux E, et al. Rheological and physiological consequences of conversion of the maternal spiral arteries for uteroplacental blood flow during human pregnancy. Placenta 2009;30(6):473–82.

16. Fisher SJ. Why is placentation abnormal in preeclampsia? Am J Obstet Gynecol 2015;213(4 Suppl):S115–22.
17. Brosens JJ, Pijnenborg R, Brosens IA. The myometrial junctional zone spiral arteries in normal and abnormal pregnancies: a review of the literature. Am J Obstet Gynecol 2002;187(5):1416–23.
18. Gellersen B, Brosens IA, Brosens JJ. Decidualization of the human endometrium: mechanisms, functions, and clinical perspectives. Semin Reprod Med 2007; 25(6):445–53.
19. Deepak V, Sahu MB, Yu J, et al. Retinoic acid is a negative regulator of sFLT1 expression in decidual stromal cells, and its levels are reduced in preeclamptic decidua. Hypertension 2019;73(5):1104–11.
20. Dunk C, Kwan M, Hazan A, et al. Failure of decidualization and maternal immune tolerance underlies uterovascular resistance in intra uterine growth restriction. Front Endocrinol (Lausanne) 2019;10:160.
21. Wikland M, Hardarson T, Hillensjo T, et al. Obstetric outcomes after transfer of vitrified blastocysts. Hum Reprod 2010;25(7):1699–707.
22. Ishihara O, Araki R, Kuwahara A, et al. Impact of frozen-thawed single-blastocyst transfer on maternal and neonatal outcome: an analysis of 277,042 single-embryo transfer cycles from 2008 to 2010 in Japan. Fertil Steril 2014;101(1):128–33.
23. Opdahl S, Henningsen AA, Tiitinen A, et al. Risk of hypertensive disorders in pregnancies following assisted reproductive technology: a cohort study from the CoNARTaS group. Hum Reprod 2015;30(7):1724–31.
24. Chen ZJ, Shi Y, Sun Y, et al. Fresh versus frozen embryos for infertility in the polycystic ovary syndrome. N Engl J Med 2016;375(6):523–33.
25. Barsky M, St Marie P, Rahil T, et al. Are perinatal outcomes affected by blastocyst vitrification and warming? Am J Obstet Gynecol 2016;215(5):603.e1-5.
26. Sites CK, Wilson D, Barsky M, et al. Embryo cryopreservation and preeclampsia risk. Fertil Steril 2017;108(5):784–90.
27. Wennerholm UB, Hamberger L, Nilsson L, et al. Obstetric and perinatal outcome of children conceived from cryopreserved embryos. Hum Reprod 1997;12(8): 1819–25.
28. Saito K, Kuwahara A, Ishikawa T, et al. Endometrial preparation methods for frozen-thawed embryo transfer are associated with altered risks of hypertensive disorders of pregnancy, placenta accreta, and gestational diabetes mellitus. Hum Reprod 2019;34(8):1567–75.
29. Redman CW, Sargent IL, Staff AC. IFPA Senior Award Lecture: making sense of pre-eclampsia - two placental causes of preeclampsia? Placenta 2014; 35(Suppl):S20–5.
30. Jeyabalan A, Stewart DR, McGonigal SC, et al. Low relaxin concentrations in the first trimester are associated with increased risk of developing preeclampsia [abstract]. Reprod Sci 2009;16(3):101A.
31. von Versen-Hoynck F, Strauch NK, Liu J, et al. Effect of mode of conception on maternal serum relaxin, creatinine, and sodium concentrations in an infertile population. Reprod Sci 2019;26(3):412–9.
32. Levine RJ, Maynard SE, Qian C, et al. Circulating angiogenic factors and the risk of preeclampsia. N Engl J Med 2004;350(7):672–83.
33. Conrad KP, Graham GM, Chi YY, et al. Potential influence of the corpus luteum on circulating reproductive and volume regulatory hormones, angiogenic and immunoregulatory factors in pregnant women. Am J Physiol Endocrinol Metab 2019; 317(4):E677–85.

34. Choux C, Ginod P, Barberet J, et al. Placental volume and other first-trimester outcomes: are there differences between fresh embryo transfer, frozen-thawed embryo transfer and natural conception? Reprod Biomed Online 2019;38(4):538–48.
35. Caughey AB, Stotland NE, Escobar GJ. What is the best measure of maternal complications of term pregnancy: ongoing pregnancies or pregnancies delivered? Am J Obstet Gynecol 2003;189(4):1047–52.
36. Xiong X, Demianczuk NN, Buekens P, et al. Association of preeclampsia with high birth weight for age. Am J Obstet Gynecol 2000;183(1):148–55.
37. Xiong X, Demianczuk NN, Saunders LD, et al. Impact of preeclampsia and gestational hypertension on birth weight by gestational age. Am J Epidemiol 2002; 155(3):203–9.
38. Dahlstrom B, Romundstad P, Oian P, et al. Placenta weight in pre-eclampsia. Acta Obstet Gynecol Scand 2008;87(6):608–11.
39. Jauniaux E, Collins S, Burton GJ. Placenta accreta spectrum: pathophysiology and evidence-based anatomy for prenatal ultrasound imaging. Am J Obstet Gynecol 2018;218(1):75–87.
40. Randall S, Buckley CH, Fox H. Placentation in the fallopian tube. Int J Gynecol Pathol 1987;6(2):132–9.
41. Sliz A, Locker KCS, Lampe K, et al. Gab3 is required for IL-2- and IL-15-induced NK cell expansion and limits trophoblast invasion during pregnancy. Sci Immunol 2019;4(38) [pii:eaav3866].
42. Conrad KP. Maternal vasodilation in pregnancy: the emerging role of relaxin. Am J Physiol Regul Integr Comp Physiol 2011;301(2):R267–75.
43. Conrad KP. G-Protein-coupled receptors as potential drug candidates in preeclampsia: targeting the relaxin/insulin-like family peptide receptor 1 for treatment and prevention. Hum Reprod Update 2016;22(5):647–64.
44. Sazonova A, Kallen K, Thurin-Kjellberg A, et al. Obstetric outcome in singletons after in vitro fertilization with cryopreserved/thawed embryos. Hum Reprod 2012; 27(5):1343–50.

When the Fetus Goes Still and the Birth Is Tragic

The Role of the Placenta in Stillbirths

Nicole Graham, MRCOG, Alexander E.P. Heazell, PhD, MRCOG*

KEYWORDS

- Placenta • Stillbirth • Perinatal death • Investigation of stillbirth • Cause of stillbirth
- Autopsy • Placental abruption • Chorioamnionitis

KEY POINTS

- Reducing stillbirth remains a significant challenge to maternity services in high-income countries (HICs).
- Pathologic conditions within the placenta are the most frequent cause of stillbirth in HICs.
- The relationship between specific placental lesions and stillbirth is less clear, due to variations in placental sampling and definitions of placental abnormalities.
- Information obtained from the placental examination reduces the likelihood of an unexplained stillbirth and provides prognostic information regarding subsequent pregnancies.
- Following stillbirth, the placenta should be sent for histopathological assessment.

INTRODUCTION

Stillbirth is defined as the death of an infant before birth. There is significant variation internationally regarding the lower gestational age limit, with the World Health Organization (WHO) using a definition of 22 weeks' gestation or a birthweight of 500 g when gestational age is unknown. However, to compare among countries, the WHO uses a definition of 28 weeks' gestation or a birthweight of 1000 g.[1] Applying this definition, there are an estimated 2.6 million stillbirths each year globally, ~98% of which occur in low and middle-income countries (LMICs).[2] However, this should not lead one to underestimate the burden of stillbirths in high-income countries (HICs). There are approximately 23,000 stillbirths per year in the United States, where stillbirth is defined as the death of an infant before birth after 20 weeks of gestation.[3]

Faculty of Biological, Medical and Human Sciences, Maternal and Fetal Health Research Centre, School of Medical Sciences, University of Manchester, Manchester Academic Health Science Centre, St. Mary's Hospital, Central Manchester University Hospitals NHS Foundation Trust, 5th Floor (Research), Oxford Road, Manchester M13 9WL, UK
* Corresponding author.
E-mail address: alexander.heazell@manchester.ac.uk

Obstet Gynecol Clin N Am 47 (2020) 183–196
https://doi.org/10.1016/j.ogc.2019.10.005
0889-8545/20/© 2019 Elsevier Inc. All rights reserved.

Applying the WHO definition for international comparison, the stillbirth rate in the United States after 28 weeks' gestation is 3.0 per 1000 stillbirths, placing the United States 27th of 49 HICs.[4] Of greater concern is that the annual rate of reduction of still-births after 28 weeks' gestation in the United States between 2000 and 2015 was only 0.4%, placing it 48th of the 49 HICs studied (**Fig. 1**A).[4] In addition, there is significant variation among states ranging from 3.37 stillbirths per 1000 live births in New Mexico up to 9.87 per 1000 total births in Mississippi (**Fig. 1**B).[3] Comparing the 5-year average stillbirth rates from 2003 to 2007 to 2013 to 2017, there is also significant variation be-tween states with regard to reduction in stillbirth, with decreases of more than 1 per 1000 births seen in New York, Louisiana, South Carolina, Virginia, West Virginia, and Connecticut, but increases greater than 0.5 per 1000 births seen in Kansas, Ore-gon, Rhode Island, Utah, Tennessee, and South Dakota (see **Fig. 1**B). As stillbirths place significant psychological, social, and economic burden on families, health ser-vices and wider society efforts are urgently needed to reduce the burden of stillbirth.[5,6] Understanding risk factors for stillbirth and the underlying pathologic processes is pro-posed as a means to reduce the stillbirth rate.

This article reviews the evidence for the role of the placenta in the etiology of still-birth, initially considering epidemiologic studies of risk factors for stillbirth and how these may mediate their effects through the placenta. We then consider placental ab-normalities reported in cases of stillbirth and how the placental etiologies change across gestation. We postulate that the presence of selective placental abnormalities is of significance in future pregnancies.

RISK FACTORS FOR STILLBIRTH IN HIGH-INCOME COUNTRIES

In HICs, stillbirths usually occur in the antepartum period, in contrast to LMICs, where approximately 50% of stillbirths occur during labor. A review of 15,840 stillbirths occurring in the United States during 2014 found that the largest proportion (30%) were unexplained.[7] Where a cause of death was reported, complications with the placenta, cord, or membranes were most the frequently cited cause (28% of deaths), followed by maternal complications (14%) and congenital abnormalities (10%). Impor-tantly, these classifications incorporated findings from autopsy in only 11.7% of cases and histopathological examination of the placenta in 47.7% of cases, which may ac-count for the high proportion of "unexplained" stillbirths.[7] Factors associated with still-birth have been extensively investigated using a variety of epidemiologic methods, including large retrospective cohort and prospective case-control studies, in some cases there have been sufficient numbers of studies to undertake meta-analyses. In the United States, the Stillbirth Collaborative Research Network (SCRN) has under-taken and published a case-control study on a well-characterized group of 614 still-births and 1816 live births.[8] In this study, examples of factors occurring before pregnancy that were independently associated with stillbirth are shown in **Table 1** with their respective adjusted odds ratios (aORs). However, these factors are present in only 19% of stillbirths, indicating that the bulk of stillbirths occur in women who do not have risk factors present in early pregnancy.[8]

Analysis of stillbirths in other HICs confirms the relationship between these factors and stillbirth. Systematic reviews coupled with large meta-analyses suggest the odds ratio (OR) for stillbirth in women with a previous stillbirth is 4.83 (95% confidence in-terval [CI] 3.77–6.18),[9] for women ≥40 years of age it is 2.12 (95% CI 1.86–2.42),[10] and with cigarette smoking the OR is 1.43 (95% CI 1.32–1.54).[11] These meta-analyses suggest that the data from the SCRN study are consistent with information from many studies performed across a variety of international settings.

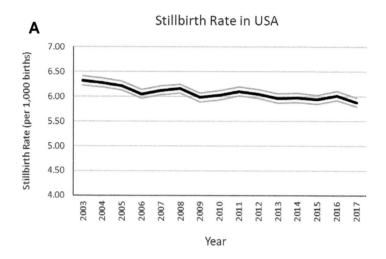

A

Stillbirth Rate in USA

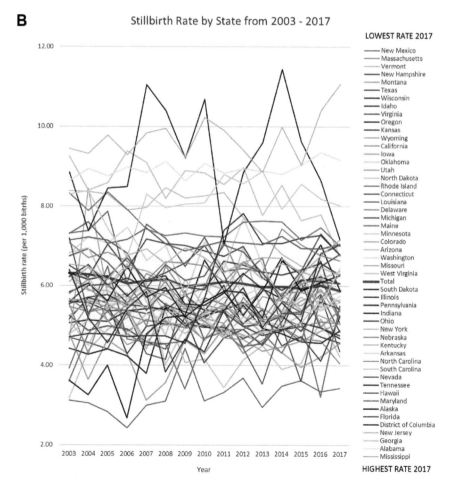

B

Stillbirth Rate by State from 2003 - 2017

LOWEST RATE 2017

New Mexico
Massachusetts
Vermont
New Hampshire
Montana
Texas
Wisconsin
Idaho
Virginia
Oregon
Kansas
Wyoming
California
Iowa
Oklahoma
Utah
North Dakota
Rhode Island
Connecticut
Louisiana
Delaware
Michigan
Maine
Minnesota
Colorado
Arizona
Washington
Missouri
West Virginia
Total
South Dakota
Illinois
Pennsylvania
Indiana
Ohio
New York
Nebraska
Kentucky
Arkansas
North Carolina
South Carolina
Nevada
Tennessee
Hawaii
Maryland
Alaska
Florida
District of Columbia
New Jersey
Georgia
Alabama
Mississippi

HIGHEST RATE 2017

Studies examining the impact of risk factors that develop during pregnancy have shown consistent associations between a small for gestational age (SGA) fetus and stillbirth (relative risk [RR] 8.0, 95% CI 6.5–9.9; aOR 6.22, 95% CI 3.79–0.23),[12] as well as the development of hypertensive disorders of pregnancy/preeclampsia (RR 2.8, 95% CI 1.5–5.1; adjusted RR 1.45, 95% CI 1.20–1.76)[12,13] and maternal perception of reduced fetal movements and stillbirth (RFM; aOR 3.54, 95% CI 2,44–5.15).[14] In particular, the association between SGA fetuses and stillbirth are thought to reflect fetal growth restriction (FGR), where the fetus does not achieve its genetic growth potential. There are also relationships between FGR and hypertensive disorders of pregnancy and FGR and RFM.

The risk factors presented here for stillbirth in HICs provide some initial clues to the relationship between placental dysfunction and stillbirth. Many of the risk factors for antepartum stillbirth described here, including obesity,[15] maternal age $\geq$40,[16] cigarette smoking,[17] reduced fetal movements,[18] FGR,[19] and hypertensive disorders of pregnancy,[20] are associated with abnormalities of placental structure and/or function. Although a detailed review of these ex vivo studies is beyond the scope of this article, a significant body of work has described changes in placental morphology, cell proliferation, cell death, and inflammation in the presence of these risk factors. Placental dysfunction, culminating in a failure to meet the oxygen and nutrient requirements of the fetus, may be a common pathway linking epidemiologic risk factors to stillbirth.[21]

Further evidence regarding the important role of the placenta in stillbirth and pregnancy loss can be inferred from the increased rate of stillbirth and SGA infants seen in confined placental mosaicism (CPM). CPM is a condition in which the placenta has a numerical or structural chromosomal abnormality, whereas the fetus has normal chromosomes. Analysis of 115 cases of CPM identified by prenatal testing compared with 230 unaffected controls found an increased rate of SGA infants (15% compared with 5%),[22] and a review of cases of CPM reported before 2011 found that 9.3% were associated with FGR and 7.2% of cases ended in stillbirth or spontaneous miscarriage.[23] This finding suggests that even when abnormalities are restricted to the placenta, they exert an important effect on fetal growth and survival.

ASSOCIATION BETWEEN PLACENTAL ABNORMALITIES AND STILLBIRTH

Placental size is routinely measured as part of the macroscopic assessment of the placenta during histopathological examination, and placental weight relative to birthweight is associated with stillbirth. A large cohort study found that placental weight is lower in stillbirths than in live births at all gestational ages. The proportion of stillbirths with fetal:placental weight ratio in the top 10% for gestational age, increased with advancing weeks' gestation, from 29% of stillbirths between 25 and 26 weeks' gestation to 36% between 39 to 40 weeks' gestation.[24] Two smaller studies provide

Fig. 1. (A) The stillbirth rate ($\geq$20 weeks' gestation) for all reported births in the United States from 2003 to 2017 showing an overall annual rate of reduction of 0.28% per year. Light grey lines indicate 95% confidence interval. (B) The stillbirth rates for individual states from 2003 to 2017, ranging from those with the lowest to highest rates in 2017 demonstrating wide variation in stillbirth rates throughout the country. For comparison, the average stillbirth rate for the United States is shown in red. (Data from Centers for Disease Control and Prevention (CDC). National Center for Health Statistics. Vital Statistics Online Data Portal. Available at: https://www.cdc.gov/nchs/data_access/vitalstatsonline.htm. Accessed Sept 30 2019.)

Table 1
Characteristics in early pregnancy and their association with stillbirth

Characteristic (Comparison)	Adjusted Odds Ratio (95% Confidence Interval)
Non-Hispanic black ethnicity (vs non-Hispanic white)	2.12 (1.41–3.20)
Previous stillbirth (vs previous live birth)	5.91 (3.18–11.00)
Diabetes (vs no diabetes)	2.50 (1.39–4.48)
Obesity ($\geq$35 kg/m^2) (vs. appropriate weight)	1.73 (1.23–2.45)
Maternal age $\geq$40 (vs 20–24 y)	2.41 (1.24–4.70)
Cigarette smoking $\geq$10 per day (vs nonsmoker)	1.55 (1.02–2.35)
History of drug misuse (vs none)	2.08 (1.12–3.88)

Data from Stillbirth Collaborative Research Network Writing Group. Association between stillbirth and risk factors known at pregnancy confirmation. JAMA 2011;306(22):2469-2479.

conflicting data as to whether or not placental weight is related to the recorded cause of stillbirth. The first study of 126 singleton stillbirths found the placental weight was less than 10th percentile in 57% of cases; the fetal:placental weight ratio was in the top decile in 58% of stillbirths due to FGR, 57% due to placental insufficiency, and in 47% of stillbirths from unknown cause.[25] In contrast, another study of 145 singleton stillbirths found that placental weight was reduced only in stillbirths associated with placental pathology, but not other causes.[26] Therefore, whether or not placental size predisposes to stillbirth, or is simply an indicator of underlying placental dysfunction, remains unknown.

A systematic review to determine the likelihood of diagnosing a cause of stillbirth from placental examination identified 41 studies that met the inclusion criteria.[27] There was considerable variation among included studies, as 63% were retrospective, sample sizes varied between 5 and 750 participants, and diagnostic criteria were specified in only 29% of studies. In the 13 studies of 3636 cases that investigated the frequency that placental lesions caused stillbirth, there was a large variation in conditions reported as placental causes of stillbirth, with more than 30 different "causes" recorded. Placental abruption was the most frequently attributed placental cause of death, although this was reported in only 10 (77%) of 13 studies and placental abruption accounted for 7% to 14% of deaths in these studies. Other frequently reported placental causes of stillbirth included infarction (54% of studies), chorioamnionitis, and villous dysmaturity (both reported by 38% of studies).[27] The lack of comparability between the recording of placental pathology and the classification system used meant that the proportion of stillbirths attributed to a placental cause of death varied considerably from 11% to 65%. There was a relationship between the number of categories of placental disease in the classification system and the proportion of cases determined as having a placental cause of death, which indicates that the ability of the classification system to record placental conditions may affect the cause of death attributed. In addition, a further 5 studies of 934 cases found that placental abnormalities, including placental abruption, praevia, vasa praevia, placental insufficiency, and other placental abnormalities, were associated with 17% of stillbirths. This study highlighted the need for consensus in the definition of placental lesions and application of classification systems that facilitate recording of placental pathology.[27]

Drawing conclusions about whether a placental abnormality caused or was associated with stillbirth can be challenging. In a series of analyses of live births, Pathak and colleagues[28] described that histopathological abnormalities of the placenta, including ascending genital tract infection, chronic placental underperfusion, intervillous thrombus, and villitis of unknown etiology, could be seen in apparently uncomplicated pregnancies (in 11.3%, 7.7%, 5.0%, and 3.7% of cases, respectively; **Table 2**). Other abnormalities, such as massive perivillous fibrin deposition, were seen more frequently in pregnancies complicated by hypertensive disorders of pregnancy (4%) or SGA (2%) infants compared with uncomplicated pregnancies (0.2%), suggesting these disorders may be more specific to adverse outcomes.[28]

To address the issue that placental pathology is seen in apparently healthy placentas, both case and control groups within the SCRN study were used to determine the frequency of placental abnormalities in stillbirth, reducing the potential for selection bias. Pinar and colleagues[29] reported findings from 518 singleton stillbirths and 1200 live births that found a similar proportion of live births reported chorioamnionitis to the study by Pathak and colleagues[28] (12%). However, all reported placental abnormalities were found more frequently in stillbirths (see **Table 2**). The most frequently reported abnormalities in stillbirth were acute chorioamnionitis of the free membranes (30%) or chorionic plate (23%), retroplacental hematoma (24%), and fetal vascular thrombi in the chorionic plate (23%).[29] Importantly, Pinar and colleagues[29] examined the relative frequency of placental lesions across gestation and found that lesions associated with infection, including chorioamnionitis and funisitis, were most common in births before 24 weeks' gestation, and were more common in live births than stillbirths before 31 weeks' gestation. In contrast, retroplacental hematoma was seen in equal proportions of live births and stillbirths before 24 weeks' gestation, but after that time, such hematomas were always more common in stillbirths. Although these disorders were most common at earlier gestations, distal villous immaturity, villous infarction, and fetal vascular thrombi were more frequent in cases of stillbirth after 32 weeks' gestation.[29] Thus, the placental lesion should be considered in the context of the gestation of the stillbirth and the clinical information surrounding the fetal death.

Man and colleagues[30] provide further information about the differing frequency of placental lesions in 946 cases of fetal death and stillbirth, of which 32% were deemed to have a placental cause of death. A placental cause of death was more common after 24 weeks' gestation compared with earlier losses. Of the 307 cases with a placental cause of death, the most frequent observation was ascending genital tract infection, chorioamnionitis, which was evident in 57% of cases (see **Table 2**). Man and colleagues[30] also reported the frequency of placental abnormalities (55/307) that were felt to have direct significance for the cause of death, most frequently maternal vascular malperfusion and fetal vascular occlusion, with rare causes including massive perivillous fibrin deposition and chronic histiocytic intervillositis. In addition, there were 54 cases in which placental lesions were seen (eg, focal villitis of unknown etiology) but were of uncertain clinical significance. As with Pinar and colleagues,[29] this cohort study also demonstrated variation in the frequency of lesions across gestation, with maternal vascular malperfusion noted to be more common in stillbirths occurring between 24 and 30 weeks' gestation compared with cases after 35 weeks' gestation. Later losses (>35 weeks' gestation) were more likely to have either no placental abnormalities or have the presence of lesions of uncertain significance.

These 2 large-scale studies of placental morphology after stillbirth clearly show that a diverse range of placental pathologies may be seen in stillbirth. Ptacek and colleagues[27] identified a total of 20 studies including 1447 cases of stillbirths that investigated the role of specific lesions in stillbirth, including chorioamnionitis, cord abnormalities, delayed villous maturation, fetal thrombotic vasculopathy, hemorrhagic endovasculitis and villitis of unknown etiology. Most studies (89%) replicated the

Table 2
Frequency of placental lesions in 3 large studies: Stillbirth Collaborative Research Network (SCRN) case-control study, a UK single-center cohort study of stillbirths, and a single UK center cohort study of live births

Lesion Type	Placental Feature	SCRN Study[29]		Man et al,[30] 2016	Pathak et al,[28] 2011
		Stillbirth, %, n = 518	Liveborn Control, %, n = 1200	Stillbirth, %, n = 946	Healthy Live Birth, %, n = 935
Infective	Acute chorioamnionitis (membranes)	30.4	12.0	—	—
Infective	Acute chorioamnionitis (chorionic plate)	23.2	11.9	—	—
Infective	Ascending genital tract infection	—	—	18.6	11.3
Vascular	Placental abruption/retroplacental hematoma	23.8	4.5	4.0	Study stated this lesion would be examined but none reported
Vascular	Multifocal or diffuse parenchymal infarction	13.7	4.5	—	—
Vascular	Chronic maternal underperfusion	—	—	4.4	7.7
Inflammatory	Chronic diffuse villitis/villitis of unknown etiology	1.6	0.5	Not specified	3.7
Inflammatory	Chronic histiocytic intervillositis	—	—	0.3	0.2
Inflammatory	Massive perivillous fibrin deposition	9.2	1.5	0.6	0.2
None	Normal histology	—	—	35.5	71.6

The SCRN study was a case-control study, so the frequency of lesions between stillbirth (case) and livebirth (control) could be directly compared, as the descriptions of abnormalities by individual studies showed minor differences. Data shown as % of participants within each column. -, no data reported regarding the lesion in this study.

finding of Pinar and colleagues that placental lesions were more commonly seen in cases of stillbirth. Yet, none of the lesions seen were either specific to stillbirth or a specific cause of stillbirth. This is best exemplified by fetal thrombotic vasculopathy, which was reported in association with various possible causes of death, including cytomegalovirus infection and umbilical cord accidents or abnormal cord coiling.[31–33]

Exploring the reported associations between rare placental lesions and stillbirths can be challenging because of the large sample sizes required. Useful information has been obtained from aggregate data in systematic reviews for chronic histiocytic intervillositis (CHI) and villitis of unknown etiology (VUE). By pooling data from 67 cases Contro and colleagues[34] demonstrated that CHI was associated with FGR in 66.7% of cases and the rate of live birth was 53.6%. Derricott and colleagues[35] reported the findings of VUE described in 10 studies including 2527 women with VUE and 20,590 controls; VUE was seen more frequently in cases of SGA and stillbirth, but only SGA demonstrated a significantly higher frequency of VUE compared with unaffected controls (28.6% vs 15.6%, $P<.001$), although this may be because of a lack of statistical power to detect a difference in stillbirths compared with live births (7.1% vs 5.1; $P = .14$). Critically, most of the placental lesions described in the preceding paragraphs are made following qualitative examination of the placenta by perinatal pathologists who not only identify lesions but grade their severity. As noted earlier, many studies do not include or refer to definitions of placental lesions and may also not obtain samples from the placenta in a standardized manner, limiting the comparability of data between studies. To address this, a multidisciplinary group was convened in Amsterdam in 2014 to agree to a standardized method for placental sampling and definitions of commonly occurring placental lesions.[36] To date, this document has been cited by more than 230 publications and hopefully, standardizing definitions of placental abnormalities will improve the accuracy of reporting of placental lesions and the generalizability of study findings.

CLINICAL UTILITY OF PLACENTAL EXAMINATION AFTER STILLBIRTH

Not surprisingly, examination of the placenta is recommended in clinical practice guidelines for the investigation of stillbirth. The systematic review of placental pathology in stillbirth found that in 9 studies of 1779 cases, the proportion of stillbirths with evidence of useful placental pathology ranged from 31.5% to 84.0% and the proportion of placental causes that were diagnosed from information found in the placenta ranged from 15.4% to 87.0%.[27] A study of 144 cases of stillbirth from a single center in the United States found that clinical and laboratory investigations found a cause of death in 24% of cases, placental examination increased the proportion with a probable cause to 61% of cases, and addition of autopsy results gave a probable cause in a total of 74% of cases.[37] Thus, placental examination had the largest incremental value in identifying the probable cause of death (with a rise of 37%). Importantly, this study found the information available altered clinical management in 36% of cases. A small study of 71 cases of stillbirth was used to determine the contribution of histopathological examination of the placenta to the classification of the cause. This study found placental assessment significantly reduced the likelihood of stillbirth being classified as unexplained (OR 0.17; 95% CI 0.04–0.70).[38] The findings of placental investigation were included in the classification of stillbirth in 47% of cases and in 16% the cause of death was determined primarily by placental examination. A study of 125 stillbirths from Scotland found that 79 (61%) showed placental changes that were considered to have caused death and a further 21 (16%) showed findings likely to influence the management of subsequent pregnancies. Interestingly, this article compared the frequency of detection of placental lesions with that of genetic abnormalities that were present in 3% of cases.[39] Although these 3 studies are comparatively small single-center cohorts, their findings are similar, indicating that placental examination is the investigation most likely to identify a cause of stillbirth. Consequently, histopathological investigation of the placenta is one of the most cost-effective tests to identify information regarding the cause of stillbirth and may influence care in subsequent pregnancies.

The clinical utility of the findings of placental histopathological examination is dependent on how the information obtained is integrated into the clinical care for women whose infants are stillborn. First, as Miller and colleagues[37] highlight, some causes of stillbirth may be apparent from maternal history and clinical observations. Cases in point include a massive placental abruption presenting with abdominal pain or vaginal bleeding, or a pregnancy with a high level of suspicion of FGR from antenatal ultrasound scans. This information should be passed on to the pathologist so they can interpret histopathological observations in the correct clinical context.[40] Second, the clinical meaning of placental lesions should be conveyed; for example, increased syncytial knots or syncytial nuclear aggregates are indicative of accelerated villous maturation, Such lesions are seen in maternal vascular malperfusion, which may be of particular relevance in the presence of FGR or preeclampsia.[41,42] One proposal from Turowski and colleagues[43] is a clinically orientated classification that combines individual placental findings into 9 clinically informative categories: (1) placenta with normal morphology, according to gestational age; (2) placenta with chorioamnionitis; (3) placenta with villitis and intervillositis; (4) placenta with maternal circulatory disorders (decidual vasculopathy); (5) placenta with fetal circulatory disorders; (6) placenta with delayed villous maturation; (7) placenta with findings suggestive of genetic aberration; (8) placenta with implantation disorders; and (9) placenta with other lesions. Applying this system to 315 placentas from pregnancies that ended in stillbirth found good levels of interobserver agreement (0.79). In this cohort, chorioamnionitis was a relatively rare diagnosis (3.8%), with the largest group comprising maternal circulatory disorders (75.9%); in agreement with other studies reported here, villitis/intervillositis and features suggestive of genetic aberrations were rare (frequencies of 1.9% and 1.3%, respectively), suggesting that this classification produces information that is consistent with other studies and has good interobserver reliability. A subsequent analysis of view from 62 obstetricians and maternal-fetal medicine consultants believed that implementing the reporting system would aid interpretation of placental pathology reports, which can then be used by mothers to plan future pregnancies with the help of health care professionals.[44]

There is a paucity of studies that have examined the effect of placental causes of stillbirth on the outcome of subsequent pregnancies. A large meta-analysis of 16 studies of 3,412,079 pregnancies found women who had a history of stillbirth had an independently high risk of stillbirth in a subsequent pregnancy (aOR 4.83%, 95% CI 3.77–6.18) with an absolute risk of 2.5%.[9] As few studies separated their analysis depending on the cause of stillbirth, the reasons for this increased risk are unclear. However, placental conditions likely have a role, as placental abruption, preeclampsia, and low-birthweight infants, all of which relate to placental dysfunction, are more common in pregnancies after stillbirth.[45] Two smaller studies have attempted to identify whether specific placental conditions increase the risk of adverse pregnancy outcomes after stillbirth. A study of 163 women in the Netherlands who had a pregnancy loss after 16 weeks' gestation described a further loss in a subsequent pregnancy in 11 cases.[46] Clinical information identified a cause for 7 of the subsequent stillbirths; these included placental conditions such as massive perivillous fibrin deposition, placental bed pathology/failure of conversion of spiral arteries, prelabor rupture of membranes, and, in 2 cases, neither the cause of the index or subsequent stillbirth could be determined.[46] A larger study of 273 women from 3 Italian hospitals found a frequency of adverse outcome (perinatal death, FGR, preterm birth <34 weeks' gestation, respiratory distress) in late pregnancy was 24.5%, including 2 further perinatal deaths.[47] Monari and colleagues[47] found that adverse neonatal outcome was more frequent in women who had maternal vascular malperfusion in their index stillbirth compared with those who had an unexplained stillbirth or other causes (aOR 2.1, 95% CI 1.2–3.8), this study also found maternal obesity was independently associated with increased risk of perinatal outcome (aOR 2.1, 95% CI 1.1–4.3).

Preliminary data from a detailed comparison of placental structure in index stillbirths (n = 10 in each group) found that syncytial nuclear aggregates were increased in index stillbirths and subsequent pregnancies compared with gestation age–matched controls, whereas other features, such as villous vascularity, returned to normal levels in subsequent pregnancies (Ganguly, unpublished data, 2017). This ex vivo evidence is consistent with persistence of maternal vascular malperfusion in a proportion of cases. The recurrence risk of other related placental conditions also has been explored in pregnancies that did not necessarily end in stillbirth or adverse pregnancy outcomes. Again, there is strong evidence that placental conditions may recur in subsequent pregnancies. Placental abruption is much more common in women with a history of placental abruption compared with unaffected index pregnancies (aOR 93, 95% CI 62–139).[48] Contro and colleagues[34] described that CHI is associated with a recurrence risk of 80%, and only 50% of pregnancies result in the birth of a liveborn infant and a single-center study found high-grade VUE recurred in 7 (37%) of 19 cases, and in those who had recurrent VUE, 3 were SGA (43%).[49] This provides evidence that histopathological findings from the index pregnancy can provide information regarding the prognosis of a subsequent pregnancy.

USING KNOWLEDGE ABOUT THE PLACENTA TO PROVIDE CARE IN A PREGNANCY AFTER STILLBIRTH

Given the evidence regarding the risk of recurrence of placental conditions in pregnancies after stillbirth, additional measures should be implemented to maximize placental health; for example, stop cigarette smoking, optimize maternal weight, and consideration should be given to giving aspirin to reduce the risk of placental disease.[50] There is very little evidence originating from studies of women with prior stillbirth to support a recommendation of aspirin,[51] but it extrapolates from a large systematic review that found commencing aspirin at a prophylactic dose before 16 weeks' gestation reduced the risk of perinatal death in late pregnancy (RR 0.41 vs 0.93).[52] Other novel treatment regimens are also now being established for other placental conditions, including CHI, which may improve outcomes.[53] However, these approaches should be regarded as empirical and further intervention studies are needed.

Because of the increased risk of an SGA fetus in a pregnancy following stillbirth, additional screening should be put in place to ensure normal fetal growth until birth. In addition to routine assessment of fetal growth, ultrasound also has been used to assess placental structure. Importantly, abnormal uterine or umbilical artery flow with a thickened placental disc may reflect the underlying disease process (eg, maternal vascular malperfusion or placental bed disorders), and these observations are associated with complications such as FGR and stillbirth.[54] Toal and colleagues[55] examined the predictive accuracy of a combination of maternal serum screening (16–18weeks), second trimester uterine artery Doppler, and placental morphologic condition (shape and/or texture), and found there were no cases of unexpected still-birth in the cohort, and no cases of severe early-onset FGR after a normal placental profile. Combining $\geq$2 abnormal components of the test predicted 14 of 19 pregnan-cies that developed severe early-onset intrauterine growth restriction (sensitivity 74%) and 15 of 22 pregnancies that ended in stillbirth (sensitivity 68%). This approach could allow antenatal surveillance to be directed to women who have the greatest chance of adverse pregnancy outcomes, as this is informed by the possibility of recurrent placental disease. Further studies are needed to determine how information about the placenta in the index stillbirth can be combined with assessment of placental morphology in a subsequent pregnancy to predict neonatal outcome.

SUMMARY

Because of the crucial role the placenta plays in determining the outcome of preg-nancy, its pivotal role in stillbirth is expected. A wide range of placental abnormalities have been reported in cases of stillbirth, and although for some of these features there is a clear relationship to the cause of death (eg, placental abruption), for others further work is needed to understand the pathophysiology and how other factors including gestation, maternal ethnicity, and health behaviors may interact to produce the placental phenotype and lead to stillbirth. Importantly, translating the findings from histopathological investigation of the placenta into clinical practice reduces the pro-portion of unexplained stillbirths and provides information that informs care of subse-quent pregnancies. Consequently, sending the placenta for histopathological examination after stillbirth or perinatal death is essential to provide valuable informa-tion for bereaved parents that may be of benefit in subsequent pregnancies.

DISCLOSURE

The authors had no financial relationships with any organizations that might have an interest in the submitted work in the previous 3 years and have no other relationships or activities that could appear to have influenced the submitted work.

REFERENCES

1. World Health Organization. Stillbirths. 201. Available at: https://www.who.int/maternal_child_adolescent/epidemiology/stillbirth/en/. Accessed July 14, 2019.
2. Lawn JE, Blencowe H, Waiswa P, et al. Stillbirths: rates, risk factors, and acceler-ation towards 2030. Lancet 2016;387(10018):587–603.
3. National Center for Health Statistics. Birth statistics 2003-2017. 2018. Available at: https://www.cdc.gov/nchs/data_access/vitalstatsonline.htm. Accessed September 30, 2019.
4. Flenady V, Wojcieszek AM, Middleton P, et al. Stillbirths: recall to action in high-income countries. Lancet 2016;387(10019):691–702.
5. de Bernis L, Kinney MV, Stones W, et al. Stillbirths: ending preventable deaths by 2030. Lancet 2016;387(10019):703–16.
6. Heazell AE, Siassakos D, Blencowe H, et al. Stillbirths: economic and psychoso-cial consequences. Lancet 2016;387(10018):604–16.
7. Hoyert DL, Gregory ECW. Cause of fetal death: data from the fetal death report, 2014. Hyattsville (MD): National Center for Health Statistics; 2016.
8. Stillbirth Collaborative Research Network Writing Group. Association between stillbirth and risk factors known at pregnancy confirmation. JAMA 2011; 306(22):2469–79.

9. Lamont K, Scott NW, Jones GT, et al. Risk of recurrent stillbirth: systematic review and meta-analysis. BMJ 2015;350:h3080.

10. Lean SC, Derricott H, Jones RL, et al. Advanced maternal age and adverse pregnancy outcomes: a systematic review and meta-analysis. PLoS One 2017;12(10): e0186287.

11. Marufu TC, Ahankari A, Coleman T, et al. Maternal smoking and the risk of still birth: systematic review and meta-analysis. BMC Public Health 2015;15:239.

12. Gardosi J, Madurasinghe V, Williams M, et al. Maternal and fetal risk factors for stillbirth: population based study. BMJ 2013;346:f108.

13. Harmon QE, Huang L, Umbach DM, et al. Risk of fetal death with preeclampsia. Obstet Gynecol 2015;125(3):628–35.

14. Heazell AEP, Budd J, Li M, et al. Alterations in maternally perceived fetal movement and their association with late stillbirth: findings from the Midland and North of England stillbirth case-control study. BMJ Open 2018;8(7):e020031.

15. Higgins L, Mills TA, Greenwood SL, et al. Maternal obesity and its effect on placental cell turnover. J Matern Fetal Neonatal Med 2013;26(8):783–8.

16. Lean SC, Heazell AEP, Dilworth MR, et al. Placental dysfunction underlies increased risk of fetal growth restriction and stillbirth in advanced maternal age women. Sci Rep 2017;7(1):9677.

17. Zdravkovic T, Genbacev O, McMaster MT, et al. The adverse effects of maternal smoking on the human placenta: a review. Placenta 2005;26(Suppl A):S81–6.

18. Warrander LK, Batra G, Bernatavicius G, et al. Maternal perception of reduced fetal movements is associated with altered placental structure and function. PLoS One 2012;7(4):e34851.

19. Burton GJ, Jauniaux E. Pathophysiology of placental-derived fetal growth restriction. Am J Obstet Gynecol 2018;218(2S):S745–61.

20. Amaral LM, Wallace K, Owens M, et al. Pathophysiology and current clinical management of preeclampsia. Curr Hypertens Rep 2017;19(8):61.

21. Heazell AE, Worton SA, Higgins LE, et al. IFPA gabor than award lecture: recognition of placental failure is key to saving babies' lives. Placenta 2015;36(Suppl 1):S20–8.

22. Baffero GM, Somigliana E, Crovetto F, et al. Confined placental mosaicism at chorionic villous sampling: risk factors and pregnancy outcome. Prenat Diagn 2012; 32(11):1102–8.

23. Goodfellow LR, Batra G, Hall V, et al. A case of confined placental mosaicism with double trisomy associated with stillbirth. Placenta 2011;32(9):699–703.

24. Haavaldsen C, Samuelsen SO, Eskild A. Fetal death and placental weight/birthweight ratio: a population study. Acta Obstet Gynecol Scand 2013;92(5):583–90.

25. Worton SA, Heazell AEP. Decreased placental weight centile and increased birthweight:placental weight ratios in stillbirths suggests placental insufficiency even in stillbirths of "unknown" cause. Placenta 2014;35:A15.

26. Pasztor N, Sikovanyecz J, Kereszturi A, et al. Evaluation of the relation between placental weight and placental weight to foetal weight ratio and the causes of stillbirth: a retrospective comparative study. J Obstet Gynaecol 2018;38(1):74–80.

27. Ptacek I, Sebire NJ, Man JA, et al. Systematic review of placental pathology reported in association with stillbirth. Placenta 2014;35(8):552–62.

28. Pathak S, Lees CC, Hackett G, et al. Frequency and clinical significance of placental histological lesions in an unselected population at or near term. Virchows Arch 2011;459(6):565–72.

29. Pinar H, Goldenberg RL, Koch MA, et al. Placental findings in singleton stillbirths. Obstet Gynecol 2014;123(2 Pt 1):325–36.

30. Man J, Hutchinson JC, Heazell AE, et al. Stillbirth and intrauterine fetal death: role of routine histopathological placental findings to determine cause of death. Ultrasound Obstet Gynecol 2016;48(5):579–84.
31. Parast MM, Crum CP, Boyd TK. Placental histologic criteria for umbilical blood flow restriction in unexplained stillbirth. Hum Pathol 2008;39(6):948–53.
32. Iwasenko JM, Howard J, Arbuckle S, et al. Human cytomegalovirus infection is detected frequently in stillbirths and is associated with fetal thrombotic vasculopathy. J Infect Dis 2011;203(11):1526–33.
33. Ernst LM, Minturn L, Huang MH, et al. Gross patterns of umbilical cord coiling: correlations with placental histology and stillbirth. Placenta 2013;34(7):583–8.
34. Contro E, deSouza R, Bhide A. Chronic intervillositis of the placenta: a systematic review. Placenta 2010;31(12):1106–10.
35. Derricott H, Jones RL, Heazell AE. Investigating the association of villitis of unknown etiology with stillbirth and fetal growth restriction - a systematic review. Placenta 2013;34(10):856–62.
36. Khong TY, Mooney EE, Ariel I, et al. Sampling and definitions of placental lesions: Amsterdam placental workshop group consensus statement. Arch Pathol Lab Med 2016;140(7):698–713.
37. Miller ES, Minturn L, Linn R, et al. Stillbirth evaluation: a stepwise assessment of placental pathology and autopsy. Am J Obstet Gynecol 2016;214(1):115.e1-6.
38. Heazell AE, Martindale EA. Can post-mortem examination of the placenta help determine the cause of stillbirth? J Obstet Gynaecol 2009;29(3):225–8.
39. Campbell J, Armstrong K, Palaniappan N, et al. In a genomic era, placental pathology still holds the key in the nondysmorphic stillbirth. Pediatr Dev Pathol 2018; 21(3):308–18.
40. Turowski G, Tony Parks W, Arbuckle S, et al. The structure and utility of the placental pathology report. APMIS 2018;126(7):638–46.
41. Calvert SJ, Jones CJ, Sibley CP, et al. Analysis of syncytial nuclear aggregates in preeclampsia shows increased sectioning artefacts and decreased inter-villous bridges compared to healthy placentas. Placenta 2013;34(12):1251–4.
42. Spinillo A, Gardella B, Bariselli S, et al. Placental histopathological correlates of umbilical artery Doppler velocimetry in pregnancies complicated by fetal growth restriction. Prenat Diagn 2012;32(13):1263–72.
43. Turowski G, Berge LN, Helgadottir LB, et al. A new, clinically oriented, unifying and simple placental classification system. Placenta 2012;33(12):1026–35.
44. Walsh CA, McAuliffe FM, Turowski G, et al. A survey of obstetricians' views on placental pathology reporting. Int J Gynaecol Obstet 2013;121(3):275–7.
45. Black M, Shetty A, Bhattacharya S. Obstetric outcomes subsequent to intrauterine death in the first pregnancy. BJOG 2008;115(2):269–74.
46. Nijkamp JW, Korteweg FJ, Holm JP, et al. Subsequent pregnancy outcome after previous foetal death. Eur J Obstet Gynecol Reprod Biol 2013;166(1):37–42.
47. Monari F, Pedrielli G, Vergani P, et al. Adverse perinatal outcome in subsequent pregnancy after stillbirth by placental vascular disorders. PLoS One 2016;11(5): e0155761.
48. Ruiter L, Ravelli AC, de Graaf IM, et al. Incidence and recurrence rate of placental abruption: a longitudinal linked national cohort study in the Netherlands. Am J Obstet Gynecol 2015;213(4):573.e1-8.
49. Feeley L, Mooney EE. Villitis of unknown aetiology: correlation of recurrence with clinical outcome. J Obstet Gynaecol 2010;30(5):476–9.
50. Ladhani NNN, Fockler ME, Stephens L, et al. No. 369-management of pregnancy subsequent to stillbirth. J Obstet Gynaecol Can 2018;40(12):1669–83.

51. Wojcieszek AM, Shepherd E, Middleton P, et al. Care prior to and during subsequent pregnancies following stillbirth for improving outcomes. Cochrane Database Syst Rev 2018;(12):CD012203.
52. Roberge S, Nicolaides KH, Demers S, et al. Prevention of perinatal death and adverse perinatal outcome using low-dose aspirin: a meta-analysis. Ultrasound Obstet Gynecol 2013;41(5):491–9.
53. Mekinian A, Costedoat-Chalumeau N, Masseau A, et al. Chronic histiocytic intervillositis: outcome, associated diseases and treatment in a multicenter prospective study. Autoimmunity 2015;48(1):40–5.
54. Toal M, Chan C, Fallah S, et al. Usefulness of a placental profile in high-risk pregnancies. Am J Obstet Gynecol 2007;196(4):363.e1-7.
55. Toal M, Keating S, Machin G, et al. Determinants of adverse perinatal outcome in high-risk women with abnormal uterine artery Doppler images. Am J Obstet Gynecol 2008;198(3):330.e1-7.

Placental Magnetic Resonance Imaging
A Method to Evaluate Placental Function In Vivo

Anne Sørensen, MD, PhD[a,b,*], Marianne Sinding, MD, PhD[a,b]

KEYWORDS

- Placental dysfunction • Fetal growth restriction • Magnetic resonance imaging (MRI)
- Placental MRI • T2*-weighted MRI • Relaxation time • T2* relaxation

KEY POINTS

- Currently, there is no antenatal clinical method to directly evaluate placental function. Therefore, the antenatal screening of placental dysfunction focuses on fetal size.
- Placental dysfunction is associated with placental hypoxia. Hence, measurement of placental hypoxia may serve as a marker of placental dysfunction in vivo.
- Placental hypoxia may be estimated using magnetic resonance imaging because the quantitative transversal relaxation time (T2*) provides noninvasive measurements of placental morphology and oxygenation.
- Placental T2* relaxation is reduced in the dysfunctional placenta, and therefore T2* is a potential clinical tool to identify placental dysfunction in vivo.

INTRODUCTION

Placental dysfunction remains one of the great challenges in modern obstetrics. Placental dysfunction may compromise the fetal supply of oxygen, leading to fetal growth restriction, hypoxia, and acidosis.[1] Accordingly, placental dysfunction provides an increased risk of stillbirth,[2] neonatal mortality and morbidity,[3] and long-term negative consequences, such as adult metabolic and cardiovascular disease.[4,5]

Currently, there is no antenatal clinical method to directly evaluate placental function. Hence, in clinical practice, the antenatal screening of placental dysfunction is based on fetal weight estimates, because being small for gestational age (SGA) is considered an antenatal marker of placental dysfunction. Women with SGA fetuses are admitted for further examination to evaluate fetal well-being, including serial ultrasound fetal weight estimates and Doppler flow measurements of the umbilical cord, the fetal circulation, and the uterine arteries.[6] Fetal prognosis is highly dependent

[a] Department of Obstetrics and Gynecology, Aalborg University Hospital, Reberbansgade 15, Aalborg 9000, Denmark; [b] Department of Clinical Medicine, Aalborg University, Sdr. Skovvej 15, Aalborg 9000, Denmark
* Corresponding author.
E-mail address: anns@rn.dk

Obstet Gynecol Clin N Am 47 (2020) 197–213
https://doi.org/10.1016/j.ogc.2019.10.009
0889-8545/20/© 2019 Elsevier Inc. All rights reserved.

on timely delivery, which is a compromise between ultrasound signs of intrauterine fetal distress and the risk of prematurity.[7] Particularly during late gestation, however, the ultrasound Doppler flow measurements may be normal even in pregnancies complicated by placental dysfunction.[8]

The current antenatal screening of placental dysfunction based on fetal weight estimates is limited by low sensitivity and a high number of false-negative cases because intrauterine estimates of fetal weight is rather imprecise.[9,10] This is a major clinical issue, because false SGA cases have an increased number of unnecessary obstetric interventions,[11] and unidentified SGA cases have a 4-fold increase in adverse neonatal outcomes due to fewer obstetric interventions compared with identified SGA cases.[12] SGA is a strong marker of placental dysfunction, but placental dysfunction also may occur among fetuses of adequate weight and not all SGA fetuses suffer from placental dysfunction.[13–15] Therefore, even a perfect antenatal detection of all SGA fetuses would not lead to a perfect antenatal detection of placental dysfunction. In order to substantially improve the antenatal screening of placental dysfunction, new methods should focus directly on placental function rather than fetal size.

The pathophysiology of placental dysfunction is believed to rely on abnormal transformation of the uterine spiral arteries into low-resistance vessels. This process is initiated by trophoblast invasion of the vascular endothelium in the first trimester as a part of the normal placentation and the vessels usually are fully dilated at mid-gestation.[16] In the dysfunctional placenta, this process is impaired, which leads to maternal hypoperfusion of the intervillous space.[17] Controversies exist regarding models to explain the pathway from maternal hypoperfusion to placental dysfunction. Several factors may contribute to this process, such as oxidative stress due to hypoxia and cycles of ischemia-reperfusion injury,[18] mechanical damage to the fetal villous tree due to the abnormal high-velocity pulsatile blood flow of the spiral arteries,[19] and acute atherosclerotic changes of the spiral arteries.[20] Regardless of cause, placental hypoxia is a key marker of placental dysfunction, and this may be useful in the antenatal detection of this condition.

Over the past decade, placental magnetic resonance imaging (MRI) has emerged from being used mainly as a research tool to use as a potential clinical tool for evaluating human placental function in vivo. MRI provides a wide range of quantitative measurements that may be used in the noninvasive assessment of the human placenta. Each of these measurements is sensitive to specific aspects of placental function, including hypoxia and morphologic changes. In the human placenta, tissue relaxation times are the most well described. In this article, the authors aim to describe the use of these relaxation times in the assessment of placental function. T2*-weighted placental MRI, which has been the main area of the authors' research over the past decade, is focused on. The rationale behind T2*-weighted placental MRI, the main findings reported in the literature, and directions for future research and clinical applications of this method are discussed.

CONTENT

MRI relaxation times are tissue-specific constants, which describe the time for the observed MRI signal to decay. The relaxation times depend on multiple biological and physiologic features of the tissue, because they are determined by the molecular environment of the protons within the tissue. Tissue relaxation occurs by 2 independent processes: longitudinal (T1) relaxation and transversal (T2) relaxation. In theory, T1 is longer in solid tissue and shorter in fluids where protons are free. For T2, it is the opposite because T2 is longer in fluids and shorter in solid tissue. T2* is related to T2; however, in addition to tissue morphology, this relaxation time is sensitive to magnetic field inhomogeneities as created by, for instance, the presence of deoxyhemoglobin, which makes T2* particularly sensitive to tissue hypoxia and thereby placental dysfunction. In the human placenta, the origin of the changes in the relaxation time remains a matter of debate, because the exact correlation between specific tissue characteristics and tissue relaxation remains unknown. From a clinical perspective, however, the placental relaxation times may serve as valuable markers of placental dysfunction.

T1 and T2 Relaxation

During the past 2 decades, placental T1 and T2 have been investigated in several human studies. In 1998, Gowland and colleagues[21] investigated the T1 relaxation in 41 normal placentas, and they demonstrated a negative correlation between placental T1 and gestational age. Subsequently, this finding was supported in additional 2 studies[22,23]; however, in later studies, the finding was not reproduced.[24–27] Differences in MRI sequence parameters may explain the inconsistency of these results. In placental dysfunction, 3 studies have demonstrated a low T1 value.[21,22,26] This finding may be explained by changes in tissue morphology and in tissue oxygenation. In T1, the association with tissue oxygenation is related to tissue Po_2, which is in contrast to T2*, where the association with tissue oxygenation is related to deoxyhemoglobin. Changes in placental T1 during maternal hyperoxia also have been investigated. In the normal placenta, the hyperoxic T1 is significantly increased,[25–27] which is thought to represent an increase in Po_2 in the blood and tissue. In the dysfunctional placenta, this response is significantly higher.[26,27]

Regarding the normal placenta, an initial study published in 1998 on placental T2 by Gowland and colleagues[21] found a negative correlation between placental T2 and gestational age. Subsequently, this finding was reproduced in 3 studies,[22,23,28] whereas a study by Derwig and colleagues[29] did not support the finding. In the latter study, however, only a narrow range of gestational age was investigated (24–29 weeks' gestation). The correlation between T2 and gestational age may be explained by the normal placental maturation, which includes morphologic changes, such as growth of the villous and vascular surface area and macromolecular deposition, as, for instance, fibrin.[23,30] Placental T2 in the dysfunctional placenta has been investigated in 3 studies.[21,22,29] In these studies, the placenta is characterized by a low T2 value, which may be related to altered tissue morphology, including, for instance, the presence of infarction, necrosis, and fibrosis.

T2* Relaxation

In T2*-weighted MRI, differences in T2* relaxation are the primary source of tissue contrast. In the placenta, the T2* relaxation depends on morphologic features, such as the villous structure, the blood volume fractions, the deposition of fibrin, and presence of infarctions and fibrosis, which affects the more fundamental T2 relaxation, as described previously, and thereby the T2* relaxation. Moreover, the T2* relaxation depends on the placental oxygen saturation (sO_2). Because deoxyhemoglobin is a paramagnetic molecule, it induces local constant magnetic field inhomogeneities, which shorten the T2* decay. Therefore, T2*-weighted imaging is sensitive to tissue sO_2, and changes in tissue sO_2 lead to changes in the T2*-weighted MRI signal. This effect is also known as the blood oxygen level–dependent (BOLD) effect.[31]

Changes in T2*-weighted MRI signals during hyperoxia/hypoxia have been demonstrated in several MRI studies with direct measurements of changes in oxygen content.[32-35] During oxygen challenge, the oxygen content of the blood rises. Because arterial blood is nearly fully saturated during normoxia, oxygen challenge increases the arterial P_{O_2} whereas it has little impact on arterial sO_2 according to the oxygen–hemoglobin dissociation curve.[36] Thus, the T2*-weighted MRI signal of arterial blood is sparsely affected during oxygen challenge. On the contrary, in venous low-saturated blood, the additional oxygen binds to deoxyhemoglobin, thereby increasing the venous sO_2 whereas the change in venous P_{O_2} is relatively small. Thus, during oxygen challenge, the increased T2*-weighted MRI signal primarily arises from increased sO_2 of venous low saturated blood.

T2*-weighted MRI may provide 2 different estimates: the BOLD signal intensity (S) and the T2* value. These estimates are explained separately.

The Blood Oxygen Level–Dependent Signal Intensity

The T2*-weighted MRI signal intensity (S) can be described as in Equation (1), in which M_0 is the relaxed magnetization, TE is the echo time, and T2* is the transversal relaxation time:

$$S \propto M_0\ e^{\left(-TE/T2^*\right)}$$

(1)

The M_0 depends on multiple factors, including (1) technical factors, such as the magnetic field strength, MRI sequence parameters, the MRI shimming effects, distance to the receiver coil, and so forth, and (2) baseline physiologic factors, such as tissue temperature, blood flow, blood volume, hematocrit, hydration, oxygenation, and tissue compositions.[37,38] These factors may vary between individuals; therefore, the *absolute* BOLD signal cannot be compared between individuals, neither can it be directly inferred into tissue sO_2. Dynamic changes in the signal, however, as can be induced by maternal oxygen challenge, varying the tissue sO_2 and thereby the T2* value in Equation (1), are comparable between individuals. Thus, *relative* BOLD signal changes, given as a percentage of the baseline BOLD signal, are comparable between individual.

The T2* Value

The transversal relaxation time, given as the T2* value in Equation (1), can be measured using a multiecho gradient-recalled echo (GRE) sequence, in which additional opposing gradients are applied, creating multiple echo signals at varying echo times (TEs). The T2* value of the placenta can be estimated as follows: for each TE, the mean MRI signal of a placental region of interest (ROI) is plotted, and the monoexponential decay function (see Equation [1]) is created, as illustrated in **Fig. 1**.[39] Using the multiple values of signal S at the varying TE, Equation (1) can be solved for T2* using a nonlinear least squares fitting algorithm.[40] Because this T2* value is calculated based on multiple signals at varying TEs, with M_0 being a free parameter, T2* does not depend on the M_0 and, therefore, T2* can be compared between individuals. Like the placental BOLD signal, however, the placental T2* value cannot directly be inferred into tissue sO_2 because the T2* value also depends on elements of tissue composition (the intrinsic T2 value).

Practical Aspects of the T2* Method

In placental MRI, most often a field strength of 1.5T has been used. This field strength gives sufficient information for standard placental evaluation. Nevertheless, in many

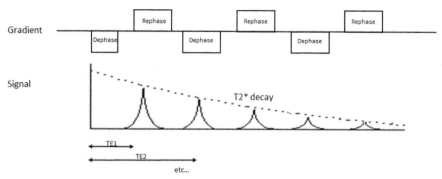

Fig. 1. The monoexponential decay function achieved using a multiecho MRI sequence (5 TEs are illustrated). (*From* Sinding MM. Placental function estimated by T2*-weighted magnetic resonance imaging. Aalborg University Publishers 2017; with permission.)

centers, 3T systems are replacing 1.5T systems. In 3T systems, the sensitivity increases; however, 3T systems may be more prone to signal inhomogeneities and susceptibility artifacts.[41] There are several ways to obtain T2*-weighted imaging of the placenta, including fast GRE sequence or gradient-echo echo planar imaging sequences, run in either single-echo or multiecho model. How the authors obtain and analyze placental T2*-weighted imaging is described.

The authors' placental MRI studies use a 1.5T system. In dynamic BOLD studies, a dynamic single-echo GRE MRI sequence is used, with the following parameters: repetition time (TR) = 8000 ms, TE = 50 ms, flip-angle = 90°, field of view of 36 cm × 36 cm, and matrix of 128 × 128, which results in an in-plane spatial resolution of 3.6 mm × 3.6 mm. Using this sequence, the authors obtain multiple slices (thickness of 6 mm, no spacing) covering the entire uterus; thus, the number of slices varies according to the size of the uterus. Each slice is repeated every eighth second. During the initial 5-minute BOLD MRI, the women breathe normoxic air. Then a non-rebreather facial mask (Hudson Respiratory Care, Durham, North Carolina) is applied while the women remain in the same position on the board, followed by a medical 10-minute oxygen challenge (100% O_2) delivered at a flow rate of 12 L/min. In order to achieve steady state hyperoxic levels in dysfunctional placentas, a minimum of 10 minutes of oxygen challenge is needed. In placental T2* studies, the authors use a multiecho GRE sequence with the following parameters: TR = 70.9 ms; 16 echoes ranging from 3.0 ms to 67.5 ms in steps of 4.3 ms; flip-angel = 30°, field of view of 350 mm × 350 mm, and matrix of 256 mm × 128 mm. The size of the matrix results in an in-plane spatial resolution of 1.37 mm × 2.73 mm. The use of 16 echoes improves the T2* fits, whereas the use of a maximum TE of 67.5 ms reduces the risk of susceptibility artifacts. The T2* value is obtained from 3 central placental slices with a slice gap of approximately 2 cm. Each slice is acquired in a single breath-hold of 12 seconds.

The authors suggest that pregnant women are placed in the MRI scanner in a left lateral position (10°–15° tilt) in order to avoid aortocaval compressions, which may reduce the maternal blood flow to the uterus[42] and thereby affect the placental T2* value. In order to reduce the presence of placental susceptibility artifacts, the authors recommend placing the placenta isocentric within the MRI scanner. Moreover, the authors recommend using a transaxial imaging plane in order to assure coverage of both the maternal and fetal compartments of the placenta, as demonstrated in **Fig. 2**.[39]

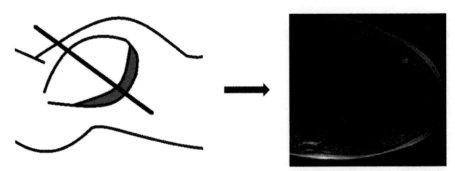

Fig. 2. (*Left*) Placement of a placental slice. (*Right*) T2*-weighted image. Placenta marked in red (ROI). (*From* Sinding MM. Placental function estimated by T2*-weighted magnetic resonance imaging. Aalborg University Publishers 2017; with permission.)

T2*-Weighted Analysis

In dynamic BOLD studies, the authors analyze the BOLD signal in 3 placental slices from each time frame. Within each slice, an ROI covering the entire placenta is drawn (see **Fig. 2**). In each image, this ROI is adjusted in order to correct for maternal movements. BOLD signal versus time curves are made and the relative change in BOLD signal (*ΔBOLD response*) is then calculated as an average of 3 slices using the normoxic steady state BOLD signal levels ($S_{baseline}$) as a reference stated in Equation (2):

$$\Delta\text{BOLD response} = (S_{\text{hyperoxic}} - S_{\text{baseline}})/S_{\text{baseline}} \times 100\% \qquad (2)$$

In baseline T2* studies, the placental ROIs are drawn in 3 placental slices at TE. The placental T2* value is calculated as an average of 3 slices, which increases the reproducibility of the T2* value.[43] Because the placenta has varying fractions of maternal and fetal compartments, the authors have considered if division of the MRI ROI into 2 layers would improve the accuracy of the method. In the T2*-weighted images, however, it is difficult to distinguish between the 2 compartments, especially in dysfunctional placentas and in early normal pregnancy. Thus, the authors have experienced that including the total placenta in the ROI increases the accuracy of the method.

The Dynamic Blood Oxygen Level–Dependent Studies

Initially, the correlation between changes in T2* signal intensity (BOLD signal) and direct measurement of fetal oxygenation was described in a sheep model by the use of internal oxygen sensors placed in the fetal liver[44] and fetal arterial blood derived from the carotid artery.[33] These studies were followed by hyperoxic BOLD studies of the human placenta in which the hyperoxic BOLD response was extensively investigated. During maternal oxygen breathing, the placental response was clearly visible as the placenta became markedly brighter and less heterogeneous, as demonstrated in **Fig. 3**.[45] In order to understand this finding, a study was performed in the rhesus macaque comparing the dynamic hyperoxic BOLD scans with contrast-enhanced MRI.[46] This study provided important information regarding the correlation between the placental anatomy and the hyperoxic BOLD response. It was demonstrated that the brighter areas in the T2*-weighted BOLD image corresponded with the oxygen-rich center of the intervillous space. During maternal oxygen breathing, the changes in the BOLD image was seen mainly at the margins of the intervillous space. This

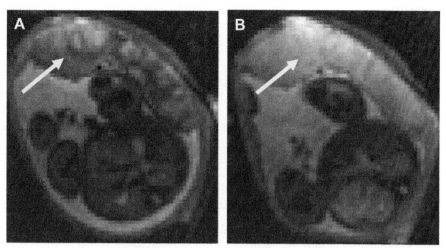

Fig. 3. Placenta T2*-weighted MRIs in a normal pregnancy. Cross-section through the central part of the placenta (*arrow*) during normoxia (*A*) and during maternal oxygen-challenge (*B*). (*From* Sørensen A, Peters D, Fründ E, et al. Changes in human placental oxygenation during maternal hyperoxia as estimated by blood oxygen level-dependent magnetic resonance imaging (BOLD MRI). Ultrasound Obstet Gynecol 2013;42(3):311; with permission.)

finding corresponds well with the hypothesis that during maternal hyperoxia the signal intensity is increased mainly at the margins of the intervillous space, where the maternal venous blood drains back into the maternal circulation. Because of the great similarities of the 2 scan types, it was concluded that in the T2*-weighted placental MRI, oxygen can be regarded as an intrinsic contrast agent. Subsequently, the hyperoxic BOLD response was investigated in a larger number of 49 normal placentas, and the positive hyperoxic response was a consistent finding.[47] In addition, a positive correlation with gestational age was demonstrated (**Fig. 4**).[47]

In the dysfunctional placenta, the hyperoxic BOLD response has been investigated in 3 human studies. The first case report of 4 dysfunctional placentas was inconclusive regarding the hyperoxic BOLD response when using only 5 minutes of oxygen challenge.[48] Then a larger case-control study of 13 dysfunctional placentas and 49 controls was performed using 10 minutes of oxygen challenge, and this study demonstrated that the BOLD response was increased in the dysfunctional placentas (see **Fig. 4**).[47] In addition, this study revealed that the time to reach the hyperoxic steady state plateau was increased in the dysfunctional placentas (**Fig. 5**),[47] which also was demonstrated in a study of monochorionic twins.[49] These studies focus attention on the time included for oxygen challenge. If the time for oxygen challenge is too short, the hyperoxic response of the dysfunctional placenta may not increase above normal. Revisiting the case report previously published by the authors' group,[48] the short oxygen challenge may explain the nonresponder presented in this report. In order to understand the increased hyperoxic BOLD response observed in dysfunctional placenta, it should be remembered that the hyperoxic BOLD response is a relative measurement (see Equation 2). Any increase in the BOLD response may be due to an increase in absolute signal intensity and/or a reduction in the absolute baseline signal intensity. Therefore, in order to understand and interpret the hyperoxic BOLD response, the authors conducted a BOLD study, including baseline T2* and hyperoxic T2* values.[47] It was demonstrated that the increased hyperoxic BOLD response

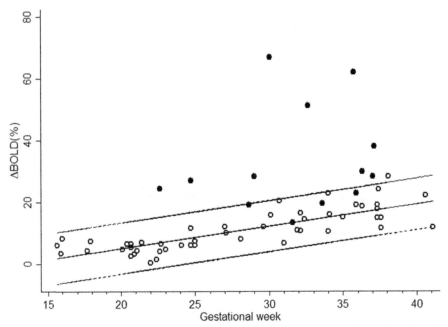

Fig. 4. The association between placental hyperoxic BOLD response and gestational age in normal pregnancies (*open circles*). Black lines indicate the least squares fit and dashed lines indicate 95% PI. Closed circles indicate 13 cases of pregnancies complicated by placental dysfunction. (*From* Sinding M, Peters DA, Poulsen SS, et al. Placental baseline conditions modulate the hyperoxic BOLD-MRI response. Placenta 2018;61:21; with permission.)

observed in pregnancies complicated by placental dysfunction, merely reflected a low baseline T2* value as the increase in T2* value during oxygen challenge (ΔT2*) did not differ between normal and dysfunctional placentas (**Fig. 6**),[47] which is also demonstrated by Ingram and colleagues.[26] Similarly, the positive correlation between the

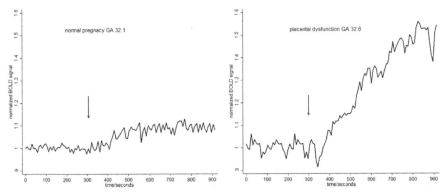

Fig. 5. Normalized BOLD signal intensity curves in a normal pregnancy (*left*) and in a pregnancy complicated by placental dysfunction (*right*). Arrows mark the start of oxygen challenge. GA, gestational age. (*From* Sinding M, Peters DA, Poulsen SS, et al. Placental baseline conditions modulate the hyperoxic BOLD-MRI response. Placenta 2018;61:21; with permission.)

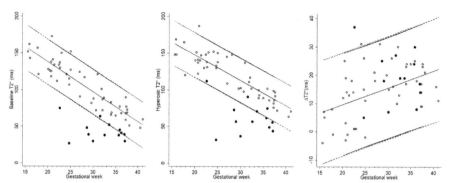

Fig. 6. The association between placental baseline T2* measurements (*left*), hyperoxic T2* (*middle*), ΔT2* (*right*), and gestational age in normal pregnancies (*open circles*) and in cases of placental dysfunction (*closed circles*). Black lines indicate least squares fit and dashed lines indicate 95% PI. (*From* Sinding M, Peters DA, Poulsen SS, et al. Placental baseline conditions modulate the hyperoxic BOLD-MRI response. Placenta 2018;61:22; with permission.)

hyperoxic BOLD response and gestational age in normal pregnancy was explained by a decreasing baseline T2*.[47] These findings are in accordance with previous BOLD studies, demonstrating that baseline conditions, which affect the baseline signal, such as baseline oxygenation, blood flow, blood volume, tissue morphology, and so forth, modulate the BOLD response amplitude.[37,38,50]

Limitations of the Blood Oxygen Level–Dependent Method

In the authors' dynamic BOLD studies, several obstacles were experienced with the method. One major limitation is the long acquisition time (15 minutes) in which even a 10-minuteoxygen-challenge may not be enough in order to reach steady state levels in the very dysfunctional placentas. If the BOLD signal does not reach the steady state level, the BOLD response may be underestimated leading to false negative results. Moreover, the authors experienced that spontaneous subclinical uterine contractions often interfere with the MRI signal (**Fig. 7**),[51] and therefore they excluded 20% of the participants.[47] Finally, the extremely time-consuming MRI analysis of the dynamic BOLD scans, including ROI drawings at multiple timeframes (1 frame for every 12 seconds), is a major limitation of the method.

Given these limitations of the dynamic BOLD method and the fact that the increased hyperoxic BOLD response of the dysfunctional placentas merely reflects a low baseline T2* value, the authors decided to continue the placental T2*-weighted MRI studies using the easier obtained and highly robust placental baseline T2* value.

The Baseline T2* Studies

In the first placental T2* study on 24 normal pregnancies, the authors demonstrated that the T2* value was reduced as gestational age advanced.[43] This finding could be explained by reduced placental oxygenation within both the intervillous blood and the fetoplacental blood as demonstrated by previous invasive studies.[52,53] Nonetheless, the maturation of the normal placenta, including the continuous development of the trophoblast throughout gestation and the deposition of fibrin, may reduce the intrinsic T2 value[21,23,30] and thereby reduce the placental T2* value. The findings were in contrast to a small study by Huen and colleagues,[25] who could not demonstrate any correlation between placental T2* and gestational age in 14 uncomplicated pregnancies at 23 weeks' to 37 weeks' gestation. Later, however, 3 large placental

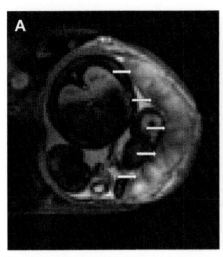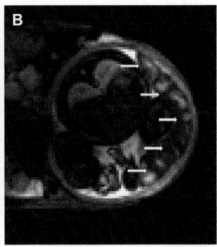

Fig. 7. T2*-weighted MR images during uterine relaxation (*A*) and uterine contraction (*B*). Placenta marked with white arrows. During the contraction, the placenta appears darker (signal intensity is reduced). (*From* Sinding M, Peters DA, FrøkjærJB, et al. Reduced placental oxygenation during subclinical uterine contractions as assessed by BOLD MRI. Placenta 2016;39:18; with permission.)

T2* studies supported the strong negative correlation between placental T2* values and gestational age (see **Fig. 6**).[47,54,55] Moreover, Ingram and colleagues[26] found a nonsignificant negative correlation. The negative correlation is also in accordance with previous MRI studies demonstrating reduced placental T2 values[21,23] and reduced placental perfusion fractions[56,57] as gestational advances.

The authors investigated the reproducibility of the T2* method and found the T2* method to be reasonable robust regarding within sessions, between sessions, and interobserver reproducibility, with the 95% limits of agreement for within-session and between-session variation for a single-slice placental T2* measurement being −2.1 ms ± 10.4 ms and −0.6 ms ± 22.6 ms, respectively.[43] Averaging 2 slices improved the reproducibility considerably (for the mean value of 2 slices the limits of 95% agreements were −1.1 ms ± 7.0 ms and −0.0 ms ± 17.8 ms), which most likely reflects the heterogeneous nature of the placenta.[43] Based on this observation, the authors recommend averaging of 2 or more slices in placental T2* studies. Likewise, at 3T, Hutter and colleagues[55] have demonstrated that the within-session and between-session variations of T2* were 1.83 ms ± 2.42 ms and 1.91 ms ± 1.60 ms, respectively.

In pregnancies complicated by placental dysfunction, baseline placental T2* values have been investigated in 4 human studies.[26,43,47,54] In these studies, placental dysfunction was defined by low birth weight[43,54] or by a combination of low birthweight and abnormal Doppler flows[26] or low birthweight and abnormal placental pathologic findings postpartum.[47] The initial T2* study included 4 cases of severe fetal growth restriction.[43] In 3 of these cases, the T2* values were significantly reduced compared with normal, and postpartum placental examination revealed signs of placental vascular malperfusion. The fourth case had a normal placental T2* value and a normal placental pathologic examination (**Fig. 8**).[43] Later, the child was diagnosed with Silver-Russell syndrome, which is a distinct syndromic growth disorder in which prenatal and postnatal growth failure are associated with other characteristic

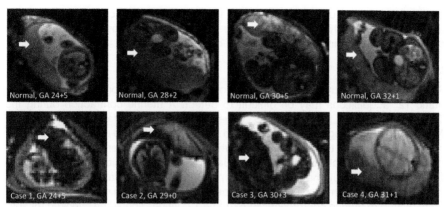

Fig. 8. T2*-weighted MRIs of placenta (*arrows*) in normal pregnancies (*upper row*) and in cases of fetal growth restriction (*lower row*). Cases 1 to 3: fetal growth restriction due to placental dysfunction (low T2* value). Case 4: fetal growth restriction due to a genetic disorder, Silver Russel syndrome (normal T2* value). (*From* Sinding M, Peters DA, Frøkjaer JB, et al. Placental magnetic resonance imaging T2* measurements in normal pregnancies and in those complicated by fetal growth restriction. Ultrasound Obstet Gynecol 2016;47(6):753; with permission.)

features, including relative macrocephaly at birth, protruding forehead in early life, body asymmetry, and substantial feeding difficulties.[58] Thus, in this case, fetal growth restriction was not caused by placental dysfunction. This initial study was followed by 3 studies, which also demonstrated a significantly reduced placental T2* values in dysfunctional placentas compared with normal.[26,47,54] In a prospective study of 97 pregnant women, it was demonstrated that the T2* value may be a strong predictor of low birthweight. In this study, placental T2* was directly compared with uterine artery Doppler performed at the time of MRI, and it was demonstrated that T2* performed significantly better than the uterine artery prediction interval (PI) in the prediction of low birth.[54] These results, however, need to be validated in larger cohorts. A major strength of this prospective study was the inclusion of placental pathologic examination, and the T2* results were highly in accordance with placenta pathologic findings.[54] Finally, a recent pilot study in dichorionic twin pregnancies has demonstrated that placental T2* difference may be a predictor of intertwin birthweight difference, irrespective of fetal size.[59]

In the T2*-weighted MRI of the dysfunctional placenta, the low T2* value is striking as the placenta appears significantly darker than normal, as presented in **Fig. 8.**[43] The low T2 may be explained by placental hypoxia and abnormal tissue morphology associated with placental dysfunction. As previously described, it is well known that the sO_2 of the fetoplacental blood may be reduced in placental dysfunction.[1,60,61] Controversies exist, however, regarding the sO_2 of the maternal blood. In addition to placental hypoxia, placental morphologic changes, such as infarction and fibrosis, may reduce the intrinsic T2 relaxation[62] and thereby the T2* value. Previous studies have demonstrated lower placental T2 values in fetal growth restriction pregnancies.[21,22,29] Moreover, the tissue fraction of blood volume also may affect the T2* value. Opposing results, however, are presented in the literature regarding the fraction of blood volume in dysfunctional placentas.[63,64] Thus, because the ROIs cover the entire placenta in transverse section, the low T2* value may reflect abnormal placental morphology, low sO_2 of maternal blood, and low sO_2 of the fetoplacental blood. Which of these parameters contributes the most to the low T2* value cannot be elucidated from the current analysis. Even so, for the purpose of a diagnostic test of placental dysfunction, this distinction may not be of clinical interest.

Limitations of the T2* Method

As opposed to the dynamic BOLD method, uterine contractions during the rather static T2* acquisitions may be difficult to detect. A uterine contraction during the T2* acquisition may reduce the T2* value, thereby creating false-positive results. MRI-compatible tocography might be used in order to detect the uterine contractions; however, it remains to be investigated whether such equipment would be able to detect these low-amplitude contractions. Because the T2 acquisition time is very short (12 seconds per slice), the authors recommend that the T2* measurement should be repeated at least 3 times with a minimal spacing of 3 minutes in order to identify artifacts related to uterine contractions.[51] Extreme T2* values should be checked for susceptibility artifacts, movement artifacts (maternal and fetal), or contractions and excluded from the analysis.

SUMMARY AND PERSPECTIVES

T2*-weighted placental MRI has the potential to be used as a clinical tool in the in vivo assessment of placental function. As demonstrated by the literature, the placental T2* value is an easily obtained and robust measurement, which can discriminate between the normal and the dysfunctional placenta. Current knowledge on T2*-weighted placental MRI is based on case-control studies and a few rather small prospective cohort studies. Larger prospective studies on well-defined populations of clinical interest should be conducted to evaluate the predictive value of placental T2*. The outcome of these studies should focus on not only fetal size but also placental dysfunction. The authors suggest including postnatal histopathologic examination, becuase placental dysfunction may occur among apparently normal weight fetuses.

Standard protocols for 1.5T and 3T should be agreed on in order to compare and combine data between centers. Getting larger data sets will allow developing individualized T2* values adjusted for multiple potential confounders. At this stage, gestational age at MRI is the only well-described confounder, and the authors suggest adjusting for differences in gestational age at MRI in any comparison of placental T2* between groups. Various MRI techniques constantly are being developed and technically improved. Combining placental T2* with other easily obtained MRI markers of placental function, such as baseline T1 and T2, may further improve the antenatal detection of placental dysfunction. From a clinical perspective, however, it is necessary to keep the MRI acquisition time below 30 minutes for patient comfort, and the MRI analysis should be easy to use and accessible for routine implementation. MRI remains at high cost and limited availability in most centers. This may change in the near future. The authors do not see placental MRI, however, as a first-line screening method. In a potential clinical setting, placental MRI should be provided mainly for selected high-risk pregnancies. There are several specific areas in which placental MRI could improve the antenatal care considerably, such as screening for placental dysfunction, late-onset fetal growth restriction, and pregnancies complicated by maternal diabetes. Each of these areas is discussed briefly.

A high proportion of false-positive cases limits the current screening for placental dysfunction based on ultrasound estimates of fetal weight. Placental MRI may identify the true cases of placental dysfunction among the high-risk pregnancies identified by ultrasound. This would lead to a more rational use of resources in antenatal care because the extensive fetal monitoring should focus on the true cases of placental dysfunction, which may be less than one-fifth of screen positives.[10] Another area of interest would be late-onset fetal growth restriction. In regard to early-onset placental dysfunction, ultrasound provides valuable insights in fetal well-being because Doppler measurements of umbilical and fetal blood flow is closely related to fetal hypoxia and acidosis.[6] In late-onset fetal growth restriction, fetal distress cannot be as accurately identified by ultrasound Doppler flow measurements, because Dopplers often remain normal even in severe cases of placental dysfunction.[8] Therefore, in these cases, placental T2* may provide a valuable addition to ultrasound, which could direct the clinical decision on when to deliver these high-risk babies. Lastly, pregnancies complicated by maternal diabetes also may benefit from additional placental MRI. In diabetes, placental function may be compromised[65] and the fetal metabolic demand may be increased due to macrosomia,[66] both leading to an increased risk of intrauterine fetal distress and stillbirth.[67] Unfortunately, ultrasound Doppler flow measurements are not as reliable in diabetic pregnancies as in normal pregnancies.[68] Therefore, pregnancies complicated by maternal diabetes are a group of high-risk pregnancies in which additional information of placental function would be highly clinical relevant.

In general, proper identification of placental dysfunction will improve the neonatal outcome through timely delivery. A more fundamental improvement in antenatal care, however, would be to identify placental dysfunction in early pregnancy, when there is still a chance to improve placental function by aspirin treatment. The authors have limited experience, however, in placental MRI at early gestation, and, prior to 16 weeks of gestation, there currently are no studies of T2*-weighted placental MRI.

In conclusion, placental MRI has emerged into a promising tool to be used in the in vivo assessment of placental function. Among the quantitative relaxations times, T2* relaxation is of particular interest because of its sensitivity to tissue oxygenation. T2*-weighted placental MRI has the ability to discriminate between the normal and the dysfunctional placenta, because the dysfunctional placenta is characterized by a low baseline T2* value. In addition, placental T2* is fast to obtain and easy to analyze, qualities which are essential in a clinical perspective. The authors have enjoyed the past decade of placental research in the area of T2*-weighted MRI and look forward to the next decade, which hopefully will bring this promising method into the clinic to improve the outcome for future high-risk pregnancies.

DISCLOSURE

The authors have nothing to disclose.

REFERENCES

1. Nicolaides KH, Economides DL, Soothill PW. Blood gases, pH, and lactate in appropriate- and small-for-gestational-age fetuses. Am J Obstet Gynecol 1989; 161(4):996–1001.
2. Froen JF, Gardosi JO, Thurmann A, et al. Restricted fetal growth in sudden intrauterine unexplained death. Acta Obstet Gynecol Scand 2004;83(9):801–7.
3. Lees C, Marlow N, Arabin B, et al. Perinatal morbidity and mortality in early-onset fetal growth restriction: cohort outcomes of the trial of randomized umbilical and fetal flow in Europe (TRUFFLE). Ultrasound Obstet Gynecol 2013;42(4):400–8.
4. Hales CN, Barker DJ, Clark PM, et al. Fetal and infant growth and impaired glucose tolerance at age 64. BMJ 1991;303(6809):1019–22.

5. Barker DJ, Gluckman PD, Godfrey KM, et al. Fetal nutrition and cardiovascular disease in adult life. Lancet 1993;341(8850):938–41.

6. Baschat AA. Fetal growth restriction - from observation to intervention. J Perinat Med 2010;38(3):239–46.

7. Baschat AA. Neurodevelopment following fetal growth restriction and its relationship with antepartum parameters of placental dysfunction. Ultrasound Obstet Gynecol 2011;37(5):501–14.

8. Oros D, Figueras F, Cruz-Martinez R, et al. Longitudinal changes in uterine, umbilical and fetal cerebral Doppler indices in late-onset small-for-gestational age fetuses. Ultrasound Obstet Gynecol 2011;37(2):191–5.

9. Bakalis S, Silva M, Akolekar R, et al. Prediction of small-for-gestational-age neonates: screening by fetal biometry at 30-34 weeks. Ultrasound Obstet Gynecol 2015;45(5):551–8.

10. Sovio U, White IR, Dacey A, et al. Screening for fetal growth restriction with universal third trimester ultrasonography in nulliparous women in the Pregnancy Outcome Prediction (POP) study: a prospective cohort study. Lancet 2015; 386(10008):2089–97.

11. Gabbay-Benziv R, Aviram A, Hadar E, et al. Pregnancy outcome after false diagnosis of fetal growth restriction. J Matern Fetal Neonatal Med 2017;30(16): 1916–9.

12. Lindqvist PG, Molin J. Does antenatal identification of small-for-gestational age fetuses significantly improve their outcome? Ultrasound Obstet Gynecol 2005; 25(3):258–64.

13. Parra-Saavedra M, Crovetto F, Triunfo S, et al. Placental findings in late-onset SGA births without Doppler signs of placental insufficiency. Placenta 2013; 34(12):1136–41.

14. Poon LC, Volpe N, Muto B, et al. Birthweight with gestation and maternal characteristics in live births and stillbirths. Fetal Diagn Ther 2012;32(3):156–65.

15. Hendrix M, Bons J, Alers N, et al. Maternal vascular malformation in the placenta is an indicator for fetal growth restriction irrespective of neonatal birthweight. Placenta 2019;87:8–15.

16. Kaufmann P, Black S, Huppertz B. Endovascular trophoblast invasion: implications for the pathogenesis of intrauterine growth retardation and preeclampsia. Biol Reprod 2003;69(1):1–7.

17. Kingdom JC, Kaufmann P. Oxygen and placental villous development: origins of fetal hypoxia. Placenta 1997;18(8):613–6.

18. Myatt L, Cui X. Oxidative stress in the placenta. Histochem Cell Biol 2004;122(4): 369–82.

19. Burton GJ, Woods AW, Jauniaux E, et al. Rheological and physiological consequences of conversion of the maternal spiral arteries for uteroplacental blood flow during human pregnancy. Placenta 2009;30(6):473–82.

20. Labarrere CA, DiCarlo HL, Bammerlin E, et al. Failure of physiologic transformation of spiral arteries, endothelial and trophoblast cell activation, and acute atherosis in the basal plate of the placenta. Am J Obstet Gynecol 2017;216(3): 287.e1-16.

21. Gowland PA, Freeman A, Issa B, et al. In vivo relaxation time measurements in the human placenta using echo planar imaging at 0.5 T. Magn Reson Imaging 1998; 16(3):241–7.

22. Duncan KR, Gowland P, Francis S, et al. The investigation of placental relaxation and estimation of placental perfusion using echo-planar magnetic resonance imaging. Placenta 1998;19(7):539–43.

23. Wright C, Morris DM, Baker PN, et al. Magnetic resonance imaging relaxation time measurements of the placenta at 1.5 T. Placenta 2011;32(12):1010–5.

24. Huen I, Morris DM, Wright C, et al. Absence of PO2 change in fetal brain despite PO2 increase in placenta in response to maternal oxygen challenge. BJOG 2014; 121(13):1588–94.

25. Huen I, Morris DM, Wright C, et al. R_1 and R_2* changes in the human placenta in response to maternal oxygen challenge. Magn Reson Med 2013;70(5):1427–33.

26. Ingram E, Morris D, Naish J, et al. MR Imaging measurements of altered placental oxygenation in pregnancies complicated by fetal growth restriction. Radiology 2017;285(3):953–60.

27. Ingram E, Hawkins L, Morris DM, et al. R1 changes in the human placenta at 3 T in response to a maternal oxygen challenge protocol. Placenta 2016;39:151–3.

28. Kameyama KN, Kido A, Himoto Y, et al. What is the most suitable MR signal index for quantitative evaluation of placental function using Half-Fourier acquisition single-shot turbo spin-echo compared with T2-relaxation time? Acta Radiol 2018;59(6):748–54.

29. Derwig I, Barker GJ, Poon L, et al. Association of placental T2 relaxation times and uterine artery Doppler ultrasound measures of placental blood flow. Placenta 2013;34(6):474–9.

30. Cameron IL, Ord VA, Fullerton GD. Characterization of proton NMR relaxation times in normal and pathological tissues by correlation with other tissue parameters. Magn Reson Imaging 1984;2(2):97–106.

31. Ogawa S, Lee TM, Nayak AS, et al. Oxygenation-sensitive contrast in magnetic resonance image of rodent brain at high magnetic fields. Magn Reson Med 1990;14(1):68–78.

32. Wedegartner U, Popovych S, Yamamura J, et al. DeltaR2* in fetal sheep brains during hypoxia: MR imaging at 3.0 T versus that at 1.5 T. Radiology 2009; 252(2):394–400.

33. Wedegartner U, Tchirikov M, Schafer S, et al. Functional MR imaging: comparison of BOLD signal intensity changes in fetal organs with fetal and maternal oxyhemoglobin saturation during hypoxia in sheep. Radiology 2006;238(3):872–80.

34. Kennan RP, Scanley BE, Gore JC. Physiologic basis for BOLD MR signal changes due to hypoxia/hyperoxia: separation of blood volume and magnetic susceptibility effects. Magn Reson Med 1997;37(6):953–6.

35. Li D, Wang Y, Waight DJ. Blood oxygen saturation assessment in vivo using T2* estimation. Magn Reson Med 1998;39(5):685–90.

36. Collins JA, Rudenski A, Gibson J, et al. Relating oxygen partial pressure, saturation and content: the haemoglobin-oxygen dissociation curve. Breathe (Sheff) 2015;11(3):194–201.

37. Cohen ER, Ugurbil K, Kim SG. Effect of basal conditions on the magnitude and dynamics of the blood oxygenation level-dependent fMRI response. J Cereb Blood Flow Metab 2002;22(9):1042–53.

38. Lu H, Zhao C, Ge Y, et al. Baseline blood oxygenation modulates response amplitude: Physiologic basis for intersubject variations in functional MRI signals. Magn Reson Med 2008;60(2):364–72.

39. Sinding MM. Placental function estimated by T2*-weighted magnetic resonance imaging. 2017. Available at: https://doi.org/10.5278/VBN.PHD.MED.00094

40. Marquardt DW. An algorithm for least-squares estimation of nonlinear parameters. J Soc Ind Appl Math 1963;11(2):431–41.

41. Bernstein MA, Huston J 3rd, Ward HA. Imaging artifacts at 3.0T. J Magn Reson Imaging 2006;24(4):735–46.

42. Humphries A, Mirjalili SA, Tarr GP, et al. The effect of supine positioning on maternal hemodynamics during late pregnancy. J Matern Fetal Neonatal Med 2018;32(23):3923–30.

43. Sinding M, Peters DA, Frokjaer JB, et al. Placental T2* measurements in normal pregnancies and in pregnancies complicated by fetal growth restriction. Ultrasound Obstet Gynecol 2016;47(6):748–54.

44. Sorensen A, Pedersen M, Tietze A, et al. BOLD MRI in sheep fetuses: a non-invasive method for measuring changes in tissue oxygenation. Ultrasound Obstet Gynecol 2009;34(6):687–92.

45. Sorensen A, Peters D, Frund E, et al. Changes in human placental oxygenation during maternal hyperoxia as estimated by BOLD MRI. Ultrasound Obstet Gynecol 2013;42(3):310–4.

46. Schabel MC, Roberts VHJ, Lo JO, et al. Functional imaging of the nonhuman primate Placenta with endogenous blood oxygen level-dependent contrast. Magn Reson Med 2016;76(5):1551–62.

47. Sinding M, Peters DA, Poulsen SS, et al. Placental baseline conditions modulate the hyperoxic BOLD-MRI response. Placenta 2018;61:17–23.

48. Sorensen A, Sinding M, Peters DA, et al. Placental oxygen transport estimated by the hyperoxic placental BOLD MRI response. Physiol Rep 2015;3(10) [pii: e12582].

49. Luo J, Abaci Turk E, Bibbo C, et al. In vivo quantification of placental insufficiency by BOLD MRI: a human study. Sci Rep 2017;7(1):3710–3.

50. Buxton RB. The physics of functional magnetic resonance imaging (fMRI). Rep Prog Phys 2013;76(9):096601.

51. Sinding M, Peters DA, Frokjaer JB, et al. Reduced placental oxygenation during subclinical uterine contractions as assessed by BOLD MRI. Placenta 2016;39: 16–20.

52. Jauniaux E, Watson A, Burton G. Evaluation of respiratory gases and acid-base gradients in human fetal fluids and uteroplacental tissue between 7 and 16 weeks' gestation. Am J Obstet Gynecol 2001;184(5):998–1003.

53. Fujikura T, Yoshida J. Blood gas analysis of placental and uterine blood during cesarean delivery. Obstet Gynecol 1996;87(1):133–6.

54. Sinding M, Peters DA, Frokjaer JB, et al. Prediction of low birth weight: Comparison of placental T2* estimated by MRI and uterine artery pulsatility index. Placenta 2017;49:48–54.

55. Hutter J, Slator PJ, Jackson L, et al. Multi-modal functional MRI to explore placental function over gestation. Magn Reson Med 2019;81(2):1191–204.

56. Sohlberg S, Mulic-Lutvica A, Lindgren P, et al. Placental perfusion in normal pregnancy and early and late preeclampsia: a magnetic resonance imaging study. Placenta 2014;35(3):202–6.

57. Moore RJ, Issa B, Tokarczuk P, et al. In vivo intravoxel incoherent motion measurements in the human placenta using echo-planar imaging at 0.5 T. Magn Reson Med 2000;43(2):295–302.

58. Wakeling EL, Brioude F, Lokulo-Sodipe O, et al. Diagnosis and management of Silver–Russell syndrome: first international consensus statement. Nat Rev Endocrinol 2017;13(2):105–24.

59. Poulsen SS, Sinding M, Hansen DN, et al. Placental T2* estimated by magnetic resonance imaging and fetal weight estimated by ultrasound in the prediction of birthweight differences in dichorionic twin pairs. Placenta 2019;78:18–22.

60. Pardi G, Cetin I, Marconi AM, et al. Diagnostic value of blood sampling in fetuses with growth retardation. N Engl J Med 1993;328(10):692–6.

61. Zhu MY, Milligan N, Keating S, et al. The hemodynamics of late-onset intrauterine growth restriction by MRI. Am J Obstet Gynecol 2016;214(3):367.e1-17.
62. Gowland P. Placental MRI. Semin Fetal Neonatal Med 2005;10(5):485–90.
63. Ong SS, Tyler DJ, Moore RJ, et al. Functional magnetic resonance imaging (magnetization transfer) and stereological analysis of human placentae in normal pregnancy and in pre-eclampsia and intrauterine growth restriction. Placenta 2004;25(5):408–12.
64. Mayhew TM, Ohadike C, Baker PN, et al. Stereological investigation of placental morphology in pregnancies complicated by pre-eclampsia with and without intrauterine growth restriction. Placenta 2003;24(2–3):219–26.
65. Taricco E, Radaelli T, Rossi G, et al. Effects of gestational diabetes on fetal oxygen and glucose levels in vivo. BJOG 2009;116(13):1729–35.
66. Casey BM, Lucas MJ, Mcintire DD, et al. Pregnancy outcomes in women with gestational diabetes compared with the general obstetric population. Obstet Gynecol 1997;90(6):869–73.
67. Lauenborg J, Mathiesen E, Ovesen P, et al. Audit on stillbirths in women with pregestational type 1 diabetes. Diabetes Care 2003;26(5):1385–9.
68. Salvesen D, Higueras M, Mansur C, et al. Placental and fetal Doppler velocimetry in pregnancies complicated by maternal diabetes mellitus. Am J Obstet Gynecol 1993;168(2):645–52.

Printed and bound by CPI Group (UK) Ltd, Croydon, CR0 4YY

03/10/2024

01040401-0002